P9-DMI-914

CT Review

CT Review

Edited by

Janet E. S. Husband

CHURCHILL LIVINGSTONE
EDINBURGH LONDON MELBOURNE AND NEW YORK 1989

CHURCHILL LIVINGSTONE
Medical Division of Longman Group UK Limited

Distributed in the United States of America by Churchill Livingstone Inc., 1560 Broadway, New York, N.Y. 10036, and by associated companies, branches and representatives throughout the world.

First published 1989

ISBN 0-443-04179-2

British Library Cataloguing in Publication Data
CT Review
1. Man. Diagnosis. Tomography. Applications of computer systems
I. Husband, Janet E. S.
616.07'572

Library of Congress Cataloging in Publication Data
CT Review/edited by Janet E. S. Husband.
p. cm.
Based on a series of lectures given at the First International London Advanced Course in Whole Body Computed Tomography, held at the Gleneagles Hotel, Scotland from 19 to 23 March 1989.
Includes index.
ISBN 0-443-04179-2
1. Tomography—Diagnostic use—Congresses. I. Husband, Janet E. S. II. International London Advanced Course in Whole Body Computed Tomography (1st: 1989: Auchterarder, Scotland)
[DNLM: 1. Tomography, X-Ray Computed—congresses. WN 160 C1043 1989]
RC78.7.T6C7 1989
616.07'572—dc19

Printed in Great Britain at The Bath Press, Avon

Preface

During recent years the applications of computed tomography (CT) have widened, image quality has improved and scanning techniques have become more sophisticated. Furthermore, a wealth of experience has been gained which has helped to define the advantages and limitations of CT compared with those of other techniques. During the early days controversies arose regarding the best uses of CT and although many of these have been resolved new issues are continually arising which promote discussion and reappraisal. Our knowledge and understanding of CT is, therefore, ever changing and it is important for radiologists practising CT to keep abreast of current concepts and new approaches in this challenging area of radiology.

CT Review is based on the series of lectures to be given at the first International London Advanced Course in Whole Body Computed Tomography to be held at Gleneagles Hotel, Scotland from 19 to 23 March 1989. Selected topics are covered which should be of interest to radiologists specializing in CT as well as to those with only a general interest in the subject who wish to keep up to date and be acquainted with current views. The idea of producing a text of the proposed lectures was conceived in July 1988 and the book is due for publication on 19 March 1989. The credit for this achievement is largely due to the commitment of the lecturers who have all provided their contributions in record time. To all these colleagues and friends I extend my warmest gratitude, for without their support the idea for the *CT Review* would never have been realized.

I would also like to take this opportunity of putting on record my appreciation of everyone who has been involved in the preparation of the manuscripts. Janice O'Donnell and I edited and assembled the text on a remote island and final thanks must go to Dave, the skipper of the small fishing boat *Nemo*, who saved the word processor and all the text from rough seas off the shores of the Isles of Scilly.

London 1989 Janet E. S. Husband

To Janice O'Donnell for her enthusiasm and tireless dedication to the International London Course in Whole Body Computed Tomography 1982–1989

Contributors

Dr Graham R. Cherryman
Department of Radiology, Royal Marsden Hospital, Downs Road, Sutton, Surrey SM2 5PT, UK

Dr Adrian Dixon
Department of Radiology, Addenbrooke's Hospital, Hills Road, Cambridge CB2 2QQ, UK

Professor N. Reed Dunnick
Department of Diagnostic Imaging, Duke University Medical Centre, Durham, North Carolina 27710, USA

Dr T. H. M. Falke
Department of Radiology, University Hospital, Rijnsburgerweg 10, 2333 AA Leiden, Holland

Dr C. D. R. Flower
Department of Radiology, Addenbrooke's Hospital, Hills Road, Cambridge CB2 2QQ, UK

Dr Harvey S. Glazer
Mallinckrodt Institute of Radiology, 510 South Kingshighway Boulevard, St Louis, Missouri 63110, USA

Dr Stephen J. Golding
Oxford Regional Computed Tomography Unit, The Churchill Hospital, Headington, Oxford OX3 7LJ, UK

Dr Jay P. Heiken
Mallinckrodt Institute of Radiology, 510 South Kingshighway Boulevard, St Louis, Missouri 63110, USA

Dr Janet E. S. Husband
Department of Radiology, Royal Marsden Hospital, Downs Road, Sutton, Surrey SM2 5PT, UK

Dr Brian Kendall
Department of Radiology, National Hospital, Queen Square, London WC1N 3BG, UK

Dr Rodney H. Reznek
Department of Radiology, St Bartholomew's Hospital, West Smithfield, London EC1A 7BE

Dr David H. Stephens
Department of Radiology, Mayo Clinic, Rochester, Minnesota 55901, USA

Dr A. P. van Seters
Department of Endocrinology, University Hospital, Rijnsburgerweg 10, 2333 AA Leiden, Holland

Professor James W. Walsh
Department of Diagnostic Radiology, Medical College of Virginia, Richmond, Virginia 23298, USA

Dr Michael P. Williams
Department of Radiology, Royal Marsden Hospital, Downs Road, Sutton, Surrey SM2 5PT, UK

CONTENTS

1. The larynx 1
James W. Walsh

2. Staging bronchial cancer 13
C. D. R. Flower and Michael P. Williams

3. The pleural space 23
C. D. R. Flower and Michael P. Williams

4. CT of pulmonary collapse 33
Harvey S. Glazer

5. Differential diagnosis of mediastinal pathology 41
Harvey S. Glazer

6. Thymic masses and hyperplasia 53
Janet E. S. Husband

7. Pancreatic neoplasms 65
Rodney H. Reznek

8. Inflammatory disease of the pancreas 77
David H. Stephens

9. Detection of liver metastases 87
Jay P. Heiken

10. Focal benign liver disease 97
David H. Stephens

11. Evaluation of colonic disease 109
Jay P. Heiken

12. Renal cystic disease 123
N. Reed Dunnick

13. Solid renal masses 137
Rodney H. Reznek

14. Adrenal imaging 151
T. H. M. Falke and A. P. van Seters

15. Blunt abdominal trauma 165
James W. Walsh

16. Interventional CT 179
N. Reed Dunnick

17. Staging of gynaecological malignancy 191
James W. Walsh

18. Staging of bladder and prostate cancer 203
Janet E. S. Husband

19. Hodgkin's and non-Hodgkin's lymphoma 217
Graham R. Cherryman

20. The spine—disc and degenerative disease 227
Brian Kendall

21. Joint disease 237
Stephen J. Golding

22. Pitfalls in CT 249
Adrian Dixon

Index 261

1. The larynx

James W. Walsh

INTRODUCTION

Since the advent of CT scanners utilizing thin sections and rapid scan times, CT has become an important imaging technique in evaluating both laryngeal carcinoma and trauma to the larynx. Direct laryngoscopy affords good visualization of mucosal surfaces and can easily detect functional impairment of the vocal cords. However, cartilaginous and deep soft-tissue involvement by tumour or trauma cannot be diagnosed by laryngoscopy. In cancer staging, CT is superior to laryngoscopy and laryngography for showing deep tumour infiltration of paralaryngeal spaces, invasion of cartilage, extension to soft tissues of the neck or subglottic space and lymph-node metastases (Mancuso & Hanafee 1979a, Archer et al 1981, Sagel 1983, Horowitz et al 1984).

CT is now recommended as the initial radiological staging procedure when additional diagnostic information is required to supplement the findings of laryngoscopy in determining the feasibility of conservation surgery (supraglottic laryngectomy, hemilaryngectomy) (Archer et al 1981, Sagel 1983). Also, CT is used to assess the glottic and subglottic regions when large fungating supraglottic tumours obscure these areas from endoscopic view.

TECHNIQUE

With the patient in the supine position, a lateral digital radiograph is obtained to localize axial sections and to achieve proper gantry angulation perpendicular to the long axis of the neck. The patient's neck is extended and chin lifted to make the larynx as parallel and the vocal cords as perpendicular to the table top as possible. Contiguous 5 mm thick sections are taken from the tongue base and angle of the mandible through the inferior border of the cricoid cartilage and first tracheal ring. A rapid scan time < 3 seconds is used during quiet inspiration. The patient is instructed not to swallow, move or talk. Intravenous contrast medium is used in cancer staging both to define tumour margins and extent and to differentiate blood vessels from lymph nodes. A dynamic incremental CT of the neck can be combined with intravenous contrast material given through a mechanical injector. This gives superior contrast-enhanced images.

Additional techniques can be used as options to improve the delineation of specific areas. In glottic lesions, ultrathin 1–2 mm thick sections can be used to enhance definition of the anterior commissure, true vocal cords and the arytenoid cartilages. In supraglottic tumours, a modified Valsalva manoeuvre can be performed by asking the patient to blow through a crimped straw to fill out the pyriform sinuses thereby improving delineation of the ary-epiglottic folds. Phonation scans can be used to determine vocal cord mobility but these manoeuvres require excellent patient co-operation.

NORMAL ANATOMY

Anatomically and therapeutically the larynx can be thought of as having three separate portions. The supraglottis is composed of the epiglottis, ary-epiglottic folds, arytenoids and false vocal cords. The glottis is composed of the true vocal cords and the anterior and posterior commissures. The subglottis is the region extending from the undersurface of the true cords to the lower margin of the cricoid cartilage (Sagel 1983, Silverman & Korobkin 1983).

The hyoid bone lies at the superior boundary of the larynx and consists of three bony components – a central body and two lateral cornu extending posteriorly and superiorly (Figs. 1.1 and 1.2). The epiglottis is located behind the body of the hyoid bone and forms the anterior wall of the laryngeal vestibule (Fig. 1.2). Its widest part is cephalad and then it tapers

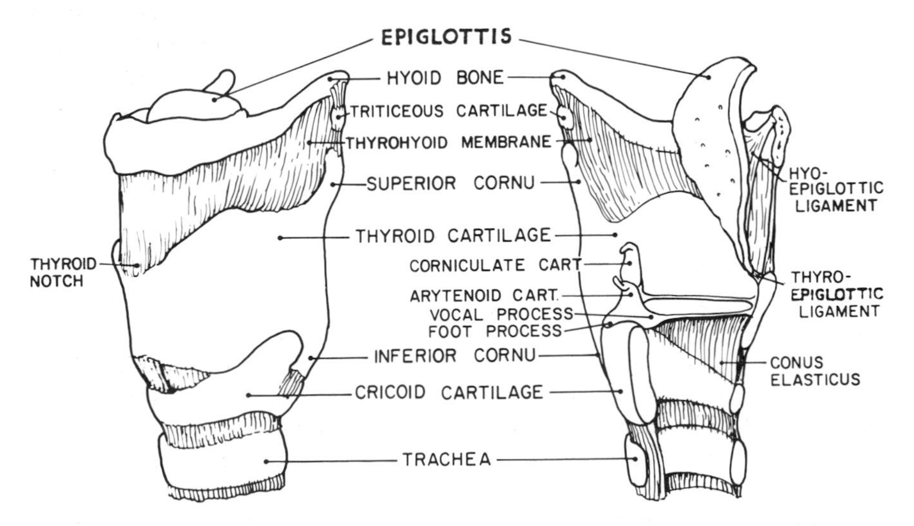

Fig. 1.1 Oblique views of major cartilaginous, ligamentous and bony structures of the larynx.

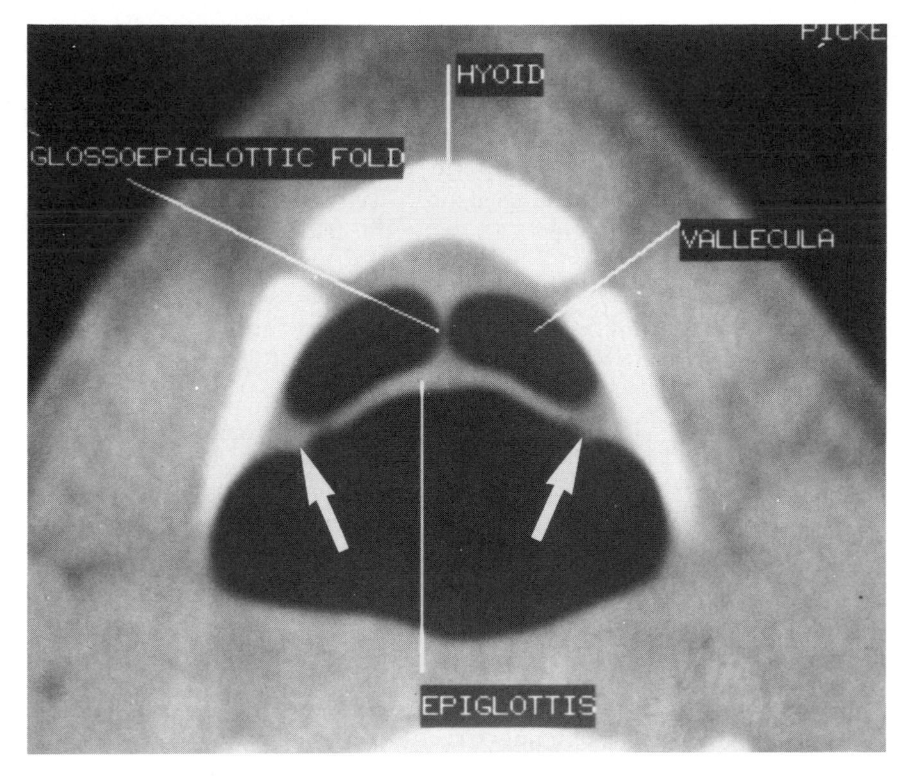

Fig. 1.2 CT scan at hyoid bone level shows the epiglottis, valleculae, the median glosso-epiglottic fold and the lateral glosso-epiglottic folds (arrows).

to its inferior tip, the petiole, where it attaches to the thyroid cartilage by the thyro-epiglottic ligament just above the anterior commissure. The epiglottis has two lateral glosso-epiglottic folds which are partly attached to the wall of the pharynx. The valleculae are two air-containing structures between the hyoid bone anteriorly and the epiglottis posteriorly and are divided by the median glosso-epiglottic fold (Fig. 1.2). The pre-epiglottic space is a mixture of fibrous and fatty tissue which extends from the valleculae superiorly to the anterior commissure inferiorly (Figs. 1.3 and 1.4). This soft-tissue space is continuous anterolaterally with the paralaryngeal space. CT is ideally suited to detect tumour extension in these spaces.

The ary-epiglottic folds are two soft-tissue bands which originate from a posterior paramedian position at the level of the arytenoids and diverge anterolaterally toward the posterior margin of the epiglottis (Figs. 1.3 and 1.4). These folds demarcate the lateral aspect of the laryngeal vestibule and form the medial walls of the pyriform sinuses. They are 2.5 mm thick superiorly and broaden to 5 mm inferiorly. The vestibule is the central portion of the laryngeal airway above the false cords. The pyriform

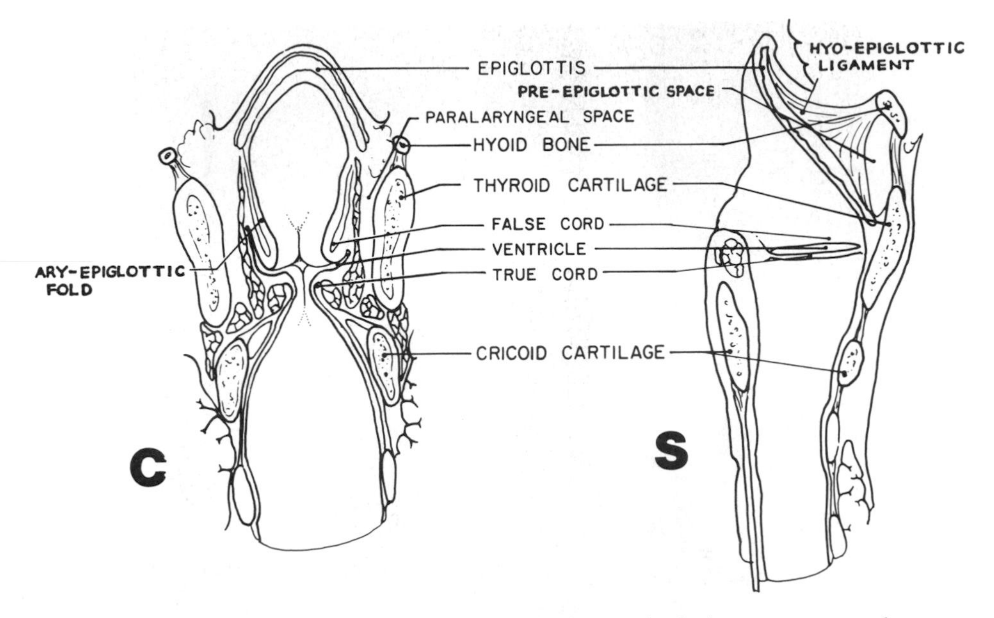

Fig. 1.3 Coronal (C) and sagittal (S) views of major laryngeal soft-tissue structures and spaces with portions of hyoid bone and thyroid and cricoid cartilages removed.

sinuses are lateral air-containing structures which bulge into the paralaryngeal space from the ary-epiglottic folds superiorly to the level of the false cords inferiorly (Fig. 1.4). The paralaryngeal space is a mixture of fibrous and fatty tissue deep to the endolarynx bounded laterally by the thyroid laminae, posteriorly by the pyriform sinuses and medially by the medial aspect of the ary-epiglottic folds.

The thyroid cartilage consists of paired laminae which extend vertically for 3 cm and fuse anteriorly (Figs. 1.1 and 1.4). The superior thyroid notch is a normal V-shaped space anteriorly between the paired thyroid laminae and should not be misinterpreted as an area of cartilaginous destruction (Fig. 1.4). The superior cornua of the thyroid cartilages are attached to the hyoid bone and their level identifies the infrahyoid portion of the pre-epiglottic space. The inferior cornua articulate with the posterolateral aspect of the cricoid cartilage to form the cricothyroid joint, which measures 1.5 mm. There is no consistency in the density or contour of the thyroid cartilage, which may be variably composed of non-calcified or calcified hyaline cartilage or bone. The cartilage calcification and/or ossification often is irregular, resulting in short segmental interruptions along both the outer and inner margins of the laminae which may simulate cancer invasion.

The cricoid cartilage is a signet-ring shaped structure with a broad posterior lamina measuring 2–3 cm in vertical height and a much narrower anterior arch measuring 5–7 mm vertically (Figs. 1.1, 1.3 and 1.5). This

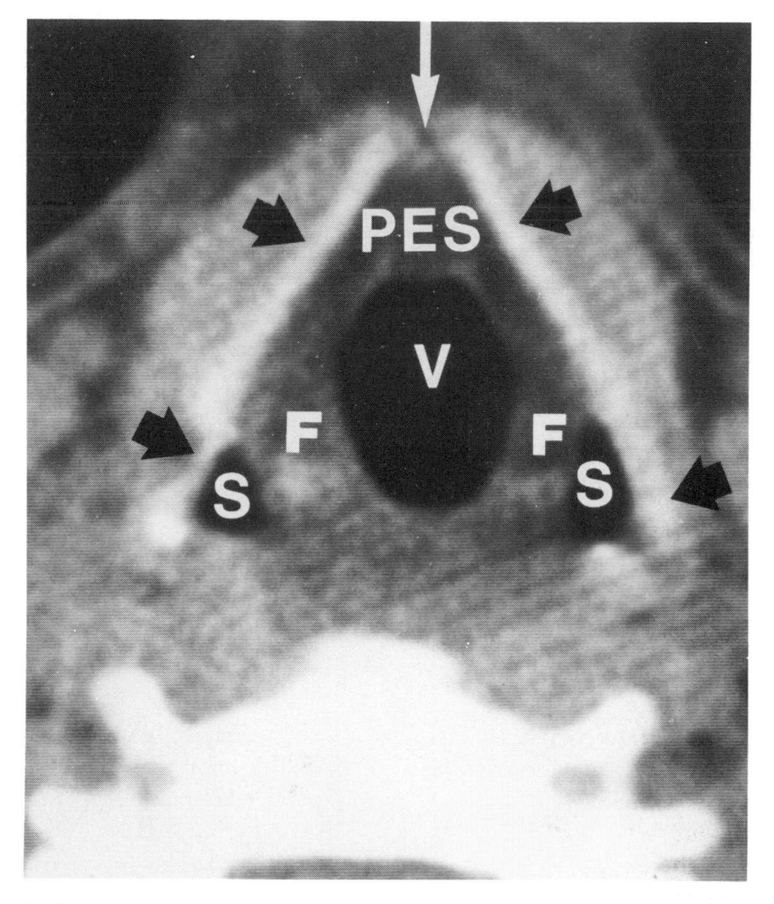

Fig. 1.4 CT scan through thyroid cartilage (black arrows) and superior thyroid notch (white arrow) showing normal fibrofatty tissue of the ary-epiglottic folds (F) and pre-epiglottic space (PES), the laryngeal vestibule (V) and the pyriform sinuses (S).

cricoid ring demarcates the subglottic space where the normal mucosa is closely adherent to the cartilaginous surface. The arytenoid cartilages are triangular structures which articulate with the superolateral borders of the posterior cricoid laminae to form the crico-arytenoid joints. The anteriorly projected vocal processes extend from the base of the arytenoids, taper into the lateral border of the airway and define the level of the true cords (Fig. 1.5). The laterally projected muscular or foot processes span a height from the base of the arytenoids to the level of the laryngeal ventricle or false cords. The muscular processes are separated from the inner surface of the thyroid cartilage by 2 mm or less.

The false cords are seen at the level of the foot processes of the arytenoid cartilage (Fig. 1.3). The laryngeal ventricle separates the false and true cords but is seen on CT in only 10–30% of normals. Each true cord is

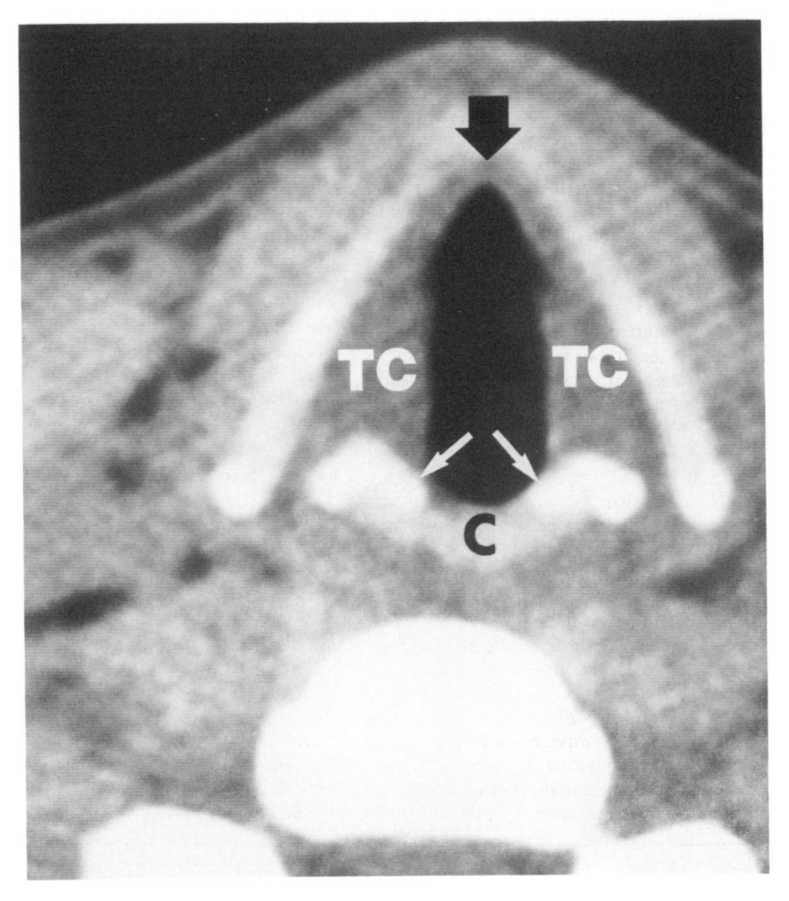

Fig. 1.5 CT scan at the level of the glottis, thyroid cartilage and top of cricoid cartilage (C) shows normal true vocal cords (TC), vocal processes of the arytenoid cartilages (white arrows) and the anterior commissure (black arrow).

composed of the vocal fold, vocal ligament, vocalis muscle and a part of the thyro-arytenoid muscle (Fig. 1.5). Each cord is thickest posteriorly (7 mm) where it inserts on the vocal process of the arytenoid at the posterior commissure. The cord tapers to 2 mm anteriorly where it meets the contralateral cord at the anterior commissure. This soft-tissue space posterior to the thyroid cartilage should be less than 2 mm thick (Fig. 1.5).

CARCINOMA

CT identifies a laryngeal tumour as a soft-tissue mass which alters the normal fibrofatty laryngeal tissues or which distorts, displaces or destroys normal laryngeal structures. CT is an excellent technique with which to evaluate the pre-epiglottic and paralaryngeal spaces that serve as a pathway

Table 1.1 TNM classification of tumours of the larynx

SUPRAGLOTTIC	
TIS	Carcinoma in situ
T1	Tumour confined to region of origin with normal mobility
T2	Tumour involves adjacent supraglottic site(s) or glottis without fixation
T3	Tumour limited to larynx with fixation and/or extension to involve postcricoid area, medial wall of pyriform sinus or pre-epiglottic space
T4	Massive tumour extending beyond the larynx to involve oropharynx, soft tissues of neck, or destruction of thyroid cartilage
SUBGLOTTIC	
TIS	Carcinoma in situ
T1	Tumour confined to the subglottic region
T2	Tumour extension to vocal cords with normal or impaired cord mobility
T3	Tumour confined to larynx with cord fixation
T4	Massive tumour with cartilage destruction or extension beyond the confines of the larynx, or both
GLOTTIC	
TIS	Carcinoma in situ
T1	Tumour confined to vocal cord(s) with normal mobility (includes involvement of anterior or posterior commissures)
T2	Supraglottic and/or subglottic extension of tumour with normal or impaired cord mobility
T3	Tumour confined to the larynx with cord fixation
T4	Massive tumour with thyroid cartilage destruction and/or extension beyond the confines of the larynx
NODAL INVOLVEMENT	
N1	Single clinically positive homolateral node less than 3 cm in diameter
N2	Single clinically positive homolateral node 3–6 cm in diameter or multiple clinically positive homolateral nodes, none over 6 cm in diameter
N3	Massive homolateral node(s), bilateral nodes, or contralateral node(s)

for the superior, anterior and inferior spread of supraglottic tumours (Table 1.1).

Supraglottic tumours may arise from the epiglottis, ary-epiglottic folds or false cords (Fig. 1.6). Also, carcinomas that arise inferiorly from the laryngeal ventricle, false vocal cords or around the arytenoid cartilages may extend superiorly into the ary-epiglottic folds. Supraglottic tumours characteristically grow in a circumferential pattern and frequently cross the midline (Fig. 1.6).

Pyriform sinus tumours are unilateral bulky tumours which characteristically exhibit a more aggressive local and cephalocaudad growth pattern than anterior (epiglottic) supraglottic lesions (Larsson et al 1981) (Fig. 1.7a). Pyriform sinus cancers extend to areas that require radical surgery for total removal and mimic the marginal tumours of the supraglottic larynx. Also, these tumours commonly involve the pre-epiglottic space, cause widening of the cricothyroid space, extend into the posterior cricoid and extralaryngeal spaces and invade the thyroid cartilage along its posterolateral margin. CT is ideally suited to demonstrate pyriform sinus

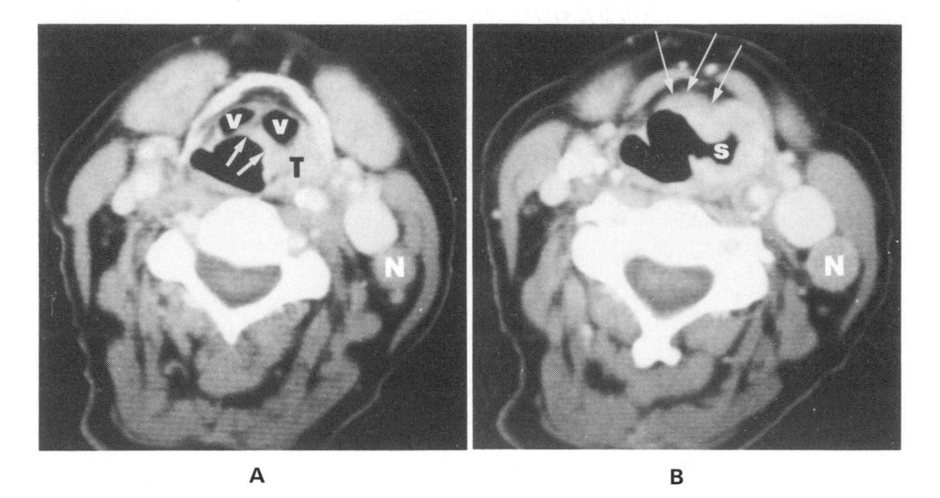

Fig. 1.6 Stage T3N3 supraglottic cancer. **A** CT scan at level of hyoid bone and valleculae (V) shows tumour mass (T) filling left pyriform sinus with extension to the epiglottis (arrows) and lymph-node metastasis (N) posterior to the left internal jugular vein. **B** CT scan 2 cm inferior shows cancer encircling left pyriform sinus (S) with tumour extension across the midline in the pre-epiglottic space (arrows) and left lymph-node metastasis (N).

tumour spread between thyroid and arytenoid cartilages or between the inferior cornu of the thyroid cartilage and the cricoid cartilage (Fig. 1.7b).

CT assessment of glottic tumours includes evaluation of cord mobility, supraglottic or subglottic extension and involvement of the anterior commissure or contralateral cord (Table 1.1; Fig. 1.8). True cord fixation may be due to:

1. Replacement of the vocalis muscle by tumour.
2. Subglottic tumour extension with fixation of the cord to the cricoid cartilage.
3. Invasion of the thyroid cartilage with cord fixation.
4. Invasion and fixation of the crico-arytenoid joint.

CT has been useful for detecting cartilaginous invasion by tumour, although some problems do exist (Mafee et al 1984, Silverman et al 1984). Only moderate to far advanced cartilaginous involvement associated with a soft-tissue tumour mass can be confidently diagnosed by CT because the normal pattern of calcification and ossification is irregular (Fig. 1.7b). When CT findings are equivocal, the surgeon should be advised to inspect and possibly biopsy the area before proceeding to total laryngectomy. Since microscopic or macroscopic (< 6 mm) cartilage invasion cannot be detected on CT, decisions regarding conservation surgery cannot be based on CT information alone (Mafee et al 1984).

Common sites of thyroid cartilage invasion are in the region of the anterior commissure ligament or at the junction of the anterior quarter and

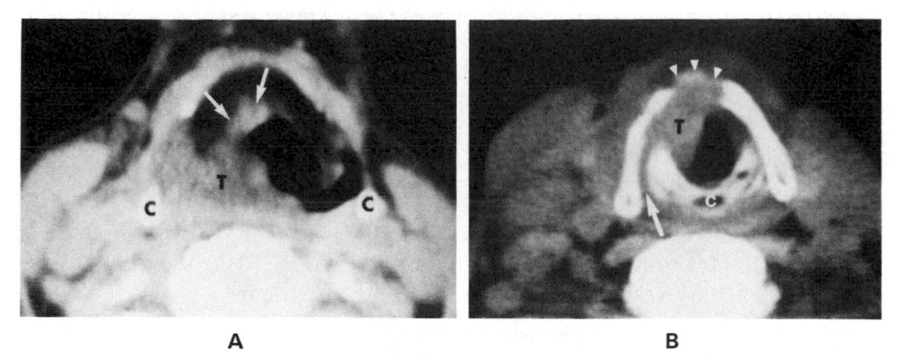

Fig. 1.7 Stage T4 pyriform sinus cancer. **A** CT scan at level of superior thyroid cornua (C) shows large tumour (T) filling right pyriform sinus with anterior spread into pre-epiglottic space (arrows). **B** CT scan at level of cricoid cartilage (C) shows inferior tumour (T) spread widening right cricothyroid joint (arrow) and associated with subglottic extension and destruction of the thyroid cartilage (arrowheads) in the area of the anterior commissure.

posterior three-quarters of the thyroid lamina (Fig. 1.7b). The initial site of invasion of the arytenoid and cricoid cartilages lies at the crico-arytenoid joint. Tumour invasion occurs at these areas because collagen fibres penetrate the perichondrium and are attached directly to the cartilage; these attachments thus serve as pathways for direct tumour spread. CT may demonstrate tumour involvement of cartilage either as areas of decreased density (chondrolysis) or areas of local increased density due to cartilage ossification (chondrosclerosis). Chondrolysis is the most common type and chondrosclerosis most frequently involves the arytenoid cartilage. This sclerosis, however, is not always due to tumour invasion but may be related to perichondritis and reactive ossification provoked by adjacent tumour.

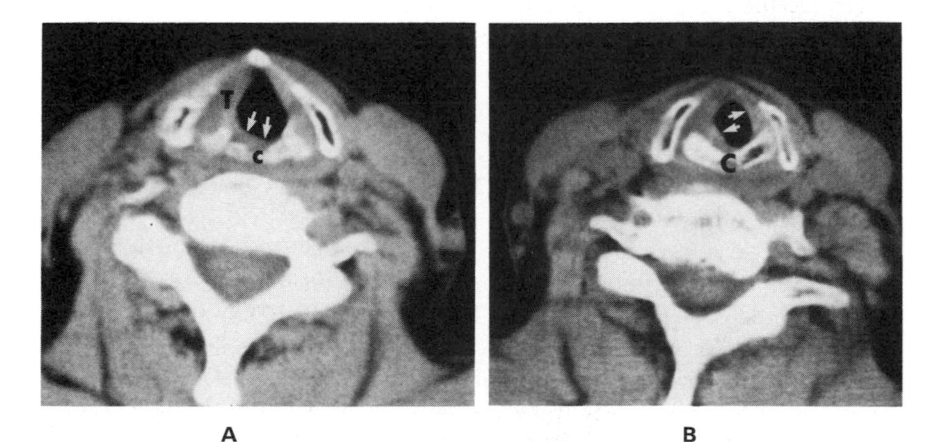

Fig. 1.8 Stage T2 cancer right vocal cord. **A** CT scan at level of vocal processes of the arytenoid cartilages shows tumour (T) thickening of right vocal cord and posterior tumour extension (arrows) in front of cricoid cartilage (C). **B** CT scan through lower cricoid cartilage (C) shows circumferential subglottic tumour extension (arrows).

LIMITATIONS OF CT

CT has several limitations in the evaluation of laryngeal cancer. CT has a limited ability to evaluate laryngeal function, especially vocal cord paresis or paralysis. This problem is partially overcome by performing CT scans during phonation. CT is unable to consistently define the laryngeal ventricle and a transition zone from the false to the true cords. Tumour spread from the true cords to supraglottic structures, or vice versa, can be very difficult to define on CT. Magnetic resonance (MR) imaging in the coronal plane may be more useful both to delineate the true ventricle and to differentiate glottic from supraglottic tumour spread. CT may overestimate tumour extent secondary to oedematous or inflammatory changes associated with a malignancy. Also, the mass effect from an adjacent bulky tumour may distort normal structures and thus mimic tumour involvement (Silverman et al 1984). Finally, CT cannot detect minor mucosal abnormalities or microscopic–macroscopic cartilage involvement and thus may underestimate tumour extent in some cases.

TRAUMA

The ability of CT to resolve minor degrees of calcification makes it ideal for demonstration of the laryngeal cartilages. In addition, the axial display of neck anatomy shows the extent of both soft-tissue and cartilaginous injury as well as the degree of resulting airway encroachment. All of these factors make CT preferable to radiography or xeroradiography in evaluating laryngeal trauma (Mancuso & Hanafee 1979b).

The injured larynx may be categorized as follows:

1. Soft-tissue injury
2. Supraglottic injury
3. Glottic injury
4. Subglottic injury
5. Tracheal injury.

Soft-tissue injuries include mucosal lacerations and haematomas of the ary-epiglottic folds or vocal cords. These injuries may be associated with cricothyroid joint dysfunction.

Supraglottic injuries consist of a fracture of the epiglottis or an avulsion of the thyro-epiglottic ligament. This may cause bleeding and oedema in the pre-epiglottic space. The second type of supraglottic injury is a transverse or vertical fracture of the thyroid cartilage. This may be associated with upward displacement of the arytenoids.

Glottic injuries are usually heralded by a midline or oblique vertical fracture of the thyroid cartilage. When the thyroid cartilages are compressed against the cervical spine, they are tethered in the parasymphyseal region and fracture vertically like a wishbone. They may also fracture obliquely or be comminuted. Thyroid cartilage fracture may be associated with true cord injury, anterior commissure disruption and cricoid fractures. While the arytenoid cartilages do not fracture as a rule, they often become dislocated at the crico-arytenoid joint. Most commonly the arytenoids are dislocated anteriorly, causing the true cords to be shortened and moved into a paramedian position.

Subglottic injuries consist of fractures of the cricoid cartilage with resultant airway narrowing by oedema, haemorrhage or chronic fibrosis. The cricoid must break in two places since it is a ring.

Tracheal injuries are characterized as fractures of the tracheal ring versus complete transection.

CONCLUSIONS

CT has made an important contribution to the assessment of patients with laryngeal carcinoma and following laryngeal trauma the technique is likely to remain a first-line investigation.

The role of MR imaging in evaluating laryngeal cancer is now evolving. The method offers great promise because of its multiplanar capability and its excellent soft-tissue contrast resolution in the detection of cartilage invasion (Lufkin & Hanafee 1986, Castelijns et al 1988). Recent work has shown that MR imaging may be superior to CT in the detection of laryngeal cartilage invasion and may therefore become the modality of choice to make this diagnosis (Castelijns et al 1988).

REFERENCES

Archer C R, Sagel S S, Yeager V L, Martin S, Friedman W H 1981 Staging of carcinoma of the larynx: comparative accuracy of CT and laryngography. American Journal of Roentgenology 136: 571–575

Castelijns J A, Gerritsen G J, Kaiser M C et al 1988 Invasion of laryngeal cartilage by cancer: comparison of CT and MR imaging. Radiology 167: 199–206

Horowitz B L, Woodson G E, Bryan R N 1984 CT of laryngeal tumours. Radiologic Clinics of North America 22: 265–279

Larsson S, Mancuso A, Hoover L, Hanafee W 1981 Differentiation of pyriform sinus cancer from supraglottic laryngeal cancer by computed tomography. Radiology 141: 427–432

Lufkin R B, Hanafee W N 1986 Imaging the laryngopharynx. Seminars in Ultrasound, CT and MR 7: 166–180

Mafee M F, Schild J A, Michael A S, Choi K H, Capek V 1984 Cartilage involvement in laryngeal carcinoma: correlation of CT and pathologic macrosection studies. Journal of Computer Assisted Tomography 8: 969–973

Mancuso A A, Hanafee W N 1979a A comparative evaluation of computed tomography and laryngography. Radiology 133: 131–138

Mancuso A A, Hanafee W N 1979b Computed tomography of the injured larynx. Radiology 133: 139–144

Sagel S S 1983 The Larynx. In: Lee J K T, Sagel S S, Stanley R J (eds) Computed Body Tomography. Raven Press, New York, pp 37–54

Silverman P M, Korobkin M 1983 High-resolution computed tomography of the normal larynx. American Journal of Roentgenology 140: 875–879

Silverman P M, Bossen E H, Fisher S R, Cole T B, Korobkin M, Halvorsen R A 1984 Carcinoma of the larynx and hypopharynx: computed tomographic-histopathologic correlations. Radiology 151: 697–702

2. Staging bronchial cancer

C. D. R. Flower and Michael P. Williams

INTRODUCTION

There are approximately 22 000 new cases of bronchial carcinoma in the United Kingdom each year and the incidence, particularly amongst women, is increasing. It accounts for approximately 12% of all malignancies. The commonest histological variants of bronchial carcinoma are squamous, adenocarcinoma, large-cell and small-cell types. From a management point of view the important division is between small-cell carcinoma and the remainder. Chemotherapy is the mainstay of treatment for small-cell carcinoma and detailed staging is not appropriate. The disease is simply classified as limited, when confined to one hemithorax and ipsilateral supraclavicular lymph nodes, or extensive. This division can be made on clinical examination, plain radiography, liver function tests and abdominal ultrasound without the need for CT.

In non-small-cell carcinoma complete surgical resection of disease at thoracotomy offers the best chance of long-term survival. Accurate staging is essential. The primary aim of staging must be to prevent unnecessary thoracotomy for those whose disease is unresectable without denying potentially curative surgery to those who may benefit. In many centres CT has become part of the presurgical staging of patients with bronchial carcinoma. CT provides exquisite axial imaging of mediastinal structures and early hopes that it would be able to demonstrate mediastinal nodes clearly have largely been fulfilled.

MEDIASTINAL LYMPH-NODE INVOLVEMENT

Normal size criteria

Studies on normal volunteers (Schnyder & Gamsu 1981, Glazer et al 1985a) and cadavers (Genereux & Howie 1984, Quint et al 1986; Kiyono et al 1988) confirm that CT scanning will demonstrate normal mediastinal lymph nodes and accurately assess their size. Nodal size at post-mortem correlates best with the short axis diameter shown on CT. Each author quotes a different normal dimension for lymph-node size depending on the region of the mediastinum under consideration. Nodes in the subcarinal and right paratracheal region tend to be the largest, whilst nodes in the left paratracheal region are smaller than on the right and may be less accurately assessed by CT. The normal values quoted for node size in the Japanese study (Kiyono et al 1988) are smaller than those in the North American work and it may be unreasonable to translate precise size ranges from one population to another. However, in general, most normal nodes shown by CT measure 5 mm or less in diameter with a small proportion, usually in the subcarinal and right paratracheal region, measuring up to 10 or 12 mm in diameter.

Technique

Careful attention to scanning technique is necessary if the CT examination and its interpretation are to yield fruitful results. It is essential that scans are contiguous, usually with 8 or 10 mm collimation and in cases of doubt it may be necessary to perform thinner sections in the 'danger areas' of the subaortic fossa and carinal region. Intravenous contrast enhancement must be used where there is doubt as to the presence or absence of nodes. In this respect it is best to perform a dynamic sequence of scans over a limited area timed to coincide with maximum intravascular opacification. Use of dynamic scanning is essential for the CT assessment of the hila and frequently raises diagnostic confidence in the assessment of the mediastinum.

Pitfalls

It is axiomatic that the radiologist has a thorough understanding of normal mediastinal anatomy and a knowledge of the potential pitfalls of CT interpretation. Anomalous vessels, such as an aberrant right subclavian artery or persistent left superior vena cava can be confused with mediastinal lymphadenopathy (Fig. 2.1). The use of intravenous contrast medium overcomes these potential problems. Other pitfalls, such as partial volume averaging from the top of the pulmonary outflow tract simulating lymphadenopathy in the aorto-pulmonary window or a superior recess of the pericardium simulating precarinal nodes, are only avoided by the use of sequential closely collimated scans.

Lymph-node metastases

Even with the knowledge of the range of normal for mediastinal lymph-node size one cannot simply equate large nodes with tumour involvement and vice versa. CT studies of the mediastinum in patients with carcinoma of the bronchus have shown that approximately 10% of nodes with a short axis diameter < 10 mm in diameter will be involved by tumour whilst approximately 15% of nodes with a diameter of > 15 mm will be

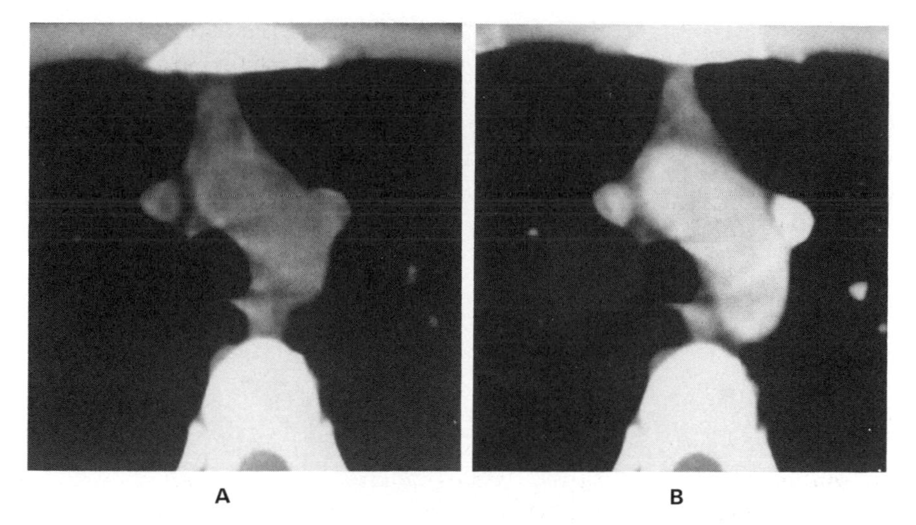

Fig. 2.1 CT scan at the level of the aortic arch. **A** Pre-contrast. **B** Post-contrast. Contrast medium was injected via the left anticubital fossa confirming that the structure lateral to the aortic arch represented a left superior vena cava.

uninvolved (Baron et al 1982, Goldstraw et al 1983, Daly et at 1984, Glazer et al 1984, McKenna et al 1985, Scott et al 1988, Staples et al 1988). Given that a high sensitivity, or negative predictive value, is required for any screening procedure, the acceptance of 'normality' as < 10 mm seems reasonable. A higher sensitivity may be obtained by lowering the criteria of 'normality' to 5 mm in diameter. This produces only a minimal gain in sensitivity for an unacceptably low specificity (Glazer et al 1985a, Staples et al 1988). Setting a size limit for normality accepts that some patients will have unexpected nodal micrometastases. However, evidence is now accumulating that for some patients with limited mediastinal nodal metastases, survival may be improved by surgical resection of tumour with ipsilateral mediastinal node clearance (Naruke et al 1978, Martini et al 1980, Pearson et al 1982).

The use of criteria which make CT a sensitive tool for the detection of mediastinal nodal metastases inevitably leads to a significant proportion of false positive results. Some will be due to normal nodes above the cut-off point of 10 mm in diameter whilst others will be due to enlarged hyperplastic or 'reactive' nodes. Such nodes are particularly likely to occur when cancer is associated with inflammatory changes in the lung or collapse of a lobe but this is not invariably the case (Whittlesey 1988). False positive diagnoses may also result from an inaccurate CT assessment of lymph-node size. A conglomeration of nodes, particularly in the subcarinal area, may be mistakenly assessed as enlargement of a single node. For all these reasons, histological sampling of CT positive nodes is mandatory.

Mediastinoscopy can sample many of the lymph-node stations at risk of

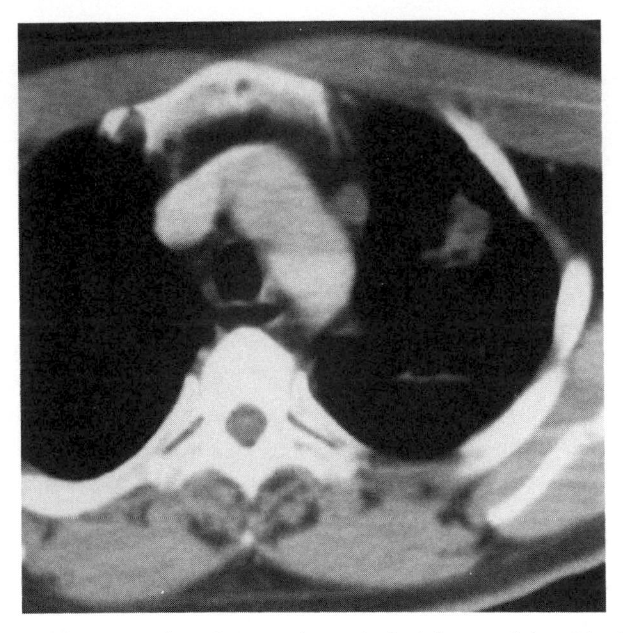

Fig. 2.2 CT scan demonstrating a 2 cm carcinoma in the left upper lobe with a 10×12 mm node lateral to the aortic arch. Such nodes may be sampled by left anterior mediastinotomy.

metastasis from bronchial carcinoma and this has been a major advance in prethoracotomy staging. Specificity is high but even at best there is a false negative rate of approximately 10% (Pearson et al 1972, Goldstraw et al 1983, Luke et al 1986, Staples et al 1988). Inevitably there are sampling errors with mediastinoscopy; not all nodes in accessible areas may be biopsied and not all nodal stations can be reached. CT may be used to guide the mediastinoscopist to enlarged nodes in accessible areas. With the CT scan used as a guide to mediastinal lymph-node exploration there should be fewer sampling errors. One study found no patients who had normal results on CT-guided mediastinal exploration to have abnormal mediastinal nodes at subsequent thoracotomy (Whittlesley 1988). CT may also indicate when other procedures are more appropriate, e.g. anterior mediastinotomy, for enlarged nodes in the subaortic fossa and lateral to the aortic arch (Fig. 2.2). Similarly, the CT demonstration of enlarged nodes in the immediate subcarinal region or posterior mediastinum may indicate a need for transbronchial needle biopsy or percutaneous needle biopsy rather than mediastinoscopy.

HILAR LYMPH-NODE INVOLVEMENT

If CT could reliably predict hilar node metastases and direct involvement of the main bronchi and pulmonary arteries by centrally placed tumours, it would provide a means for predicting whether pneumonectomy rather than

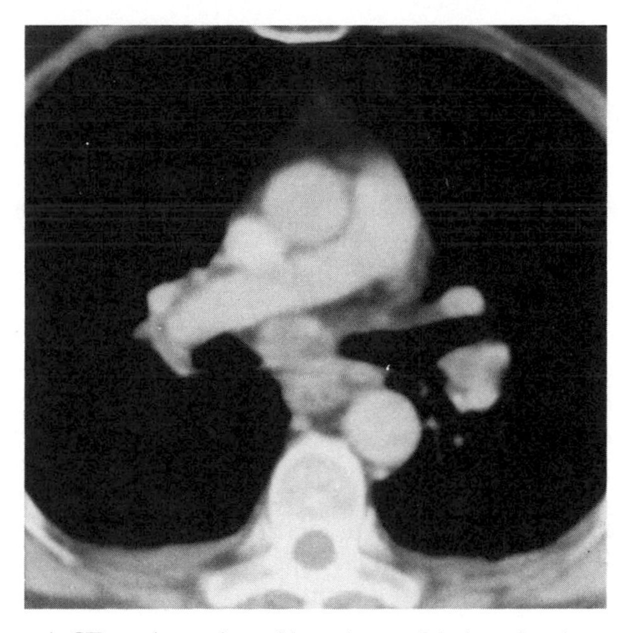

Fig. 2.3 Dynamic CT scan in a patient with carcinoma of the bronchus demonstrating a 2 × 2 cm node in the subcarinal region and a 1.5 cm node in the left hilum. Without intravenous contrast medium the hilar node may easily be confused with the left lower lobe artery.

lobectomy would be required. For the assessment of the hilum Glazer et al (1983) claimed that dynamic incremental CT was better than plain radiography or 55° posterior oblique hilar tomography (Fig. 2.3). In this study, however, there was a high prevalence of abnormal hila (69%) and the study group included patients with hilar and mediastinal lymphadenopathy which was obvious on conventional radiography. When applied to a more representative sample of patients with bronchial carcinoma being considered for surgical resection, the same authors found the overall accuracy of CT no better than 55° posterior oblique hilar tomography. Although CT was slightly more sensitive than tomography it was less specific as nodes from 1–2 cm in diameter were better identified by CT although they often did not contain tumour (Glazer et al 1985b). Other difficulties in predicting whether pneumonectomy or lobectomy is required have recently been emphasized. In a study by Quint et al (1987) the features necessitating pneumonectomy were invasion of major pulmonary arteries or veins, invasion of major bronchi and transfissural tumour spread. No assessment of hilar node status was made. Prediction of vascular invasion by CT was generally good but few patients required pneumonectomy for this reason. The main indications for pneumonectomy were invasion of the walls of major bronchi or transfissural spread and the sensitivity of CT for both these features was only approximately 50%.

DIRECT TUMOUR SPREAD

Direct mediastinal and chest wall invasion by tumour has been regarded as evidence of unresectability until recently. However, many surgeons are now prepared to resect tumours that involve the chest wall, mediastinal pleura, pericardium and diaphragm. Nevertheless, demonstration of invasion of these structures would be very useful and, in particular, unequivocal evidence of invasion of the great vessels and oesophagus would preclude operation. In general, CT has been rather disappointing in predicting both mediastinal and chest wall invasion and it is wise for radiologists to err on the conservative side. Demonstration of a tumour in contiguity with the mediastinum or pleura, even when there is associated pleural thickening, does not necessarily indicate tumour extension. Chest wall invasion can only be diagnosed reliably when there is evidence of bone destruction or frank extension into the soft tissues (Figs. 2.4 and 2.5) (Pennes et al 1985, Pearlberg et al 1987). A salutary reminder of these limitations was provided by one study which indicated that chest wall pain was as likely to predict chest wall invasion as CT! (Glazer et al 1985).

DISTANT METASTASES

The adrenals may be the only site of metastatic spread in a small proportion of patients and continuation of the CT study into the upper abdomen provides the bonus of imaging the liver and adrenals at little extra cost in time. Adrenal masses > 2 cm are usually due to metastases but smaller masses are more likely to be due to adenomas (Sandler et al 1982, Oliver et al 1984, Pagani 1984). Solitary adrenal masses should therefore be

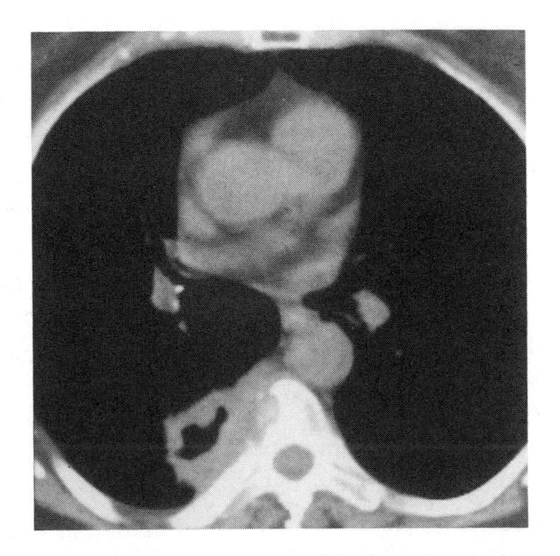

Fig. 2.4 A cavitating squamous-cell carcinoma of the bronchus is shown to be unresectable by CT because of vertebral body invasion.

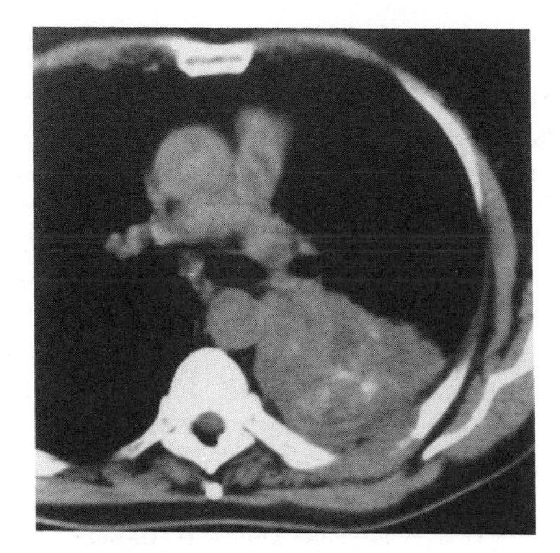

Fig. 2.5 CT in a patient with a large peripheral carcinoma confirms chest wall invasion by demonstrating tumour extension into the intercostal muscles and by showing associated rib destruction.

biopsied percutaneously and only if a cytological or histological diagnosis of a metastasis is made should the patient be denied surgery.

In non-small-cell lung cancer only a small proportion of patients will have cerebral metastases at presentation and the likelihood of this being the only site of metastatic disease is very small. It therefore seems reasonable to dispense with the additional time and cost of cranial CT unless there are specific indications.

CONCLUSIONS

Although several difficulties are encountered in attempting to assess lymph-node status and direct tumour invasion in patients with carcinoma of the bronchus, there is no doubt that CT can provide important information for the surgeon. Thus, the extent of disease demonstrated by CT may preclude surgery altogether and the demonstration of enlarged mediastinal nodes may provide a useful guide for lymph-node sampling at mediastinoscopy. CT has been relatively disappointing for staging centrally placed tumours and appears to be no better than conventional methods for predicting whether pneumonectomy or lobectomy is required.

REFERENCES

Baron R L, Levitt R G, Sagel S S, White M J, Roper C L, Marbarger J P 1982 Computed tomography in the pre-operative evaluation of bronchogenic carcinoma. Radiology 145: 727–732

Daly B D, Faling L J, Pugatch R D et al 1984 Computed tomography: an effective technique

for mediastinal staging in lung cancer. Journal of Thoracic and Cardiovascular Surgery 88: 486–494
Genereux G P, Howie J L 1984 Normal mediastinal lymph node size and number: CT an anatomic study. American Journal of Roentgenology 142: 1095–1100
Glazer H S, Duncan-Meyer J, Aronberg D J, Moran J F, Levitt R G, Sagel S S 1985 Pleural and chest wall invasion in bronchogenic carcinoma: CT evaluation. Radiology 157: 191–194
Glazer G M, Francis I R, Shirazi K K, Bookstein F L, Gross B H, Orringer M B 1983 Evaluation of pulmonary hilum: comparison of conventional radiography, 55° posterior oblique tomography and dynamic computed tomography. Journal of Computer Assisted Tomography 7: 983–989
Glazer G M, Gross B H, Aisen A M, Quint L E, Francis I R, Orringer M B 1985b Imaging of the pulmonary hilum: a prospective comparative study in patients with lung cancer. American Journal of Roentgenology 145: 245–248
Glazer G M, Gross B H, Quint L E, Francis I R, Bookstein F L, Orringer M B 1985a Normal mediastinal lymph nodes: number and size according to American Thoracic Society Mapping. American Journal of Roentgenology 144: 261–265
Glazer G M, Orringer M B, Gross B H, Quint L 1984 The mediastinum in non-small-cell cancer. American Journal of Roentgenology 142: 1101–1105
Goldstraw P, Curzer M, Edwards D 1983 Pre-operative staging of lung cancer: accuracy of computed tomography versus mediastinoscopy. Thorax 38: 10–15
Kiyono K, Sone S, Sakai F et al 1988 The number and size of normal mediastinal lymph nodes: a postmortem study. American Journal of Roentgenology 150: 771–776
Luke W P, Todd T R G, Cooper J D 1986 Prospective evaluation of mediastinoscopy for assessment of carcinoma of the lung. Journal of Thoracic and Cardiovascular Surgery 91: 53–56
McKenna R J, Libshitz H I, Mountain C E, McMurtrey M J 1985 Roentgenographic evaluation of mediastinal nodes for pre-operative assessment in lung cancer. Chest 88: 206–210
Martini N, Flehinger B J, Zaman M B, Beattie E J Jr 1980 Prospective study of 445 lung carcinomas with mediastinal lymph-node metastases. Journal of Thoracic and Cardiovascular Surgery 80: 390–399
Naruke T, Suemasu K, Ishikawa S 1978 Lymph-node mapping and curability at various levels of metastasis in resected lung cancer. Journal of Thoracic and Cardiovascular Surgery 76: 832–839
Oliver T W, Bernardino M E, Miller J I, Mansour K, Greene D, Davis W A 1984 Isolated adrenal masses in non-small-cell bronchogenic carcinoma. Radiology 153: 217–218
Pagani J J 1984 Non-small-cell lung carcinoma: adrenal metastases. Computed tomography and percutaneous needle biopsy in their diagnosis. Cancer 53: 1058–1060
Pearlberg J L, Sandler M A, Beute G, Lewis J W Jr, Madrazo B L 1987 Limitations of CT in evaluation of neoplasms involving chest wall. Journal of Computer Assisted Tomography 11: 290–293
Pearson F G, DeLarue N C, Ilves R, Todd T R, Cooper J D 1982 Significance of positive superior mediastinal nodes identified at mediastinoscopy in patients with resectable cancer of the lung. Journal of Thoracic and Cardiovascular Surgery 83: 1–11
Pearson F G, Nelems J M, Henderson R D et al 1972 The role of mediastinoscopy in the selection of treatment for bronchial carcinoma with involvement of superior mediastinal lymph nodes. Journal of Thoracic and Cardiovascular Surgery 64: 382–387
Pennes D R, Glazer G M, Wimbish K J, Gross B H, Long R W, Orringer M B 1985 Chest wall invasion by lung cancer: limitations of CT evaluation. American Journal of Roentgenology 144: 507–511
Quint L E, Glazer G M, Orringer M B, Francis I R, Bookstein F L 1986 Mediastinal lymph-node detection and sizing at CT and autopsy. American Journal of Roentgenology 147: 469–472
Quint L E, Glazer G M, Orringer M B 1987 Central lung masses: prediction with CT of need for pneumonectomy versus lobectomy. Radiology 165: 735–738
Sandler M A, Pearlberg L, Madrazo B L, Gitschlag K F 1982 Computed tomographic evaluation of the adrenal gland in the pre-operative assessment of bronchogenic carcinoma. Radiology 145: 733–736

Schnyder P A, Gamsu G 1981 CT of the pretracheal retrocaval space. American Journal of Roentgenology 136: 303–308
Scott I R, Muller N L, Miller R R, Evans K G, Nelems B 1988 Resectable Stage III lung cancer: CT, surgical and pathologic correlation. Radiology 166: 75–79
Staples C A, Muller N L, Miller R R, Evans K G, Nelems B 1988 Mediastinal nodes in bronchogenic carcinoma: comparison between CT and mediastinoscopy. Radiology 167: 367–372
Whittlesey D 1988 Prospective computed tomographic scanning in the staging of bronchogenic cancer. Journal of Thoracic and Cardiovascular Surgery 95: 876–882

3. The pleural space

C. D. R. Flower and Michael P. Williams

INTRODUCTION

Computed tomography is a relatively simple and effective method for imaging the pleura. Overlying shadows from lung densities and soft tissues which may obscure the interface between pleura and lung on plain radiography are not a problem and the cross-sectional display of CT is ideal for the demonstration of the medial, lateral, anterior and posterior aspects of the pleural surface at all levels throughout the thorax. CT is of most value when used to investigate thoracic problems which are not adequately addressed by chest radiography or ultrasound.

FLUID COLLECTIONS

Pleural effusion

CT is the most sensitive method for the detection of pleural fluid. It is generally possible to distinguish pleural fluid collections from solid pleural lesions on the basis of attenuation values. Pleural effusions usually have a density of up to 20 Hounsfield units with solid lesions having higher values. However, attenuation values are of little help in distinguishing between different causes of pleural fluid. Even an acute haemothorax may appear of water density. Most pleural effusions are free flowing and produce a sickle-shaped opacity in the most dependent part of the thorax. Loculated fluid collections are seen as lenticular opacities of fixed position. The transverse axial display of CT usually makes it easy to recognize that fluid lies in the pleural space although when pleural fluid lies in the posterior costophrenic recesses adjacent to the diaphragm it may be difficult to differentiate from ascites. A number of signs have been described to differentiate between juxtadiaphragmatic pleural effusion and ascitic fluid. The most important guide to the location of fluid is its relationship to the hemidiaphragm. Fluid which lies anterior to the hemidiaphragm and is surrounded by it is intra-abdominal whilst fluid posterior to the diaphragm is within the pleural space. Another helpful sign for distinguishing pleural fluid from ascites is lateral displacement of the diaphragmatic crura by accumulation of fluid in the pleural recesses between the crura and the spine (Dwyer 1978). An

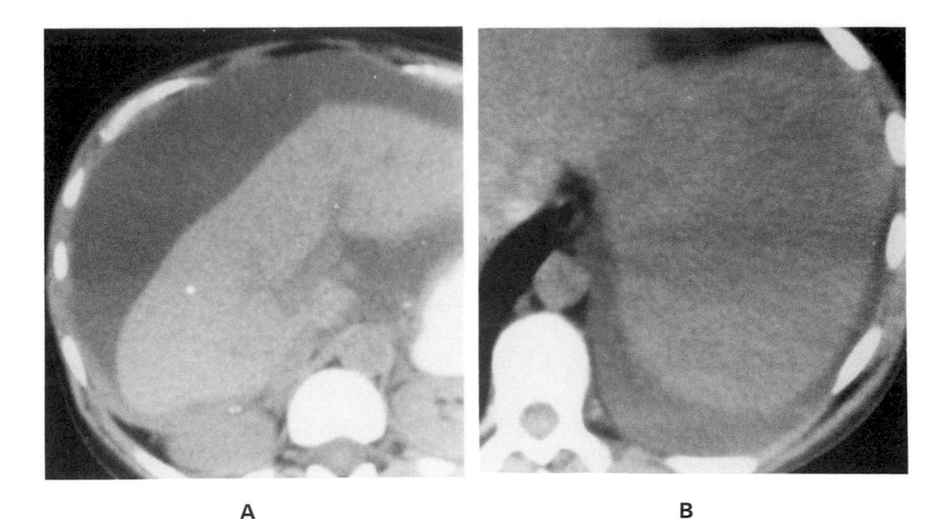

Fig. 3.1 CT sections through the juxtadiaphragmatic regions in two patients to illustrate the 'interface' sign. **A** CT scan demonstrating ascites from ovarian carcinoma. The interface between liver and ascitic fluid is sharp. Note thickening of the hemidiaphragm by peritoneal metastases and the incidental area of hepatic calcification. **B** CT scan of a lymphoma patient with splenomegaly and a left pleural effusion. The interface between spleen and effusion is hazy due to partial volume effect from diaphragm interposed between fluid and spleen.

'interface' sign has also been described (Teplick et al 1982). Pleural effusion typically shows a hazy interface between the fluid and liver and/or spleen whereas the interface between ascites and these organs is sharply demarcated (Fig. 3.1). The explanation for this sign is that in the case of pleural fluid there is always a partial volume effect from the hemidiaphragm at the apparent interface between fluid and liver or spleen. In contra-distinction, a true interface exists between ascites and the intra-abdominal organs, the margins of which thus appear sharp. The existence of the bare area of the liver can also be of some help in localization of juxtadiaphragmatic fluid as the coronary ligament, which attaches the liver to the posterior peritoneum, excludes ascites from the bare area. Ascitic fluid, therefore, cannot surround the entire postero-superior aspect of the liver, whereas a pleural effusion may appear to do so (Naidich et al 1983).

Even with these guidelines there are potential pitfalls. Probably the most common is when a pleural effusion is present but a prominent posterior parietal pleural line is mistaken for the hemidiaphragm. Fluid posterior to the true hemidiaphragm and thus in the chest, appears anterior to this false hemidiaphragm and may be mistaken for ascites. Similarly, subsegmental atelectasis can form a curvilinear band parallel to, and simulating, the true hemidiaphragm (Silverman et al 1985). Fluid anterior to the atelectatic lung gives a false impression of subdiaphragmatic peritoneal fluid.

Alterations of juxtadiaphragmatic anatomy caused by postsurgical changes or pleural adhesions will also cause difficulty, as may inversion of the hemidiaphragm which occurs with very large pleural effusions. Naidich et al (1983) suggest that parasagittal reconstructions may help in displaying the anatomy of diaphragmatic inversion but usually real-time ultrasound provides a quicker and easier method to demonstrate this phenomenon.

Pleuropulmonary disease

The accurate distinction between pulmonary and pleural disease or the demonstration that both are associated is particularly useful in clinical practice (Pugatch et al 1978). Thus, unexpected fluid collections may be seen in association with pneumonia or tumour, and underlying lung or mediastinal disease may be seen as the cause of a pleural effusion or empyema. Unravelling pleuropulmonary disease by CT is best accomplished at an early stage in the diagnostic pathway to allow prompt and accurate therapy and intervention (Fig. 3.2).

Air–fluid collections

Unexpected or unusual air–fluid collections seen on the chest radiograph, however small, should prompt CT. This will enable suppurative lung disease (abscess or bronchiectasis) to be distinguished from an empyema or

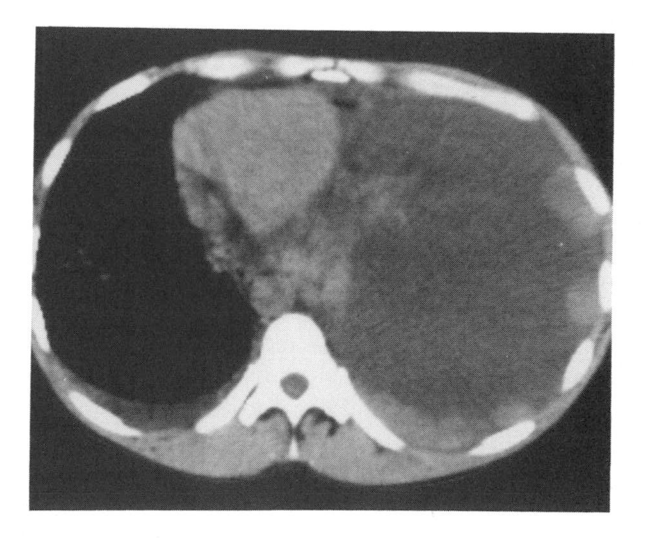

Fig. 3.2 CT scan showing bilateral effusions and extensive right-sided pleural masses in a patient in whom plain radiography demonstrated only a large left pleural effusion. CT-guided biopsy of one of these masses revealed metastatic soft-tissue sarcoma.

bronchopleural fistula. Enhancement with intravenous contrast medium improves diagnostic ability and scanning is performed at selected levels to coincide with the early tissue phase after a bolus injection (Bressler et al 1987).

Numerous features have been described to differentiate a lung abscess from an empyema (Stark et al 1983a, Proto & Merkar 1984). Separation of uniformly thickened visceral and parietal pleura, which is best demonstrated after intravenous contrast medium enhancement, is a specific sign of empyema and is not seen in cases of lung abscess. Another sign specific to empyema is compression of adjacent uninvolved lung. This may be recognized by noting distortion and bowing of bronchi and vessels around the periphery of the lesion. A lung abscess, being an intrapulmonary process, destroys vessels and bronchi within the lesion but does not affect those outside it. The characteristics of the wall of the collection are also helpful. In empyema at least a portion of the wall is usually thin, smooth and uniform, whereas a lung abscess typically has a thick irregular wall. The size and shape of the lesion and the angle with the chest wall are less reliable distinguishing signs. An abscess tends to be rounded and relatively small whereas an empyema is usually oval and rather larger. Classically, an abscess makes an acute angle with the chest wall, whereas an empyema tends to make an obtuse angle. These signs are not specific, however, and a large tense empyema may show an acute angle with the chest wall. Multiplicity of lesions, air–fluid levels within the lesion, the presence of pleural fluid and associated consolidation are unhelpful in distinguishing between an abscess and empyema. As noted by Stark et al (1983a) multiple diagnostic CT features are usually present in each case and this group were able to differentiate lung abscess from empyema in 100% of 70 cases.

Pleural drainage

The vast majority of pleural drainage procedures are undertaken for simple serous effusions and only plain radiography and clinical examination are required. In the case of known or suspected empyema, however, this may not suffice and ultrasound or CT-guided thoracocentesis may be necessary. CT and ultrasound-guided drainage of empyemas was originally undertaken only after failure of conventional tube drainage (van Sonnenberg et al 1984) but it is increasingly being used as a primary method of treatment for the diagnosis and drainage of infected pleural collections (Westcott 1985, Hunnam & Flower 1988). Failure of conventional tube drainage is usually the result of poor positioning of the chest drain which may result not only in incomplete drainage but may also cause pain, subcutaneous emphysema, leakage and chylothorax. CT has shown that tubes introduced at the bedside are often inaccurately sited (Stark et al 1983b). CT obviates incorrect placement of the tube and shows if there are multiple locules which will require more than one tube for complete drainage. CT may also demonstrate unexpected associated or causative conditions, such as perforated oesophagus, bronchopleural fistula or subphrenic collection (van Sonnenberg et al 1984).

The method of CT-guided empyema drainage is essentially similar to that for percutaneous abdominal abscess drainage. Catheters of 8.3–12 French gauge will usually suffice and only occasionally will there be such thick pus present that the tube will not drain and thoracotomy and decortication will be required. Incomplete drainage of the empyema can readily be checked by follow-up CT examination and if necessary further catheters may be introduced into undrained locules. Catheters left within an empyema cavity should be connected to water seal suction until the cavity collapses. Care should be taken to ensure that all the side holes of the catheter are within the cavity to be drained so that air does not inadvertently leak into the pleural space. As long as such simple guidelines are followed then percutaneous catheter drainage of an empyema is a safe procedure and is well tolerated by the patient.

Either CT or ultrasound may be used as a guide to localize pleural fluid collections and, most importantly, to demonstrate the level of the diaphragm prior to thoracocentesis. Ultrasound is simple to use on the larger lesions and in patients who are well enough to sit up it allows easy access to the most dependent part of the empyema cavity. CT is preferred where the lesion is small, multilocular or in close proximity to vital structures.

As a general rule percutaneous catheter drainage is employed in empyemas and avoided in lung abscesses as in the latter condition there is the possibility of contamination of adjacent lung and unaffected pleural space. Lung abscesses which are refractory to conventional therapy and which abut the pleural surface, however, may be treated successfully with CT-guided percutaneous drainage (van Sonnenberg et al 1984).

PNEUMOTHORAX

The majority of pneumothoraces are accurately demonstrated by standard chest radiography. Difficulties arise when films can only be exposed with the patients supine or semi-recumbent when the signs of the pneumothorax are subtle. Pneumothoraces which have a significant effect on ventilation may be missed in such circumstances. Such occult pneumothoraces are well shown by CT which can also be used to safely guide intercostal tube placement (Tocino et al 1984, Tocino & Miller 1987, Casola et al 1988).

SOFT-TISSUE PLEURAL LESIONS

Thickening of the pleura by fibrosis, localized plaques or tumour is usually well demonstrated and accurately defined by CT although occasionally an accompanying effusion may mask associated pleural masses. Tissue characterization of pleural tumours is impossible by CT with the exception of pleural lipomas which have the characteristic low attenuation of fat.

CT may be useful in evaluating the pleuropulmonary changes associated with asbestos exposure. CT is much more sensitive than chest radiography for the detection of pleural plaques (Katz & Kreel 1979) although it is not generally required for their diagnosis. CT can be useful, however, when there is doubt as to their presence or when they are multiple and mimic pulmonary masses on the chest radiograph. In the obese patient with prominent extrapleural fat deposits CT may be helpful for excluding the presence of pleural plaques. 'Benign' pleural thickening secondary to asbestos exposure is commonly associated with deformity of the adjacent lung; CT reveals a variety of appearances from crease-like changes, usually invisible on the chest radiograph, to round atelectasis (Heller et al 1970, Alexander et al 1981, Scott et al 1984). Recently, it has been suggested that high-resolution CT scanning using 1.5 mm thick sections viewed at wide window settings, may be even more sensitive than conventional chest CT for the detection of both pleural thickening and pleural fibrosis in patients with clinical asbestosis (Aberle et al 1988).

Another circumstance in which CT may be helpful is when there is unexplained pleural thickening on the chest radiograph. The differentiation between a malignant pleural tumour and fibrothorax is important and sometimes difficult. The history may help as some patients with a chronic fibrothorax give a history of either previous haemorrhage or empyema although in others the underlying cause remains obscure. One feature which may be helpful in distinguishing radiologically between chronic fibrothorax and mesothelioma is that in the former the normal low

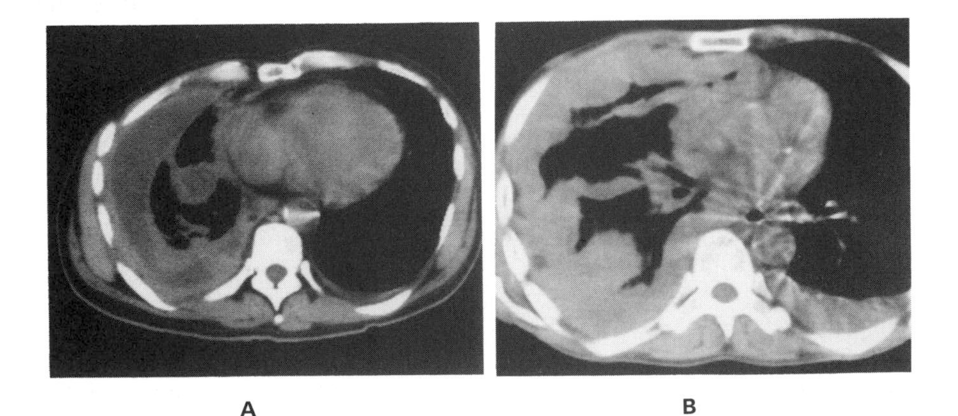

Fig. 3.3 Mesothelioma. **A** CT scan shows the lung encased by a combination of pleural fluid and solid tumour. Note crowding of the ribs on the right, pericardial thickening and loss of the extrapleural low density stripe. **B** CT scan shows a lobulated soft-tissue dense tumour encasing the right lung. Note subcarinal lymphadenopathy and contralateral effusion.

density extrapleural stripe is usually clearly visible whereas in the latter the stripe is obliterated (Fig. 3.3a).

Extensive pleural malignancy is most commonly seen in mesothelioma and in diffuse secondary adenocarcinoma. The CT appearances of these neoplastic processes are similar. Typically, there is a lobulated rind of pleural tumour encasing the lung associated with a variable amount of pleural fluid (Fig. 3.3). The distinction between the solid components and the effusion may be difficult and this may present problems when attempting to drain the pleural fluid in a symptomatic patient. In patients with mesothelioma there may be features suggestive of asbestos exposure visible in the contralateral hemithorax, e.g. pleural plaques or pleural calcification. Both mesothelioma and secondary pleural adenocarcinoma will spread along the fissures and eventually into the lung parenchyma. There may be associated mediastinal lymphadenopathy, pericardial thickening and tumour spread to the contralateral hemithorax. In advanced mesothelioma tumour may even spread through the diaphragm and into the abdomen.

The post-pneumonectomy space

CT is invaluable for the assessment of the opaque hemithorax after pneumonectomy. Plain radiography is only able to detect disease recurrence by gross mediastinal displacement. CT may detect recurrent tumour at a much earlier stage and can detect small locules of gas in an empyema not visible on plain radiography.

It is important to be aware of the expected findings on CT in patients post-pneumonectomy. In the majority of cases the fluid-filled post-pneumonectomy space persists even several years after surgery. In the remainder this space becomes obliterated by homogeneous soft tissue density material. There is an inverse relationship between over-expansion of the contralateral lung and persistence of the post-pneumonectomy space. If the contralateral lung enlarges well then the post-pneumonectomy space tends to become obliterated whilst with less marked expansion the post-pneumonectomy space tends to remain large and filled with fluid (Biondetti et al 1982). Calcification may be seen around the margins of the post-pneumonectomy space, even when it remains filled with fluid centrally. In the case of a right pneumonectomy the mediastinum rotates and the aortic arch comes to lie transversely with the left lung herniating into the right hemithorax anterior to it. In the case of a left pneumonectomy the mediastinum tends to shift laterally to the left, the aortic arch lying along the sagittal plane with the right lung herniating both anterior and posterior to the mediastinum. It is essential to recognize these normal displacements post-pneumonectomy in order not to confuse displaced vascular structures with recurrent disease.

Recurrent disease is usually shown as nodal masses within the mediastinum or as soft-tissue dense masses projecting into the fluid-filled post-pneumonectomy space. If there is any doubt as to the presence of recurrent disease then scanning through the area of interest during the infusion of intravenous contrast medium is essential.

CHEST WALL TUMOURS

The commonest tumours of the chest wall are rib deposits from metastatic carcinoma or multiple myeloma and these are best assessed by plain radiography. Focal rib destruction is not as well shown on CT as with conventional radiography. This is partly because only a small portion of the rib is seen on axial images and partly because partial volume averaging makes assessment of rib destruction difficult. CT is superior to conventional radiography for the demonstration of vertebral body involvement or erosion.

Pleural invasion, either from a primary chest wall tumour or from local spread of a tumour of the mediastinum or lung, cannot be reliably detected with CT (Pennes et al 1985, Scott et al 1988). However, CT may be helpful in the demonstration of chest wall involvement from tumour arising in internal mammary lymph nodes. Carcinoma of the breast or lymphoma may spread from these nodes to involve muscle and to destroy the anterior

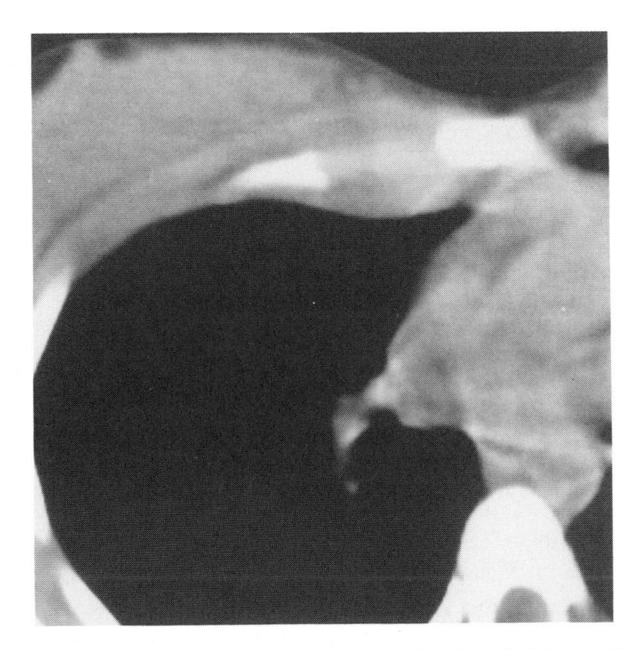

Fig. 3.4 CT scan of the chest in a patient with chest wall pain and a history of previous Hodgkin's disease. This demonstrates chest wall invasion from recurrent disease arising in an internal mammary lymph node. Plain radiography and physical examination were normal.

end of the costal cartilages but this will not be visible on plain radiography (Fig. 3.4). Primary or secondary tumours affecting the sternum are also much better evaluated with CT than with plain radiography. On occasion, CT may show subtle early abnormalities due to a chest wall tumour in a patient who presents with persistent chest wall pain.

Primary chest wall tumours which have a large soft-tissue component are well shown by CT and the technique is particularly helpful for defining the upper and lower limits of the tumour. CT frequently demonstrates more extensive disease than is apparent on clinical examination or conventional radiography.

CONCLUSION

Evaluation of pleural space pathology on conventional radiographs can be very difficult and CT offers a quick and simple method for resolving these problems. In many instances the information derived from CT has important implications for diagnosis and further management.

REFERENCES

Aberle D R, Gamsu G, Ray C S, Feuerstein I M 1988 Asbestos related pleural and parenchymal fibrosis: detection with high resolution CT. Radiology 166: 729–734

Alexander E, Clark R, Colley D 1981 CT of malignant pleural mesothelioma. American Journal of Roentgenology 137: 287–291

Biondetti P R, Fiore D, Sartori F, Colognato A, Ravasini R, Romani S 1982 Evaluation of the post-pneumonectomy space by computed tomography. Journal of Computer Assisted Tomography 6: 238–242

Bressler E L, Francis I R, Glazer G M, Gross B H 1987 Bolus contrast enhancement for distinguishing pleural from parenchymal lung disease: CT features. Journal of Computer Assisted Tomography 11: 436–440

Casola G C, van Sonnenberg E, Keightley A, Ho M, Withers C, Lee A S 1988 Pneumothorax: radiologic treatment with small catheters. Radiology 166: 89–91

Dwyer A 1978 The displaced crus: a sign for distinguishing between pleural fluid and ascites on computed tomography. Journal of Computer Assisted Tomography 2: 598–599

Heller R, Murray L, Weber A 1970 Radiological manifestations of malignant pleural mesothelioma. American Journal of Roentgenology 108: 53–59

Hunnam G R, Flower C D R 1988 Radiologically guided percutaneous catheter drainage of empyemas. Clinical Radiology 39: 121–126

Katz D, Kreel L 1979 Computed tomography in pulmonary asbestosis. Clinical Radiology 30: 207–213

Naidich D P, Megibow A J, Hilton S, Hulnick D H, Siegelman S S 1983 Computed tomography of the diaphragm: peridiaphragmatic fluid localisation. Journal of Computer Assisted Tomography 7: 641–649

Pennes D R, Glazer G W, Wimbish K J, Gross B H, Long R W, Orringer M B 1985 Chest wall invasion by lung cancer: limitations of CT evaluation. American Journal of Roentgenology 144: 507–511

Proto A V, Merkar G L 1984 Central bronchial displacement with large posterior pleural collections. Journal of the Canadian Association of Radiologists 35: 128–132

Pugatch R D, Faling L J, Robbins A H, Snider G L 1978 Differentiation of pleural and pulmonary lesions using computed tomography. Journal of Computer Assisted Tomography 2: 601–606

Scott I R, Muller N L, Miller R R, Evans K G, Nelems B 1988 Resectable Stage III lung cancer: CT, surgical and pathologic correlation. Radiology 166: 75–79

Scott W W, Scott P P, Siegelman S S 1984 Asbestos related pleural disease. In: Siegelman S (ed) Computed tomography of the chest. Churchill Livingstone, New York, pp 139–174
Silverman P M, Baker M E, Mahony B S 1985 Atelectasis and subpulmonic fluid: a CT pitfall in distinguishing pleural from peritoneal fluid. Journal of Computer Assisted Tomography 9: 763–766
Stark D D, Federle M P, Goodman P C, Podrasky A E, Webb W R 1983a Differentiating lung abscess and empyema: radiography and computed tomography. American Journal of Roentgenology 141: 163–167
Stark D D, Federle M P, Goodman P C 1983b CT and radiographic assessment of tube thoracostomy. American Journal of Roentgenology 141: 253–258
Teplick J G, Teplick S K, Goodman L R, Haskin M E 1982 Interface sign: a computed tomographic sign for distinguishing pleural and intra-abdominal fluid. Radiology 144: 359–362
Tocino I, Miller M H, Frederick P R, Bahr A L, Thomas F 1984 CT detection of occult pneumothorax in head trauma. American Journal of Roentgenology 143: 987–990
Tocino I, Miller M H 1987 Computed tomography in blunt chest trauma. Journal of Thoracic Imaging 2: 45–49
van Sonnenberg E, Nakamoto S K, Mueller P R et al 1984 CT and ultrasound-guided catheter drainage of empyemas after chest tube failure. Radiology 151: 349–353
Westcott J L 1985 Percutaneous catheter drainage of pleural effusion and empyema. American Journal of Roentgenology 144: 1189–1193

4. CT of pulmonary collapse*

Harvey S. Glazer

INTRODUCTION

The patterns of pulmonary collapse seen on the plain chest radiograph have been well described (Proto & Tocino 1980). However, the appearance may be confusing, especially if scarring or adhesions exist between the lung and adjacent pleura. Computed tomography is often helpful in clarifying that the plain film findings are secondary to collapse and it may also suggest the underlying cause and determine the presence and extent of an obstructing process (Naidich et al 1983a, b, Glazer et al 1984, Naidich et al 1984, Raasch et al 1984). In addition, the underlying mediastinum is not obscured by the collapsed lung on CT and can be easily evaluated for coexistent lymphadenopathy or direct invasion by a bronchial neoplasm. Bronchoscopy, however, still plays a vital role in the evaluation of pulmonary collapse, especially in determining the histological nature of an obstructing lesion.

GENERAL OBSERVATIONS

Both the direct (fissural displacement, hypo-aeration, vascular/bronchial crowding) and indirect (mediastinal shift, hilar displacement, compensatory hyperaeration, decreased size of hemithorax, elevation of hemidiaphragm) signs of collapse seen on plain chest radiographs can be applied to CT. This concept is important so that the CT findings are not confused with a 'mass'. Although most observations can be made on a standard CT examination (contiguous 8–10 mm sections) several additional thin sections (4–5 mm) may be helpful for identifying an obstructing mass in specific lobar or segmental bronchi. The administration of intravenous contrast material may prove useful for separating a proximal obstructing mass from distal atelectatic lung.

* Adapted in part from Sagel S S, Glazer H S CT of the lung, pleura and chest wall. In: Lee J K T, Sagel S S, Stanley R J (eds) Computed Body Tomography with MRI Correlation. Raven Press, New York (in press).

LEFT UPPER LOBE COLLAPSE

The left upper lobe (LUL) collapses predominantly in an anterosuperior direction against the anterior chest wall. Superior migration of the lung is limited somewhat by the left pulmonary artery passing over the LUL bronchus. As a result the superior segment of the left lower lobe (LLL) frequently hyperexpands towards the left lung apex. On CT, the atelectatic LUL appears as a triangular or V-shaped soft-tissue density structure that abuts the chest wall anterolaterally with the apex of the V merging with the pulmonary hilum. As the collapse increases there is less contact between the LUL and the lateral chest wall. The collapsed lobe is bordered medially by the mediastinum and posteriorly by the major fissure, which is displaced anteriorly. Although the lobe is usually of homogeneous soft-tissue density, some crowded air-filled bronchi may be seen.

Secondary signs of collapse include elevation of the left hilum with foreshortening of the aortopulmonary window and mediastinal displacement which is usually accompanied by herniation of the right lung anteriorly. The LUL bronchus, which is normally lower than the RUL bronchus, may be seen at approximately the same level when the left hilum is elevated. Moreover, the LLL bronchus may move anterolaterally. If the elevated left pulmonary artery is imaged lateral to the aortic arch, it may simulate lymphadenopathy. The hyperexpanded superior segment of the left lower lobe frequently extends between the collapsed LUL and aortic arch, accounting for the 'periaortic lucency' seen on the plain chest radiograph. Decreased size of the left hemithorax is also apparent and is often much more striking on CT than on the chest radiograph.

A proximal obstructing lesion is usually manifested by obvious bronchial

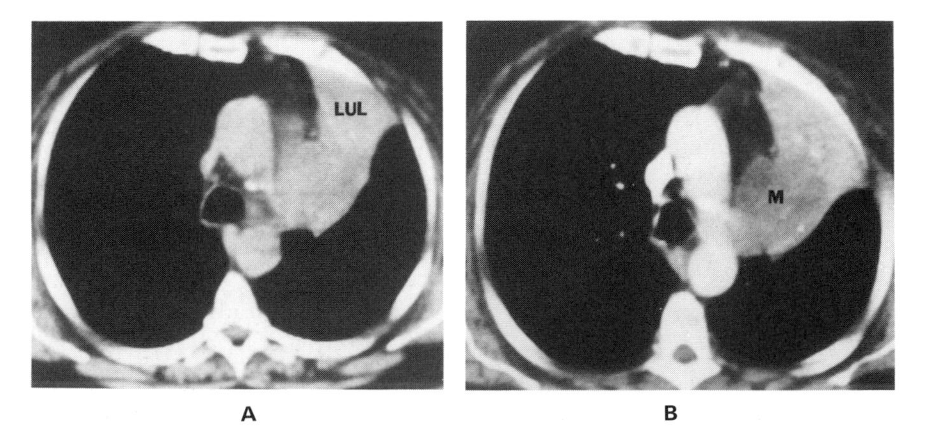

Fig. 4.1 Left upper lobe collapse. **A** Pre-contrast CT scan at level of aortopulmonary window demonstrates the collapsed left upper lobe (LUL) which bulges centrally secondary to an obstructing bronchogenic carcinoma. **B** Post-contrast CT scan showing that the lower attenuation mass (M) is more easily separated from the enhancing atelectatic lung.

narrowing or an intraluminal mass. However, it may be necessary to obtain several thin CT sections through the suspected level of obstruction to confidently identify subtle abnormalities. Careful attention to the contour of the collapsed lobe may confirm the presence of a proximal mass. In the absence of a large proximal obstructing lesion, the collapsed lobe should taper smoothly towards the hilum. If the obstructing mass, e.g. bronchogenic carcinoma or lymphadenopathy, is large enough a contour bulge may be seen. The wedge of lung will be seen to widen focally rather than taper as it extends to the hilum (Fig. 4.1). This is the CT equivalent of the 'S-sign of Golden' and may be more apparent than on plain chest radiographs. This finding, especially when focal, is highly suggestive of a mass, although a long smooth convex fissural margin can be seen occasionally in the absence of adjacent tumour (Khoury et al 1985). An abnormal contour may also be seen in patients with a drowned lung or altered anatomy secondary to scarring or thoracic deformity. Although the distinction between benign and malignant neoplasms can only be made histologically, in some cases CT can confidently identify a benign cause of obstruction, e.g. broncholithiasis.

Intravenous contrast administration may be helpful for delineating a proximal tumour and separating it from collapsed lung as well as from adjacent mediastinal structures (Figs. 4.1 and 4.2). Collapsed lung usually enhances to a greater degree than a neoplasm. Since this differential enhancement may only be apparent during certain phases of the contrast injection, it is important to obtain rapid serial images after bolus injection. However, in some cases separation may not be possible despite optimal technique. If the collapsed lung contains a large amount of water, e.g. drowned lung distal to tumour, it may not enhance more than the tumour. In addition, if the blood supply to the collapsed lobe is obstructed or if the tumour is vascular, there may be insufficient difference in the enhancement pattern to allow separation (Khoury et al 1985).

RIGHT UPPER LOBE COLLAPSE

The pattern of right upper lobe (RUL) collapse is different from that of LUL collapse because there are several anatomical differences between the two lobes. The RUL is smaller than the LUL (which incorporates the lingular division) and has two fissural borders (minor and major fissures). Furthermore, the right main stem bronchus is more apt to shift as a result of lobar collapse, because it is not fixed at the hilum by the right pulmonary artery. These differences result in the RUL collapsing superiorly and medially rather than predominantly anteriorly as in LUL collapse. On CT, the collapsed RUL is seen as a sharply-defined triangular density bordered by the minor fissure laterally and the major fissure posteriorly (Fig. 4.3). The minor fissure, which is displaced more than the major fissure, has a straight border, whereas the major fissure may have a straight, concave or convex border. With RUL collapse, there is elevation of the right hilum. As

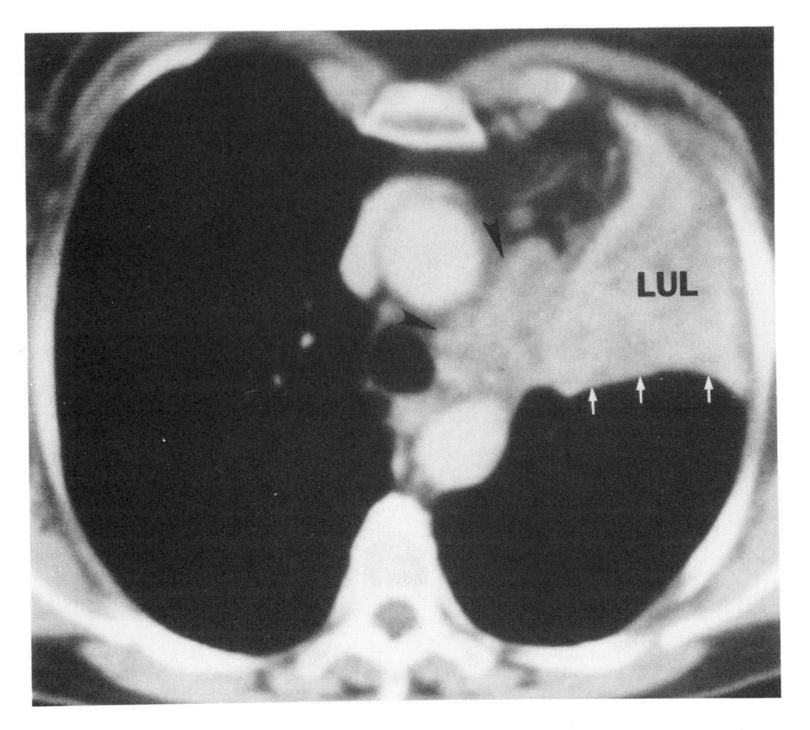

Fig. 4.2 Left upper lobe collapse. A post-contrast CT scan demonstrates aortopulmonary window lymphadenopathy (arrowheads). Note the relative enhancement of the left upper lobe (LUL) which was obstructed by a bronchogenic carcinoma seen on more caudal images. Major fissure (arrows).

a result, the right pulmonary artery may be seen at a higher level than normal. In addition, the right main stem bronchus may rotate anteriorly. Hyperexpansion of the RML and RLL also occurs. The superior segment of the RLL may extend between the mediastinum and medial border of the collapsed RUL but this is a less frequent finding than with collapse of the LUL. Moreover, anterior lung herniation is less common, probably because of the smaller size of the RUL.

RIGHT MIDDLE LOBE COLLAPSE

With collapse of the right middle lobe (RML) the minor fissure and lower half of the major fissure move closer together. On CT, the collapsed lobe is triangular or trapezoidal shaped and is demarcated by the minor fissure anteriorly and major fissure posteriorly (Fig. 4.4). The interface between the RML and RUL is often less distinct than that between the RML and the right lower lobe (RLL) because the minor fissure is more parallel to the scanning plane. The collapsed RML decreases its contact with the lateral chest wall but maintains its contact with the anterior chest wall on more

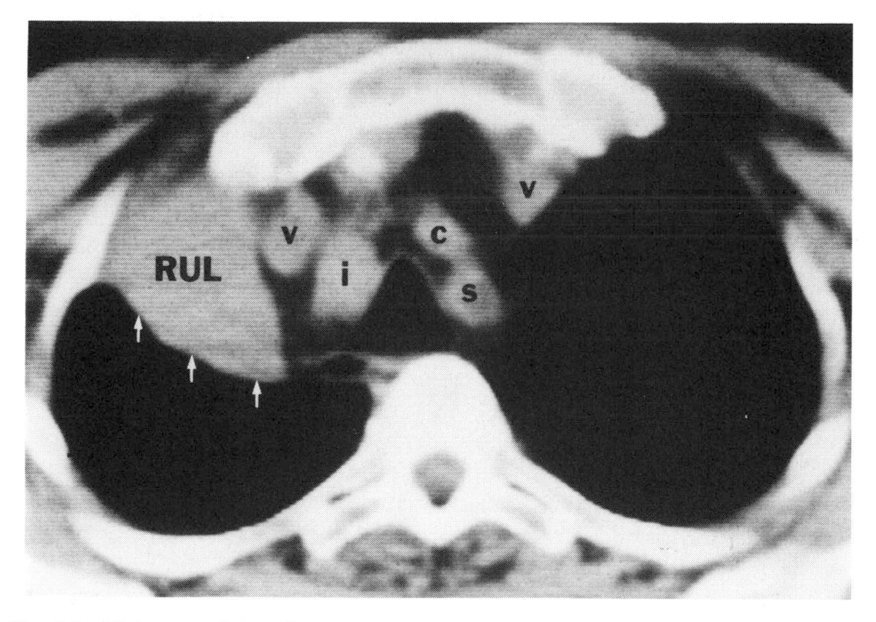

Fig. 4.3 Right upper lobe collapse. The collapsed right upper lobe (RUL) is triangular shaped and bordered posteriorly by the major fissure (arrows). Innominate artery (i), left common carotid artery (c), left subclavian artery (s), innominate veins (v).

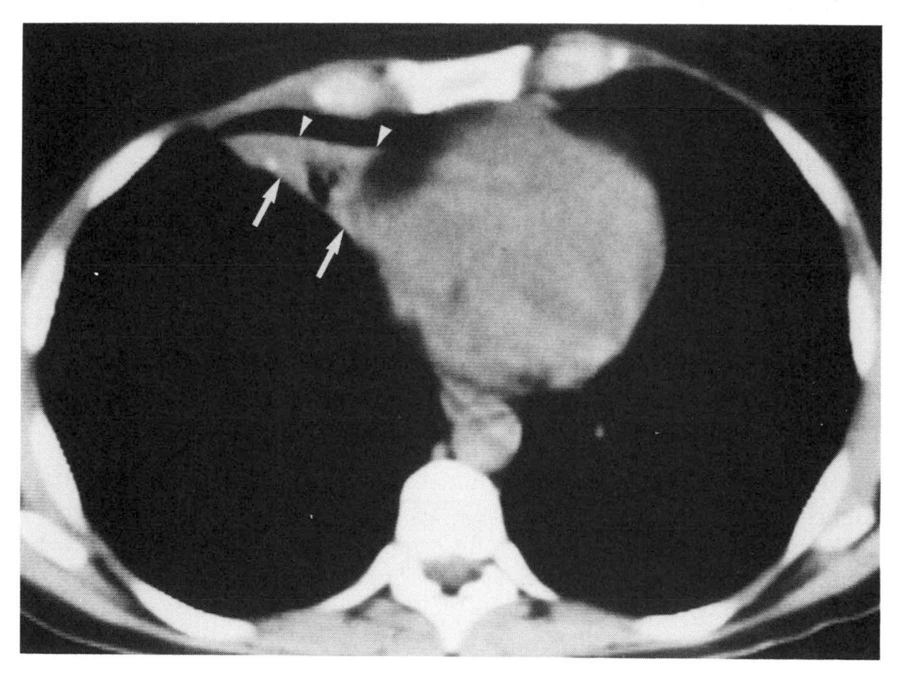

Fig. 4.4 Right middle lobe collapse. The collapsed right middle lobe abuts the right side of the heart. Major fissure (arrows), minor fissure (arrowheads).

caudal images. As the volume of the RML is small there is usually no significant mediastinal shift, compensatory hyperinflation or decreased volume of the hemithorax. If the collapsed lobe appears wider centrally rather than peripherally, a central obstructing mass is probably present. Segmental middle lobe collapse, which may be confusing on plain chest radiographs, is easily detected on CT by following the course of the middle lobe bronchus as it bifurcates into the medial and lateral segmental bronchi. The medial segment abuts the heart and anterior chest wall, whereas the lateral segment extends more posteriorly and does not contact the heart.

LOWER LOBE COLLAPSE

The pattern of collapse is similar for the RLL and the LLL. Both collapse caudally, posteriorly and medially towards the spine. On CT, the collapsed lower lobe appears as a wedge-shaped soft-tissue density structure adjacent to the spine. The major fissure, which forms the lateral border of the lobe, is displaced posteriorly. The upper border of the collapsed lobe is usually concave in the absence of a large central mass, whereas the lower border may be straight, concave or convex. The varying configurations relate to the extent of collapse, presence or absence of a central mass, degree of distal pneumonia and the anatomy of the inferior pulmonary ligament (Rost & Proto 1983). If the attachment of the pulmonary ligament to the hemi-diaphragm is incomplete, the lower lobe may collapse more completely adjacent to the spine and have a rounded appearance. Secondary signs of collapse include inferior and medial displacement of the hilum, postero-medial displacement of the lower lobe bronchus, ipsilateral mediastinal shift and hemidiaphragm elevation, compensatory hyperinflation and decreased size of the hemithorax.

COMPRESSIVE ATELECTASIS

Compressive, or passive, atelectasis most frequently occurs secondary to fluid within the pleural space. Whereas a large pleural effusion can obscure parenchymal disease on the plain chest radiograph, CT can demonstrate atelectatic lung underlying the pleural effusion. If the bronchus is patent and air bronchograms are seen throughout the lobe, proximal obstruction is unlikely. The distinction between the lower density pleural fluid and relatively higher density collapsed lung can be appreciated on non-contrast enhanced images but the difference is accentuated by intravenous contrast administration. In patients with malignant pleural disease, the lung may be compressed by tumour masses as well as by pleural fluid. In addition, neoplasm within the pleural space is more easily seen following intravenous contrast administration.

The patterns of compressive atelectasis secondary to a pleural effusion relates, in part, to the size of the pleural effusion (Paling & Griffin 1985).

With small effusions, CT may demonstrate only segmental collapse of a lower lobe which is seen anterior to the pleural effusion. The major fissure is visible anterior to the remainder of the aerated lower lobe. As the pleural effusion increases in size, most of the lower lobe becomes collapsed and the major fissure is no longer visible as a discrete structure. With larger effusions fluid can be seen extending into the major fissure anterior to the collapsed lobe. The inferior pulmonary ligament can be identified transfixing the medial border of the lower lobe to the mediastinum and dividing the medial pleural space into anterior and posterior compartments.

CICATRIZATION ATELECTASIS

Cicatrization atelectasis refers to volume loss secondary to scarring from previous inflammatory disease (Naidich et al 1983a, b). Endobronchial obstruction is not present and no central mass is seen. The degree of volume loss is usually more marked than in cases of collapse secondary to endobronchial obstruction. Associated bronchiectatic changes and pleural thickening are frequently present. The pattern of collapse may be altered, which is probably secondary to pleural adhesions and parenchymal scarring. For example, the cicatrized RUL may collapse posteriorly with posterior rotation of the carina and RUL bronchus.

ROUNDED ATELECTASIS

Rounded atelectasis is a form of non-segmental pulmonary collapse that may mimic a neoplasm. Although the plain film findings are frequently characteristic, CT can be helpful in confirming the diagnosis (Mintzer et al 1981, Doyle & Lawler 1984). The CT findings include:

1. A rounded or oval mass that forms an acute angle with thickened pleura. The pleura is usually thickest at its contact with the mass.
2. Vessels and bronchi converging in a curvilinear fashion into the lower border of the mass (CT equivalent of the 'comet sign').
3. Air bronchogram in the central portion of the mass. The periphery of the mass may be denser because it represents the area of most complete atelectasis.
4. Adjacent hyperinflated lung.

Rounded atelectasis is often associated with a history of asbestos exposure or other inflammatory processes involving the pleural space. CT frequently demonstrates pleural plaques or parenchymal fibrosis in other areas of the thorax. Rounded atelectasis usually remains stable on serial radiographic studies but occasionally very slow growth may occur. In the majority of cases, the CT findings are so characteristic that further evaluation is not usually necessary. However, if the CT findings are equivocal, percutaneous needle biopsy of the 'mass' can be very valuable for clarification.

CONCLUSIONS

The morphological patterns of pulmonary collapse are elegantly demonstrated with CT and knowledge of these patterns is essential for correct interpretation of complex pleuro-pulmonary pathology. In recent years the ability of CT to elucidate confusing appearances on conventional chest radiographs has been increasingly recognized and the technique now has an important place in the assessment of these patients.

REFERENCES

Doyle T C, Lawler G A 1984 CT features of rounded atelectasis of the lung. American Journal of Roentgenology 143: 225–228

Glazer H S, Aronberg D J, VanDyke J A, Sagel S S 1984 CT manifestations of pulmonary collapse. Contemporary Issues in Computed Tomography 4: 81–119

Khoury M B, Godwin J D, Halvorsen R A Jr, Putman C E 1985 CT of obstructive lobar collapse. Investigative Radiology 20: 708–716

Mintzer R A, Gore R M, Vogelzang R L, Holz S 1981 Rounded atelectasis and its association with asbestos-induced pleural disease. Radiology 139: 567–570

Naidich D P, Ettinger N, Leitman B S, McCauley D I 1984 CT of lobar collapse. Seminars in Roentgenology 19: 222–234

Naidich D P, McCauley D I, Khouri N F, Leitman B S, Hulnick D H, Siegelman S S 1983a Computed tomography of lobar collapse. 1. Endobronchial obstruction. Journal of Computer Assisted Tomography 7: 745–757

Naidich D P, McCauley D I, Khouri N F, Leitman B S, Hulnick D H, Siegelman S S 1983b Computed tomography of lobar collapse. 2. Collapse in absence of endobronchial obstruction. Journal of Computer Assisted Tomography 7: 758–767

Naidich D P, Zerhouni E A, Siegelman S S 1984 Computed Tomography of the Thorax. Raven Press, New York

Paling M R, Griffin G K 1985 Lower lobe collapse due to pleural effusion: a CT analysis. Journal of Computer Assisted Tomography 9: 1079–1083

Proto A V, Tocino I 1980 Radiologic manifestations of lobar collapse. Seminars in Roentgenology 15: 117–173

Raasch B N, Heitzman E R, Carsky E W, Lane E J, Berlow M E, Witwer G 1984 A computed tomographic study of bronchopulmonary collapse. Radiographics 4: 195–232

Rost R C Jr, Proto A V 1983 Inferior pulmonary ligament: computed tomographic appearance. Radiology 148: 479–483

5. Differential diagnosis of mediastinal pathology

Harvey S. Glazer

INTRODUCTION

CT is the primary tomographic imaging procedure for evaluating the mediastinum. It can determine the size, site of the origin, extent and relationship of masses to normal anatomical structures. Although CT is basically a morphological technique, determination of the relative attenuation values of a mediastinal mass improves the ability to characterize masses beyond that provided by the plain chest radiograph. In some cases, CT will permit a definitive non-invasive diagnosis.

FATTY MASSES

A lesion of pure fat density with well-defined margins is almost invariably benign. In such cases, the CT diagnosis is usually conclusive and no further diagnostic evaluation is needed. True fatty tumours of the mediastinum are not nearly as common as diffuse lipomatosis or herniations of abdominal fat through the diaphragm.

Mediastinal lipomatosis

This is a benign condition in which collections of histologically normal, unencapsulated fat are present in the mediastinum (Naidich et al 1984). It is most frequently seen with obesity or exogenous corticosteroid administration but in some patients there may be no predisposing factors.

The excess fat deposition is most prominent in the upper anterior mediastinum and may cause a gentle convex bulging of the mediastinal contour. Fat less commonly accumulates in the paraspinal areas or near the cardiophrenic angles (pericardial fat pads). The fat in mediastinal lipomatosis is of uniform low density (HU −80 to −120). If inhomogeneity is present, alternative diagnoses, such as liposarcoma, neoplastic infiltration, mediastinitis or haemorrhage, need to be considered. Small foci of residual thymic tissue in the anterior mediastinum should not be confused with infiltrated fat.

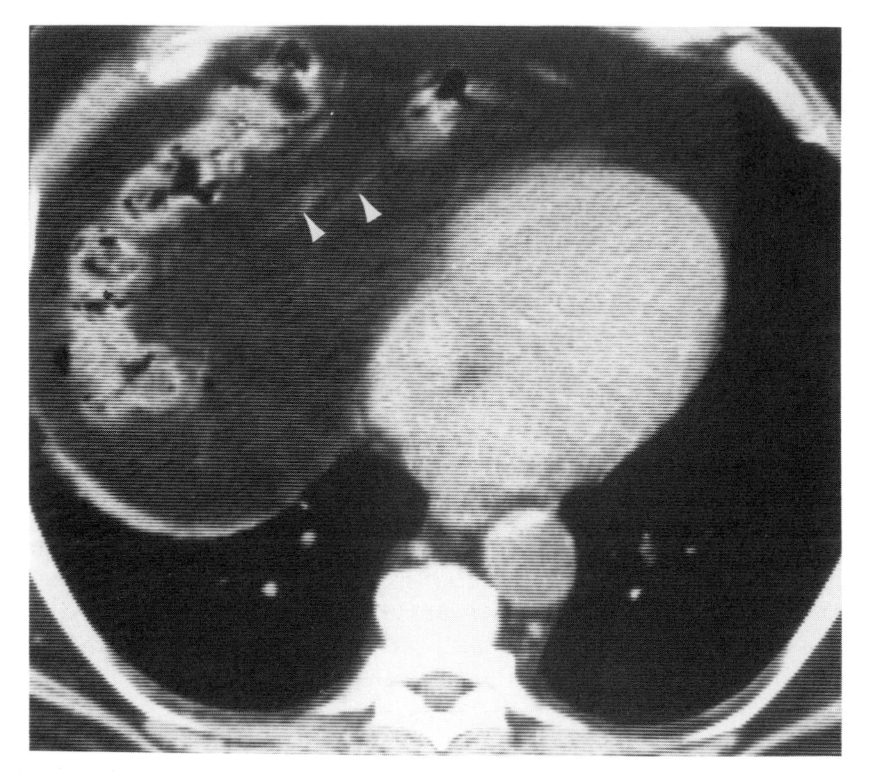

Fig. 5.1 Morgagni hernia. A large mass containing fat and transverse colon displaces the heart slightly to the left. Omental vessels (arrowheads).

Herniation of abdominal fat

Focal collections of fat in the peridiaphragmatic areas may be secondary to herniations of abdominal fat. Omental fat herniating through the foramen of Morgagni (virtually always on the right side) results in a mass in the right cardiophrenic angle (Fig. 5.1). Identification of thin linear densities within the fat, which probably represent small omental vessels, can help distinguish this from a pericardial fat pad. Fat herniation through the foramen of Bochdalek, most commonly seen posterolaterally on the left, may occasionally be located more medially and present as a mediastinal mass. Herniation of perigastric fat may occur through the oesophageal hiatus.

Neoplasms

Mediastinal lipomas are uncommon and may be seen in any part of the mediastinum, including the region of the atrioventricular grooves and along the interventricular septum (Gale & Karlinsky 1988). They are pliable, may be encapsulated and usually do not compress adjacent structures unless they are very large. Their borders are smooth and sharply defined. If the mass is inhomogeneous, containing areas of soft-tissue density or is poorly demarcated, a liposarcoma or other superimposed process should be suspected. Some liposarcomas have predominantly soft-tissue attenuation values rather than fat density.

Teratoma is a well-demarcated germ-cell neoplasm containing variable amounts of fat, fluid and soft tissue (Suzuki et al 1983). Most intrathoracic teratomas are located in the anterior mediastinum, reflecting their frequent origin from the thymus (see Ch. 6).

Thymolipomas are a rare benign mediastinal tumour that contains thymic and mature fat elements (Shirkhoda et al 1987) (see Ch. 6).

Other causes of fatty masses

Extravasation of lipid-rich hyperalimentation fluid has been described as a rare cause of a fatty mediastinal mass (Cobb & Mendelson 1987). Extra-medullary haematopoiesis may rarely contain a large fatty component in addition to soft-tissue density (Yamato & Fuhrman 1987). A clinical history of anaemia is usually present.

CYSTIC MASSES

A variety of mediastinal masses may be partially or entirely cystic. Congenital cysts, neoplasms, inflammatory processes and goitres may all demonstrate areas of near-water density on CT (Im et al 1987, McCarthy & Ross 1987). In some cases, the cystic nature of a mass may not be apparent because it contains mucoid, inflammatory or haemorrhagic fluid. Moreover, other processes may occasionally mimic a cystic mass.

Congenital cysts

Congenital mediastinal cysts can be divided into foregut cysts, pericardial cysts and thymic cysts.

Foregut cysts

Foregut cysts may be classified as bronchogenic, oesophageal or neurenteric.

Bronchogenic cysts are the most common type of foregut cyst and arise as a result of abnormal ventral budding of the tracheobronchial tree (Fig. 5.2). The wall of the cyst contains elements of the bronchial wall but may also contain elements of the oesophagus. They are most frequently located in the subcarinal or right paratracheal region but may also be seen in the hila or lung parenchyma. Approximately 50% are of homogeneous near-water density reflecting their serous nature and, if small and asymptomatic,

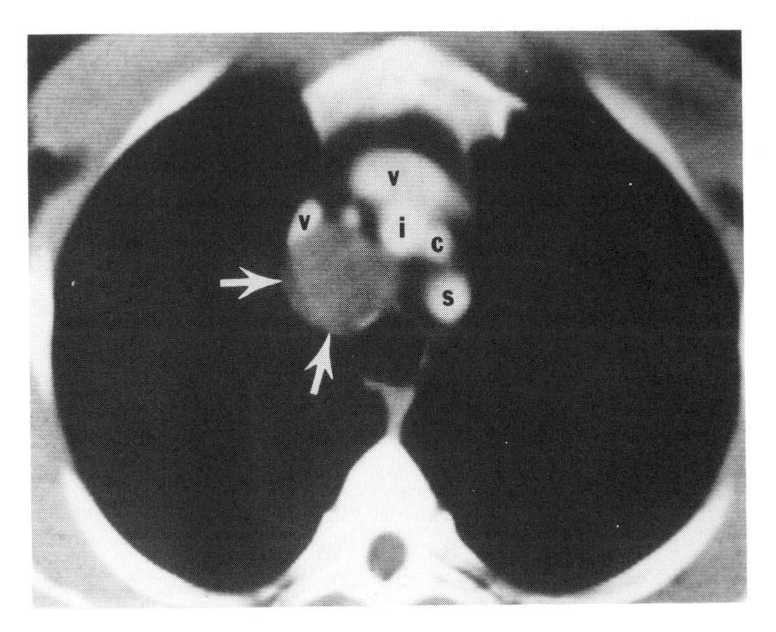

Fig. 5.2 Bronchogenic cyst. A well-defined water density mass (arrows) is seen in the right paratracheal region. Innominate artery (i), left common carotid artery (c), left subclavian artery (s), innominate veins (v).

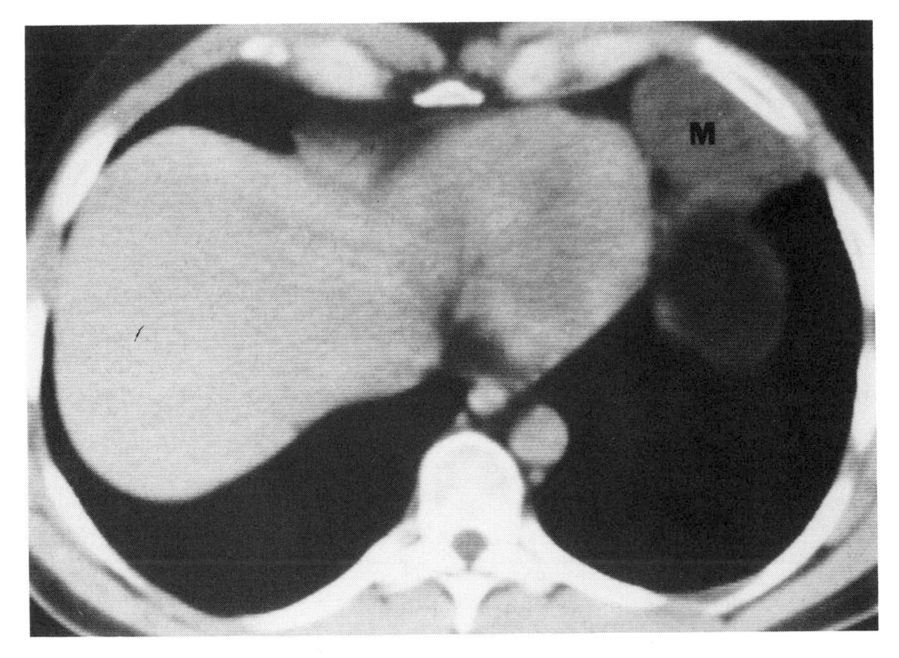

Fig. 5.3 Pericardial cyst. A well-defined homogeneous water density mass (M) is seen adjacent to the left side of the heart.

can be followed radiographically. Others may range from low soft-tissue density to that higher than muscle, either because of their viscid mucous content or because the fluid contains calcium oxalate (Nakata et al 1986, Yernault et al 1986). Occasionally calcification may develop in the wall of the cyst and air may be seen within the cyst if it develops a communication with the airway. Lesions that are greater than water density are indistinguishable from solid soft-tissue neoplasms, although their total lack of contrast enhancement may be a clue to the correct aetiology. In such circumstances, surgery (or percutaneous biopsy) is usually required for definitive evaluation.

Oesophageal cysts are located adjacent to, or within, the oesophageal wall and often protrude into the posterior mediastinum.

Neurenteric cysts may be distinguished from other mediastinal cysts by their usual association with spinal anomalies.

Pericardial cysts

Pericardial cysts are most frequently located in the cardiophrenic angles, approximately 60% at the right cardiophrenic angle and 90% adjacent to the hemidiaphragm (Fig. 5.3). The attenuation values are close to that of water. They are usually somewhat triangular in shape and, while sharply marginated, conform to surrounding structures.

Thymic cysts

Thymic cysts are secondary to persistence of the thymopharyngeal duct and thymic tissue is present in the wall of the cyst (see Ch. 6).

Neoplasms

Although most neoplasms are generally of soft-tissue density on CT, low attenuation areas may be present, representing areas of cyst formation, necrosis or old haemorrhage. These findings have been described in a variety of tumours, e.g. germ-cell neoplasms, Hodgkin's disease, thymomas. In most cases the 'cystic areas' are either thick-walled or inhomogeneous, allowing distinction from congenital cysts. There also may be other findings, e.g. lymphadenopathy, that suggest a neoplastic process. Similar low attenuation areas can be seen in neoplasms that have been treated with radiation or chemotherapy.

Low attenuation 'cystic' lymph nodes may be seen secondary to metastases, e.g. squamous-cell carcinoma. These findings, which are attributed to central necrosis, have been described elsewhere in the body, most commonly in the neck, and are more apparent after the administration of intravenous contrast material. Lymph nodes, secondary to involvement by metastatic testicular cancer, may show low attenuation values. This feature may be due to necrosis or cystic degeneration but also may reflect the intrinsic properties of the malignancy, e.g. mature teratomatous elements (Yousem et al 1986).

Nerve root tumours, e.g. Schwannomas or neurofibromas, can occur anywhere along the course of a nerve. In the mediastinum they usually arise from an intercostal nerve but the site of origin may also be the vagus or phrenic nerve. Most are sharply defined and located in the paravertebral area and in some cases smooth expansion of a vertebral foramen is seen. The attenuation values and degree of inhomogeneity depend on the relative proportion of neural tissues, fibrous elements and degree of cystic degeneration (Kumar et al 1983, Cohen et al 1986). Varying degrees of contrast enhancement may be seen and both benign and malignant neurogenic tumours can be inhomogeneous on CT. The lower density of some neural tumours has been attributed to the high lipid content of neural tissue.

Lymphangiomas are relatively uncommon benign tumours that arise from lymphoid tissue and most frequently present before two years of age as a mass posterior to the sternocleidomastoid muscle. Most mediastinal lymphangiomas arise in the neck and secondarily extend into the mediastinum. They are generally of near-water density, thin-walled and multiloculated but occasionally may appear as a solitary cyst (Pilla et al 1982). They may contain solid components if haemorrhage or infection has occurred. Although usually well-defined, these cysts may infiltrate adjacent structures and can be difficult to remove surgically.

Meningocoele

An intrathoracic meningocoele is a protrusion of the leptomeninges through an intervertebral foramen into the thoracic cavity and is associated with neurofibromatosis in approximately 75% of patients. On CT an homogeneous near-water density paravertebral mass is seen and other findings may include enlargement of intervertebral foramina, kyphoscoliosis and associated vertebral and rib anomalies. A CT myelogram or magnetic resonance (MR) imaging will confirm the diagnosis by demonstrating communication with the subarachnoid space (Weinreb et al 1984).

Inflammatory processes

A fluid-filled mediastinal mass may represent a mediastinal abscess (Carrol et al 1987). Associated CT findings, e.g. gas bubbles, contiguity or communication with an empyema or subphrenic abscess, assist in the differentiation from other processes. Percutaneous needle aspiration under CT guidance may be required to distinguish an abscess from an uninfected postoperative seroma or haematoma.

An extrapancreatic fluid collection may spread into the posterior mediastinum from the retroperitoneum via either the aortic or oesophageal hiatus in the diaphragm. Typically, these masses are of near-water density but their attenuation values may be higher if there is superimposed infection or haemorrhage. Contiguity between the mediastinal fluid collection and peripancreatic inflammatory disease can be demonstrated on serial scans.

GOITRE

In most cases, an accurate diagnosis of intrathoracic goitre can be made on CT and it is readily distinguished from numerous other mediastinal masses (Glazer et al 1982). Intrathoracic goitres are nearly always contiguous with a cervical thyroid on serial scans. They are usually well defined and often contain focal areas of calcification. The attenuation values of the soft-tissue intrathoracic component are frequently less than that of the cervical thyroid but greater than that of muscle. These appearances, however, are highly variable and relate to the iodine content of the goitre. If the iodine content is very low, the CT density may be similar to that of surrounding soft-tissue. Intrathoracic goitres often contain low attenuation areas which probably represent cystic degeneration.

While generally unnecessary for diagnosis, administration of intravenous contrast medium may result in marked enhancement, reflecting the vascularity of the mass. Prolonged enhancement, greater than two minutes after injection, may also be seen and is considered to be related to iodine uptake by the gland. The enhancement pattern is frequently inhomogeneous due to multinodularity of intrathoracic goitres and their variable iodine content.

Thyroid carcinoma with mediastinal extension may be indistinguishable from a goitre but its margins are usually ill-defined with no fat plane between the mass and the mediastinal vessels. In advanced tumours there may be direct invasion of adjacent structures. Thyroid carcinoma may be associated with cervical and/or mediastinal lymphadenopathy as well as pulmonary nodules.

Pitfalls

Various processes may occasionally mimic a cystic mediastinal mass. On a single scan, a thrombosed vein, e.g. the superior vena cava, may simulate a necrotic lymph node because it has a relatively enhancing periphery and a lower density centre. However, a correct diagnosis can be achieved by careful review of consecutive scans.

A fluid-filled oesophagus, e.g. secondary to achalasia, oesophageal diverticulum or colonic interposition, may mimic the appearance of a congenital mediastinal cyst or fluid collection. An air–fluid level is generally seen and contiguous scans will reveal that it represents part of the gastro-intestinal tract. In confusing cases, oral contrast medium may be helpful.

Loculated pleural fluid adjacent to the mediastinum or fluid within a distended pericardial recess may present a confusing picture (Shin et al 1986). Identification of pleural/pericardial fluid elsewhere in the chest will usually permit the correct diagnosis to be made.

HIGH ATTENUATION MASSES

Unenhanced masses

Masses may demonstrate diffuse or focal areas of high density prior to the administration of intravenous contrast medium because they contain calcium, have a high iodine content or contain areas of haemorrhage. Fluid collections that communicate with the oesophagus may also contain areas of high density if oral contrast medium has been given.

Calcification within lymph nodes, which frequently is more apparent on CT than on plain chest radiographs, usually denotes old healed granulomatous disease, e.g. histoplasmosis. Lymph nodes may be diffusely calcified or may only contain scattered areas of calcification. Egg shell calcification, classically described in silicosis, can also be seen in sarcoidosis, treated lymphoma and granulomatous disease. A more unusual cause of calcified lymph nodes is metastatic neoplasm, e.g. mucinous ovarian or colonic carcinoma, bronchio-alveolar cell carcinoma or papillary carcinoma of the thyroid (Naidich et al 1984, Mallens et al 1986). In general, primary tumours with a predilection to calcify also tend to produce metastases which calcify. In addition, treated lymph nodes (post-irradiation or chemotherapy) may show areas of calcification. Amyloidosis and angiofollicular lymph-node hyperplasia are other rare causes of calcified mediastinal lymph nodes. In most cases, the clinical history and other associated CT findings, e.g. history of prior malignancy, permit distinction among the various different possibilities.

Areas of calcification can occur within a variety of primary mediastinal masses which include neoplasms, e.g. teratoma, thymoma, neural tumour, goitres, aneurysms and, rarely, mediastinal cysts. Although the pattern of calcification is generally not helpful, peripheral calcification in a mass adjacent to a vascular structure is highly suggestive of an aneurysm, whereas calcification within a fatty mass is highly suggestive of a teratoma.

As described earlier, goitres may have relatively high attenuation values due to a high iodine content.

Haemorrhage can occur within any mediastinal mass. The extent of alteration in the attenuation values of the mass will depend on several factors, including the degree and age of the haemorrhage as well as the initial composition of the mass, e.g. fluid versus solid. Post-traumatic and isolated haematomas of the mediastinum may also occur (Fig. 5.4).

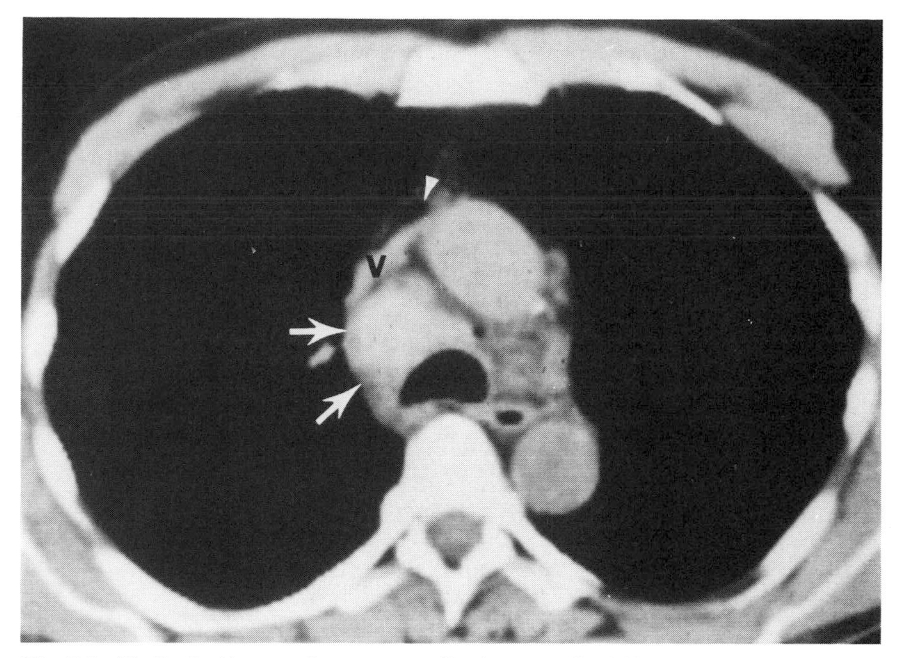

Fig. 5.4 Mediastinal haemorrhage post-mediastinoscopy. A relatively high density paratracheal mass (arrows) is seen compressing the superior vena cava (V). A small amount of air (arrowhead) is seen in the anterior mediastinum secondary to the recent mediastinoscopy.

Occasionally these may demonstrate a fluid/fluid level. Again, the attenuation values of the haematoma will vary with its age, older haematomas having lower attenuation values.

Contrast-enhancing masses

In some cases mediastinal masses may be further characterized by evaluating the response to the administration of intravenous contrast material (Spizarny et al 1987). The most common enhancing mediastinal mass is an aortic aneurysm. Although the diagnosis is generally straightforward, the appearance may be confusing when the aneurysm presents in an unusual location, when the lumen of the aneurysm is small with respect to the mural thrombus or when the injection technique is suboptimal.

Congenital vascular anomalies may occasionally mimic enlarged mediastinal lymph nodes. In most cases the correct diagnosis is apparent by reviewing consecutive scans.

Oesophageal varices may be large enough to produce a paraspinal mass but intravenous contrast medium permits a definitive diagnosis. Associated findings of cirrhosis and portal hypertension are usually present on scans through the upper abdomen.

Hypervascular neoplasms (e.g. metastatic renal-cell carcinoma or papillary carcinoma of the thyroid, paraganglioma, haemangioma, phaeochromocytoma) goitres and Castleman's disease (angiofollicular lymph-node hyperplasia) may also demonstrate significant contrast enhancement (Fiore et al 1983), Onik & Goodman 1983, Drucker et al 1987). However, with the current CT equipment, the use of bolus injection techniques and a careful review of sequential images, highly vascular lesions are unlikely to be confused with a vascular structure.

CONCLUSION

Evaluation of mediastinal masses is one of the most rewarding areas of body CT and even in the early days this superb diagnostic capability was quickly recognized. Refinements in scanning techniques, particularly with respect to the use of intravenous contrast medium, has further improved the detection and characterization of mediastinal lesions. Thus, the technique should be used as the investigation of choice in any patient requiring further evaluation of a suspected or known mediastinal mass.

REFERENCES

Carrol C L, Jeffrey R B Jr, Federle M P, Vernacchia F S 1987 CT evaluation of mediastinal infection. Journal of Computer Assisted Tomography 11: 449–454

Cobb R J, Mendelson D S 1987 CT findings in mediastinal extravasation of hyperalimentation fluid. Journal of Computer Assisted Tomography 11: 158–159

Cohen L M, Schwartz A M, Rockoff S D 1986 Benign schwannomas: pathologic basis for CT inhomogeneities. American Journal of Roentgenology 147: 141–143

Drucker E A, McLoud T C, Dedrick C G, Hilgenberg A D, Geller S C, Shepard J O 1987 Mediastinal paraganglioma: radiologic evaluation of an unusual vascular tumor. American Journal of Roentgenology 148: 521–522

Fiore D, Biondetti P R, Calabro F, Rea F 1983 CT demonstration of bilateral Castleman tumors in the mediastinum. Journal of Computer Assisted Tomography 7: 719–720

Gale M E, Karlinsky J B 1988 Computed tomography of the chest: a teaching file. Year Book Medical Publishers, Chicago

Glazer G M, Axel L, Moss A A 1982 CT diagnosis of mediastinal thyroid. American Journal of Roentgenology 138: 495–498

Im J-G, Song K S, Kang H S et al 1987 Mediastinal tuberculous lymphadenitis: CT manifestations. Radiology 164: 115–119

Kumar A J, Kuhajda F P, Martinez C R, Fishman E K, Jezic D V, Siegelman S S 1983 CT of extracranial nerve sheath tumors. Journal of Computer Assisted Tomography 7: 857–865

McCarthy M J, Ross P R 1987 Cystic lesions of the mediastinum. Presented at the Society of Thoracic Radiology, Orlando, Florida

Mallens W M C, Nijhuis-Heddes J M A, Bakker W 1986 Calcified lymph-node metastases in bronchiolo-alveolar carcinoma. Radiology 161: 103–104

Naidich D P, Zerhouni E A, Siegelman S S 1984 Computed tomography of the thorax. Raven Press, New York

Nakata, H, Sato Y, Nakayama T, Yoshimatsu H, Kobayashi T 1986 Bronchogenic cyst with high CT numbers: analysis of contents. Journal of Computer Assisted Tomography 10: 360–362

Onik G, Goodman P H 1983 CT of Castleman disease. American Journal of Roentgenology 140: 691–692

Pilla, T J, Wolverson M K, Sundaram H, Heiberg E, Shields J B 1982 CT evaluation of cystic lymphangiomas of the mediastinum. Radiology 144: 841–842

Shin M S, Jolles P R, Ho K-J 1986 CT evaluation of a distended pericardial recess presenting as a mediastinal mass. Journal of Computer Assisted Tomography 10: 860–862
Shirkhoda A, Chasen M H, Eftekhari F, Goldman A M, Decaro L F 1987 MR imaging of mediastinal thymolipoma. Journal of Computer Assisted Tomography 11: 364–365
Spizarny D L, Rebner M, Gross B H 1987 CT evaluation of enhancing mediastinal masses. Journal of Computer Assisted Tomography 11: 990–993
Suzuki M, Takashima T, Itoh H, Choutoh S, Kawamura I, Watanabe Y 1983 Computed tomography of mediastinal teratomas. Journal of Computer Assisted Tomography 7: 74–76
Weinreb J C, Arger P H, Grossman R, Samuel L 1984 CT metrizamide myelography in multiple bilateral intrathoracic meningoceles. Journal of Computer Assisted Tomography 8: 324–326
Yamato M, Fuhrman C R 1987 Computed tomography of fatty replacement in extramedullary hematopoiesis. Journal of Computer Assisted Tomography 11: 541–542
Yernault J C, Kuhn G, Dumortier P, Rocmans P, Ketelbant P, DeVuyst P 1986 'Solid' mediastinal bronchogenic cyst: mineralogic analysis. American Journal of Roentgenology 146: 73–74
Yousem D M, Scatarige J C, Fishman E K, Siegelman S S 1986 Low-attenuation thoracic metastases in testicular malignancy. American Journal of Roentgenology 146: 291–293

6. Thymic masses and hyperplasia

Janet E. S. Husband

INTRODUCTION

Until the early 1960s the thymus was an organ of mystery, its function was obscure and its radiological demonstration confined to childhood. Today, it is well established that the primary function of the thymus is to produce T lymphocytes which are concerned with cell-mediated immunity. Histologically, the thymus consists of epithelial cells and lymphoid tissue which is contained in germinal centres. These germinal centres are responsible for producing the T lymphocytes. Thymic function becomes progressively less important as age advances and hence the thymus atrophies with fatty replacement of the germinal centres.

CT is an excellent method of depicting thymic anatomy and reduction in the size of the gland, which is related to diminishing function during adult life, is well demonstrated.

ANATOMY

The thymus is a bilobed structure situated in the superior and anterior mediastinum. The gland is fused superiorly and extends from just below the thyroid gland down as far as the pericardium. The left lobe usually extends further inferiorly than the right. Posteriorly the thymus is closely related to the trachea, the left innominate vein, the branches of the aorta, the aortic arch and the ascending aorta and main pulmonary trunk.

The CT appearances of the normal thymus vary with age. In children up to the time of puberty the gland is clearly identified as a soft-tissue density structure filling the anterior mediastinum. Since young children have little mediastinal fat, distinction between the thymus and adjacent vessels may be difficult. After puberty the gland gradually regresses in volume and in young adults is usually seen as a soft-tissue triangular-shaped structure surrounded by mediastinal fat. At this time the borders of the normal thymus are flat or even concave.

After the age of about 25–30 years fatty involution occurs. On CT the gland may appear as a small nubin of soft tissue or may simply be represented by strands of soft tissue within the anterior mediastinal fat.

Over the age of about 50 years the thymus is frequently invisible. Baron et al (1982a) analysed the normal thymus in 154 patients undergoing chest CT. They found that the gland was seen in 100% of patients up to the age of 30 years but after the age of 50 years the gland was only visible in 17%.

The size of the normal gland has been correlated with age and measurements of the normal range for different age groups have been established (Baron et al 1982a). This study and that of Francis et al (1985) show that thymic thickness is a more reliable measurement than width. Up to the age of 20 years the maximum normal thickness of the gland is 1.8 cm whereas over the age of 20 years the maximum thickness is 1.3 cm (Baron et al 1982a).

THE ABNORMAL THYMUS

The introduction of CT stimulated new interest in the thymus gland. Early reports highlighted the ability of CT to detect suspected thymomas in patients with myasthenia gravis and the CT appearances of other thymic masses were also documented (Mink et al 1978, McLoud et al 1979, Baron et al 1982b). More recently attention has also been given to the demonstration of reactive thymic hyperplasia and infiltration by such conditions as Hodgkin's lymphoma (Choyke et al 1987, Kissin et al 1987).

Myasthenia gravis

In patients with myasthenia gravis the most important question is whether the syndrome is associated with a thymoma or thymic hyperplasia since distinction between these two entities determines patient management. Thymoma occurs in 8–15% of the patients with myasthenia gravis and, if detected, surgery is generally recommended because 15–35% of these tumours are malignant (Keynes 1955, Wilkins et al 1966). Other reasons for adopting a surgical approach in patients with thymoma are that the prognosis is worse in the presence of a thymoma and removal of a tumour may be accompanied by a remission of myasthenia (Keesey 1979). Although remission of myasthenic symptoms can be achieved by thymectomy whether it is associated with a thymoma or hyperplasia, in patients with hyperplasia surgery is usually reserved until medical treatment fails (Blalock et al 1941).

Thymoma

Thymomas most frequently occur in patients aged between 20 and 30 years and are considered to be tumours of epithelial origin. On CT thymomas appear as masses of homogeneous soft-tissue density situated in the superior anterior mediastinum. They enhance uniformly if intravenous contrast medium is given. A benign thymoma is usually well demarcated

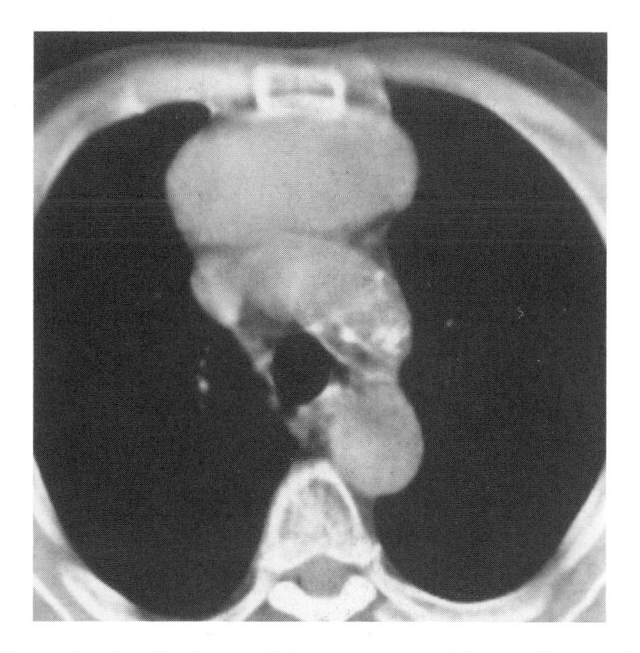

Fig. 6.1 CT scan showing the characteristic appearances of a benign thymoma in a 50-year-old male patient. Note preservation of the mediastinal fat planes.

and may be round, oval or even lobulated (Fig. 6.1). In many cases the tumour is not large enough to alter the contour of the mediastinum on a conventional chest film and this is why CT has made such an important contribution to diagnosis. Thymomas are much easier to recognize on CT in patients over the age of 40 years (Fon et al 1982). This is because there is considerable difficulty in differentiating the normal gland or hyperplasia from a small tumour in younger patients.

Malignant thymomas are locally invasive and the tumour infiltrates into the mediastinum and along pleural surfaces. On CT the mass may have an ill-defined border with obliteration of the fat planes between the tumour and great vessels (Fig. 6.2). Although obliteration of the fat planes does not consistently indicate invasion the presence of preserved fat planes does exclude macroscopic invasion. Occasionally an invasive thymoma grows through adjacent vessel walls and a mixture of thrombus and tumour produces venous obstruction. Metastases from thymomas are rare but if they do occur are found on pleural surfaces. Advanced thymomas can spread directly into the abdomen through the diaphragmatic hiatus (Zerhouni et al 1982). As in other tumours documentation of the full extent of disease is important for determining resectability and, if surgery is not possible, for defining radiotherapy portals or providing a baseline for monitoring chemotherapy response.

The accuracy of CT for detecting thymomas in patients over 40 years is

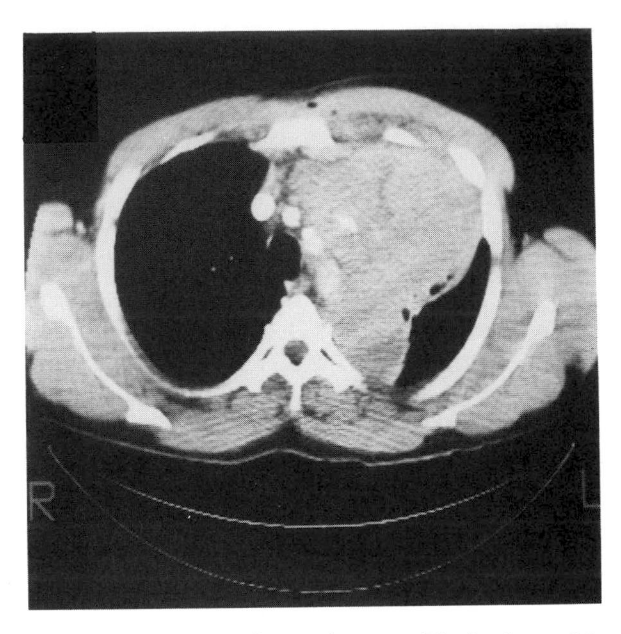

Fig. 6.2 CT scan of a patient with a malignant thymoma. The fat planes of the mediastinum are obliterated and tumour extends as far as the chest wall.

> 90%. Fon et al (1982) correctly diagnosed 14 out of 16 cases of thymoma. Of the two cases not diagnosed on CT one was a microscopic tumour and the other was a small macroscopic tumour surrounded by normal thymic tissue. In patients under the age of 40 years the accuracy of CT is considerably less due to the coexistence of normal thymic tissue and tumour. In the series by Fon et al (1982) conventional chest radiographs were abnormal in only 56% of patients, thus emphasizing the value of CT in detecting occult disease.

Thymic lymphoid (germinal) hyperplasia

Thymic hyperplasia is associated with myasthenia gravis in 65–80% of cases. Thymic lymphoid hyperplasia refers to the pathological appearance of the gland in which there is proliferation of active lymphoid germinal centres within the medulla. In addition, there is an increase in plasma cells and lymphocytes surrounding these germinal centres. The cortex of the gland shows involution. In thymic lymphoid hyperplasia the overall weight of the gland is not usually significantly increased (Castleman & Norris 1949). Thus, on CT the gland may appear entirely normal in a patient with thymic hyperplasia although in some patients the gland may appear diffusely enlarged (Baron et al 1982b). There is no difference in density between a hyperplastic gland and a normal thymus.

True thymic hyperplasia

True thymic hyperplasia involves the cortex as well as the medulla. In true hyperplasia the histological pattern reveals normal thymic elements in normal proportions. The overall size and weight of the gland are increased.

True hyperplasia is seen in association with Graves' disease, acromegaly and Addison's disease. It also occurs as a reaction to stress. During stress the gland atrophies and this is then followed by rebound hyperplasia. This phenomenon has been described in children recovering from burns, complex surgery and after the administration of oral corticosteroids (Caffey & Sibley 1960, Gelfand et al 1972, Rizk et al 1972). Thymic rebound hyperplasia has recently been described following chemotherapy for malignant disease. In a study reported from the Royal Marsden Hospital in patients treated with chemotherapy for testicular tumours we found thymic enlargement in 11.6% of patients (Kissin et al 1987). The phenomenon occurred 3–14 months after the beginning of treatment. The attenuation values of the gland did not change in association with the increase in size and overall the gland maintained its characteristic triangular shape (Fig. 6.3).

The importance of recognizing the phenomenon of reactive hyperplasia in response to chemotherapy is that an enlarging mass in the anterior mediastinum may otherwise be diagnosed as recurrent tumour. In testicular tumours the anterior mediastinum is rarely the only site of recurrence but in patients with lymphoma the distinction between relapse and reactive hyperplasia is more difficult.

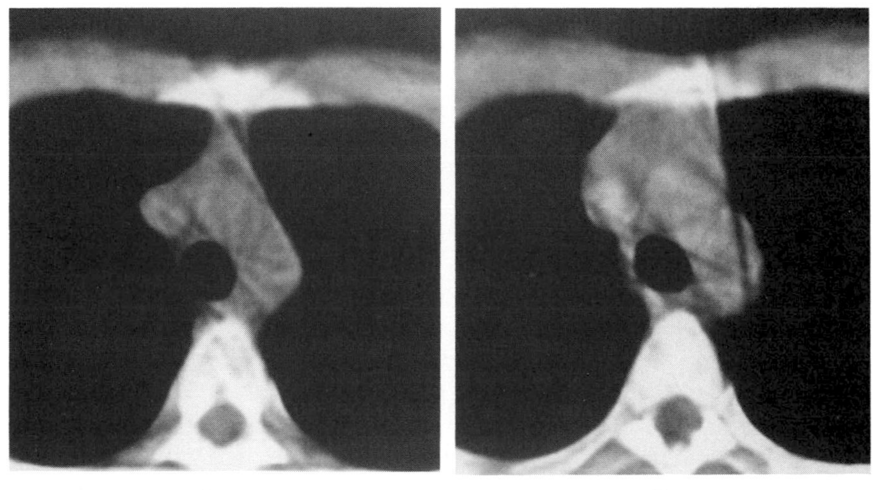

Fig. 6.3 True thymic lymphoid hyperplasia in a 23-year-old patient treated with chemotherapy for metastatic testicular teratoma. **A** Before treatment the thymus is normal in size and shape. **B** A CT scan ten months later shows considerable enlargement of the gland. (Reproduced with the kind permission of *Radiology*.)

Lymphomatous infiltration of the thymus

In Hodgkin's lymphoma an anterior mediastinal mass may represent disease in lymph nodes, infiltration of the thymus by tumour or possibly reactive hyperplasia. The characteristic shape of enlarged anterior mediastinal lymph nodes is seldom confused with an enlarged thymus on CT and the major issue is therefore the distinction between lymphomatous involvement of the thymus and reactive hyperplasia. Infiltration of the thymus by Hodgkin's lymphoma is a well-recognized feature of the disease but was rarely diagnosed before the days of CT, except at post-mortem. Diffuse infiltration produces thymic enlargement which has a uniform soft-tissue density on CT. The appearances of the gland cannot be differentiated from those of rebound hyperplasia. In a recent study of 100 patients with thoracic Hodgkin's disease, the incidence of thymic enlargement and the CT appearances of the gland at the time of primary staging and at suspected relapse (Heron et al 1988) were analysed. The data showed an overall incidence of thymic enlargement of 34% and in all cases there was concurrent lymphadenopathy. It is likely that thymic enlargement seen in this group of patients was due to tumour infiltration because regression of lymph-node size on treatment was parallelled by a reduction in the size of the thymus (Fig. 6.4). Conversely, in those patients who did not respond to treatment an increase in size of lymph-nodes was accompanied by an increase in size of the gland.

In the author's experience, thymic enlargement due to tumour infiltration is always associated with mediastinal lymph-node involvement

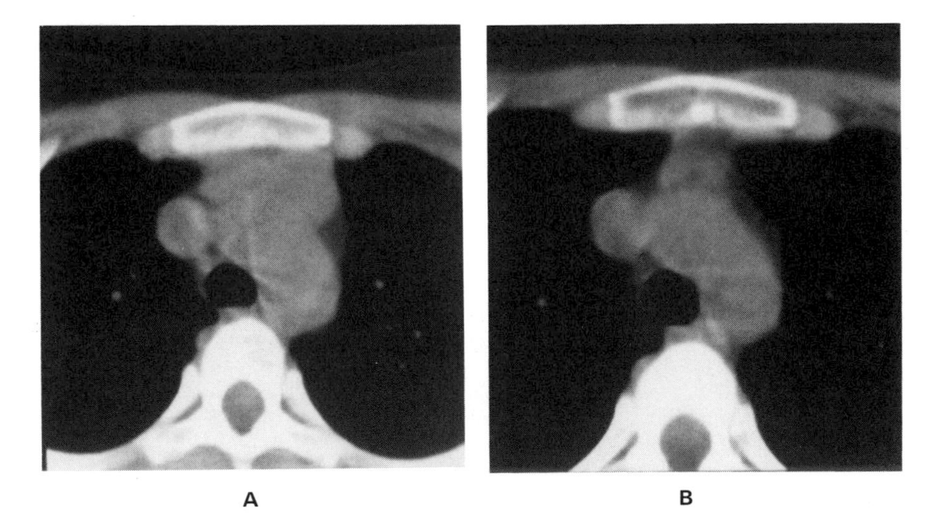

Fig. 6.4 CT scans in a patient with non-Hodgkin's lymphoma. **A** Before treatment. The thymus is enlarged. **B** Following treatment there has been considerable reduction in the size of the thymus indicating that thymic enlargement was probably due to lymphomatous infiltration. (Reproduced with the kind permission of *Radiology*.)

and if isolated thymic enlargement occurs an alternative diagnosis should be suspected. In patients previously treated with chemotherapy thymic rebound hyperplasia should be considered. There are no obvious differences in the CT appearances of thymic tumour infiltration and thymic hyperplasia. However, the timing of thymic enlargement in relation to therapy and the presence or absence of disease elsewhere may permit distinction between these two entities in the majority of patients.

In a patient who presents with an anterior mediastinal mass, differentiation between an invasive thymoma and thymic infiltration by lymphoma may be difficult since both are locally invasive. Calcification is not helpful in the differential diagnosis because it is not seen in lymphoma and is only rarely found in thymoma. As with the distinction between thymic hyperplasia and lymphomatous infiltration, the presence of coexistent enlarged nodes points to a diagnosis of lymphoma whereas pleural deposits are more likely to be seen in thymoma.

Germ-cell tumours

Germ-cell tumours comprise a large variety of benign and malignant mediastinal masses which are considered to be of thymic origin. They include dermoid cysts, benign teratomas, malignant teratomas and seminomas. The majority of germ-cell tumours are benign and of the malignant tumours, teratomas are the most common.

Dermoid cysts

On CT dermoid cysts show a classical appearance of a well-demarcated lesion situated in the anterior mediastinum. Calcification of the rim is seen in about 30% of cases and the contents of the cyst are usually of near-water density (Fig. 6.5). Spontaneous haemorrhage into the cyst may occur resulting in an increase in attenuation values.

Benign teratoma

These masses consist of a mixture of tissues including fat, fluid, soft-tissue and calcium. On CT these components are represented by various densities ranging from calcium to fat depending upon the proportion of different components. Rarely, a fat/fluid level may be seen (Seltzer et al 1984). The mass is well defined and frequently shows an enhancing rim. Distinction from a malignant teratoma may be impossible.

Malignant germ-cell tumours

Malignant teratoma is the most common primary malignant germ-cell tumour and is seen most frequently in young males. On CT these tumours

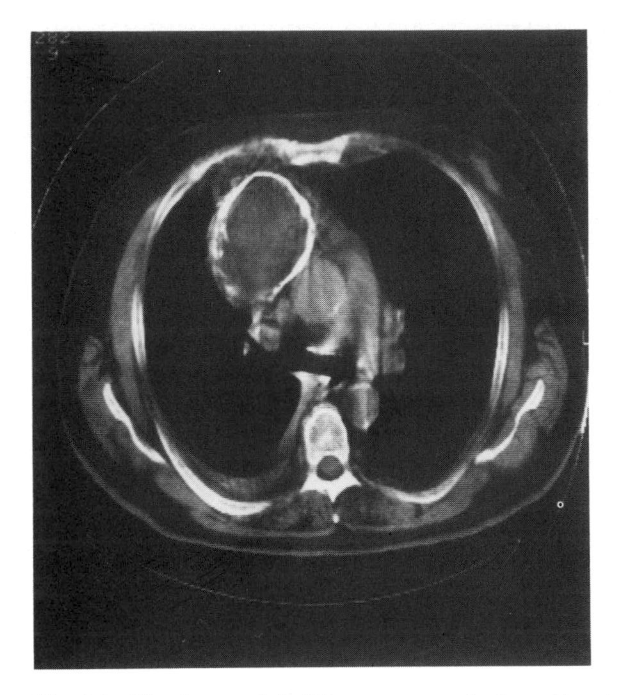

Fig. 6.5 The characteristic CT appearances of a dermoid cyst.

appear as inhomogeneous masses containing areas of soft-tissue density and water density. The soft-tissue components enhance with contrast medium and the borders of the mass are ill-defined, irregular and sometimes frankly invasive (Fig. 6.6). Malignant teratomas metastasize predominantly to the lungs and large 'cannon-ball' lung metastases are not uncommonly seen at the time of presentation.

Primary mediastinal seminomas are also malignant but very rare. On CT they are seen as large soft-tissue masses which may contain areas of lower attenuation presumably due to necrosis. There are no specific features which enable distinction to be made from malignant thymoma or lymphoma. The presence of pulmonary metastases, however, is more indicative of a seminoma than either a lymphoma or a thymoma.

Other primary malignant germ-cell tumours are very rare and insufficient information is available to determine any characteristic CT findings.

Thymic cyst

Congenital thymic cysts contain fluid which is homogeneous and of near-water density. Thymic cysts may also develop following radiotherapy to the mediastinum for Hodgkin's disease (Baron et al 1981, Heron et al 1988).

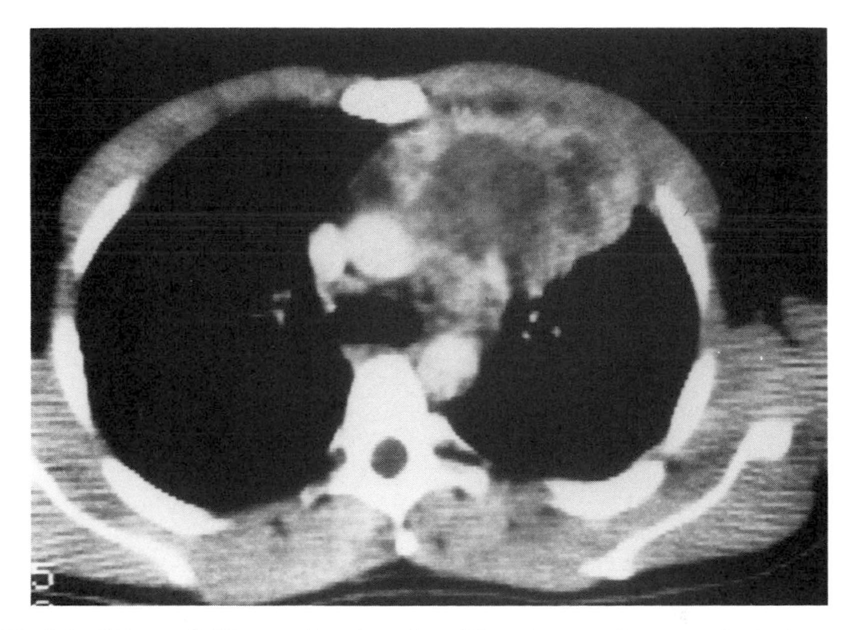

Fig. 6.6 CT scan of a 22-year-old male patient with a primary malignant mediastinal germ-cell tumour.

These cysts frequently enlarge over a relatively short period of time and may be confused with recurrence unless CT is undertaken. They may persist unchanged or may undergo slow spontaneous regression.

Other rare thymic masses

Other masses involving the thymus may occasionally be identified on CT. These include haemangiomas, lymphangiomas and thymolipomas. A thymolipoma is a rare benign mass which is usually diagnosed as an incidental finding. The tumour consists of fat elements and mature thymic tissue. The one case we have seen was a young boy of 15 years of age who presented with enlarged lymph nodes in the neck due to Hodgkin's disease. The chest radiograph showed a large mass arising from the mediastinum and CT revealed a fatty mass containing soft-tissue strands (Fig. 6.7). Thoracotomy confirmed the diagnosis of thymolipoma.

Carcinoid tumours and metastases may involve the thymus. They show heterogenic contrast enhancement and are indistinguishable from other malignant thymic lesions.

CONCLUSION

The demonstration of thymic pathology is an important aspect of mediastinal CT and the detection of occult thymomas in patients with

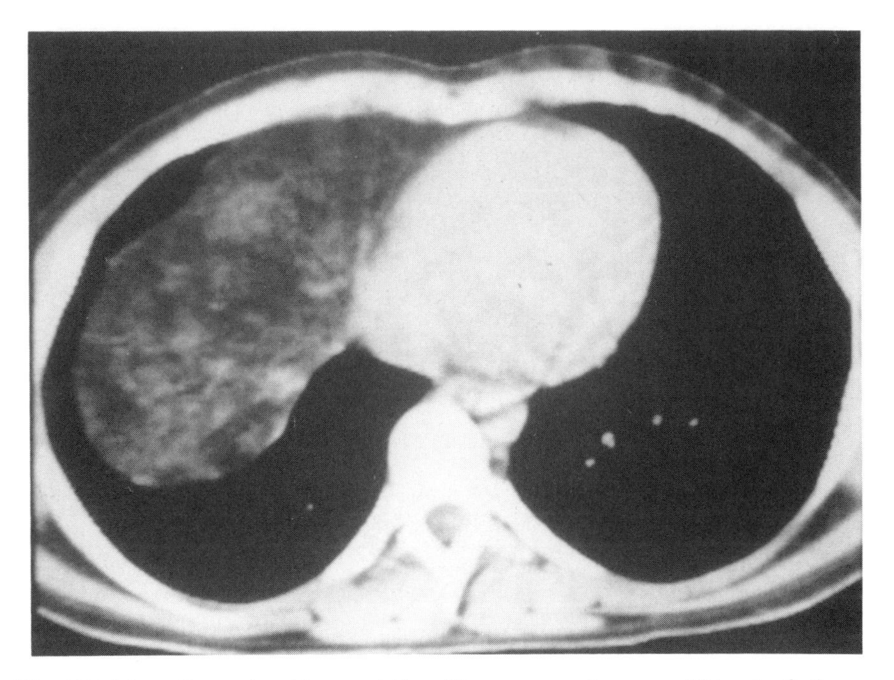

Fig. 6.7 Thymolipoma in a 15-year-old boy. The mass contains areas of fat and soft-tissue density.

myasthenia gravis has been particularly rewarding. Since effective chemotherapy is now available for several malignant tumours it is also important to be aware of the atrophic and hyperplastic changes which occur during and after chemotherapy. Primary germ-cell tumours and other masses arising in the thymus are rare but in some instances the CT appearances are sufficiently characteristic to enable a definitive diagnosis to be made.

REFERENCES

Baron R L, Lee J K T, Sagel S S, Peterson R R 1982a Computed tomography of the normal thymus. Radiology 142: 121–125

Baron R L, Lee J K T, Sagel S S, Levitt R G 1982b Computed tomography of the abnormal thymus. Radiology 142: 127–134

Baron R L, Sagel S S, Baglan R J 1981 Thymic cysts following radiation therapy for Hodgkin's disease. Radiology 141: 593–597

Blalock H, Harvey A M, Ford F R, Lilienthal J L Jr 1941 The treatment of myasthenia gravis by removal of the thymus gland: preliminary report. Journal of the American Medical Association 117: 1529–1533

Caffey J, Sibley R 1960 Regrowth and overgrowth of the thymus after atrophy induced by oral administration of corticosteroids to human infants. Pediatrics 26: 762–770

Castleman B, Norris E H 1949 The pathology of the thymus in myasthenia gravis: a study of 35 cases. Medicine 28: 27–58

Choyke P L, Zeman R K, Gootenberg J E, Greenberg J N, Hoffer F, Frank J A 1987 Thymic atrophy and regrowth in response to chemotherapy: CT evaluation. American Journal of Roentgenology 149: 269–272

Fon G T, Bein M E, Mancuso A A, Keesey J C, Lupetin A R, Wong W S 1982 Computed tomography of the anterior mediastinum in myasthenia gravis. Radiology 142: 135–141

Francis I R, Glazer G M, Bookstein F L, Gross B H 1985 The thymus: reexamination of age-related changes in size and shape. American Journal of Roentgenology 145: 249–254

Gelfand D W, Goldman A S, Law A J 1972 Thymic hyperplasia in children recovering from thermal burns. Journal of Trauma 12: 813–817

Heron C W, Husband J E, Williams M P 1988 Hodgkin disease: CT of the thymus. Radiology 167: 647–651

Keesey J C 1979 Indications for thymectomy in myasthenia gravis in plasmapheresis and immunobiology of myasthenia gravis. Houghton Mifflin, Boston pp 124–136

Keynes G 1955 Investigations into thymic disease and tumour formation. British Journal of Surgery 42: 449–462

Kissin C M, Husband J E, Nicholas D, Eversman W 1987 Benign thymic enlargement in adults after chemotherapy: CT demonstration. Radiology 163: 67–70

McLoud T C, Wittenberg J, Ferrucci J T 1979 Computed tomography of the thorax and standard radiographic evaluation of the chest: a comparative study. Journal of Computer Assisted Tomography 3: 170–180

Mink J H, Bein M E, Sukov R et al 1978 Computed tomography of the anterior mediastinum in patients with myasthenia gravis and suspected thymoma. American Journal of Roentgenology 130: 239–246

Rizk G, Cuteo L, Amplatz K 1972 Rebound enlargement of the thymus after successful corrective surgery for transposition of the great vessels. American Journal of Roentgenology 116: 528–530

Seltzer S E, Herman P G, Sagel S S 1984 Differential diagnosis of mediastinal fluid levels visualised on computed tomography. Journal of Computer Assisted Tomography 8: 244–246

Wilkins E W, Edmunds L H, Castleman B 1966 Cases of thymoma at the Massachusetts General Hospital. Journal of Thoracic and Cardiovascular Surgery 52: 322–330

Zerhouni E A, Scott W W, Baker R R, Wharam M O, Siegelman S S 1982 Invasive thymomas: diagnosis and evaluation by computed tomography. Journal of Computer Assisted Tomography 6: 92–100

7. Pancreatic neoplasms

Rodney H. Reznek

INTRODUCTION

Several imaging methods are now available for investigating patients with suspected pancreatic neoplasms. The selection of the most appropriate technique depends on the clinical indications and availability of equipment and will vary according to local preference and expertise. In recent years, because of its high diagnostic accuracy, CT has made a major impact on the approach to detecting pancreatic neoplasms. Nevertheless, in many instances, ultrasound with its low cost and ready availability is preferred as the first investigation. This chapter reviews the current role of CT in the evaluation of patients with suspected pancreatic neoplasms and describes the CT appearances in a variety of these tumours.

TECHNIQUE

Evaluation of the pancreas with CT requires optimal use of oral and intravenous contrast medium. Intravenous contrast medium should be routinely administered because it improves tumour detection and demonstrates the relationship of the tumour to adjacent vessels.

Peak enhancement of the pancreas follows that of the aorta by about three seconds and appears to be dependent on the concentration of intravascular contrast medium (Rossi et al 1982, Hosok 1983). Best results are achieved by rapidly injecting a bolus of about 50–100 ml of contrast medium and performing a dynamic scan with table incrementation (Hosok 1983). 10 mm collimation is sufficient to detect most lesions. However, 5 mm collimation is recommended for detecting islet-cell tumours. Thin slices increase the frequency of pancreatic duct visualization.

CLASSIFICATION

The most common primary pancreatic neoplasms arise from duct cells and islet cells. Tumours arising from acinar cells, connective tissue and from cells of unknown origin are extremely rare (Robbins & Cotran 1979). Primary duct cancers are either solid or cystic.

SOLID NEOPLASMS OF DUCT CELL ORIGIN

Adenocarcinoma

Duct-cell carcinoma accounts for 75% of non-endocrine malignancies of the pancreas (Cubilla & Fitzgerald 1980) and its incidence has trebled over the past 40 years (McMahon et al 1981). The tumour is localized to the head in 60% of cases, the body in about 10% and the tail in 5%. The entire gland is involved in the remaining 25% (Cubilla & Fitzgerald 1979). The prognosis remains extremely poor with a 5-year survival rate of $< 1\%$ (Gudjonsson et al 1978) but occasionally tumours < 2 cm diameter in the head of the pancreas are 'curable' (Moosa & Levin 1981).

CT appearances

Primary tumour. In most series, CT shows a pancreatic abnormality in over 99% of patients with cancer (Freeny et al 1988). A focal mass is the most common finding in pancreatic adenocarcinoma (Fig. 7.1). However, smaller masses may be diagnosed in the head of the gland particularly if they result in bile or pancreatic duct dilatation.

Reliance on absolute pancreatic measurements for detecting masses has now largely been abandoned because the normal variation in pancreatic size is too great. Most tumours distort the contour of the gland but small masses show more subtle features, e.g. the normal wedge-shaped appearance of the uncinate process may be rounded by the mass. A 'normal-sized' head in an otherwise atrophic gland may suggest a carcinoma (Fig. 7.2).

Almost all carcinomas enhance but to a lesser extent than the surrounding pancreas when dynamic scanning is used (Hosok 1983).

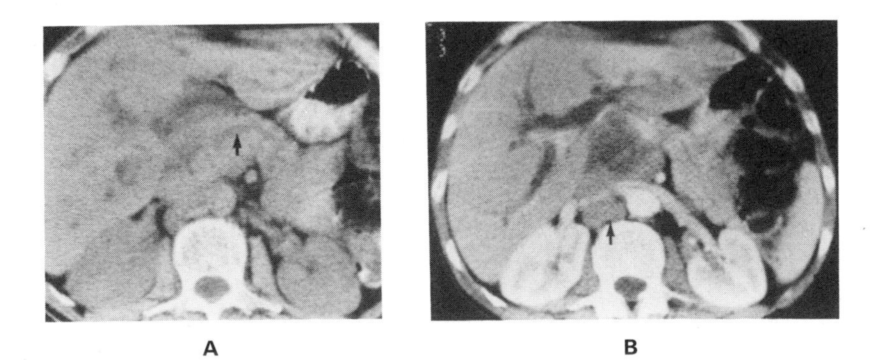

Fig. 7.1 **A** Unenhanced scan of the pancreas shows dilated intrahepatic bile ducts and dilated pancreatic ducts (arrowed). The pancreatic mass is difficult to identify with certainty. **B** Post-contrast scan at a similar level shows an obvious mass enhancing to a lesser extent than the normal pancreas. Right para-aortic lymph-node enlargement can also be seen (arrowed).

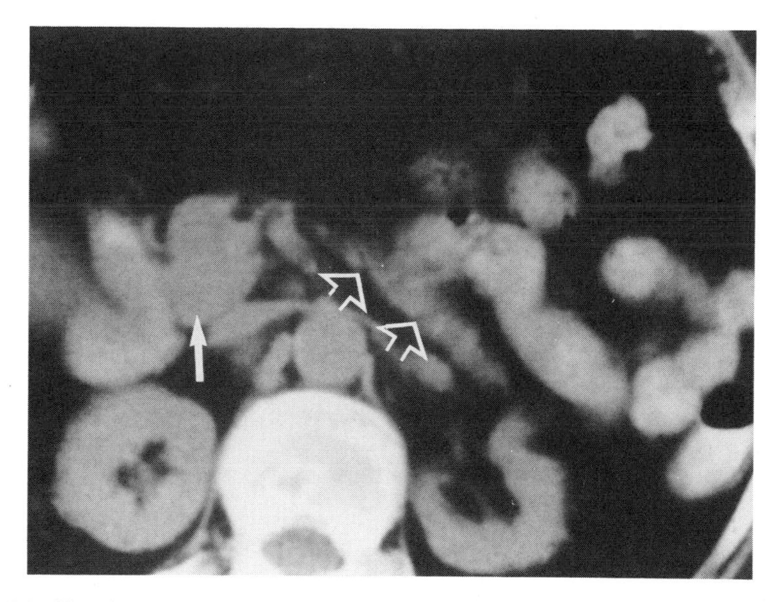

Fig. 7.2 Unenhanced scan showing atrophy of the body and tail of the pancreas (open arrow). The head of the pancreas does not appear atrophic (arrow) and contained a neoplastic mass lesion although it appeared 'normal'.

Occasionally, lucent areas are seen within the mass which may be related to associated pancreatitis rather than tumour necrosis as was previously believed.

Duct dilatation. Duct dilatation is more frequently seen if the dynamic scanning technique is employed. In carcinoma, proximal dilatation of the main pancreatic duct is seen in 50–85% of patients (Fishman & Siegelman 1983, Freeny et al 1988). The sign is particularly important for detecting a small duct-cell carcinoma of the head of the pancreas or an ampullary carcinoma because pancreatic duct dilatation may be the only abnormality on CT.

Adenocarcinoma of the head almost always causes biliary obstruction which is most frequently seen as dilatation of the common duct rather than of the intrahepatic ducts (Fishman & Siegelman 1983). Typically, CT shows a dilated common duct down to the site of the tumour but, unlike benign disease, there is a sudden transition from a dilated duct to no visible duct at all within the tumour.

Involvement of adjacent structures. Vascular encasement is seen on CT as narrowing or obliteration of the vessel lumen. A more subtle finding, which may even be present in the absence of a conspicuous pancreatic mass, is thickening of the wall of the coeliac axis or superior mesenteric artery which produces an irregular or 'club-shaped' appearance. This is thought to be due to malignant invasion of perivascular lymphatics.

Retroperitoneal extension may occur into the fat surrounding the coeliac axis or superior mesenteric artery without encasing the vessels. This may appear as streaks or strands of soft tissue adjacent to the mass. Thickening of Gerota's fascia suggests direct extension but this may also be caused by associated pancreatitis. Retroperitoneal extension is evident at presentation in 40–60% of patients with carcinoma (Fishman & Siegelman 1983).

Nodal and distant metastases. CT shows regional nodal involvement in 15–20% of patients with adenocarcinoma but some involved nodes are not enlarged and are therefore not detected by CT (Freeny et al 1988).

The liver is by far the most common site of distant metastases which are present on CT in 20–50% of cases (Fishman & Siegelman 1983, Ward et al 1983). Ascites occurs in about 10% of cases and is usually due to small peritoneal metastases rather than portal vein obstruction (Ward et al 1983).

The assessment of resectability. Preoperative assessment of resectability is desirable because about 10–15% of patients have resectable tumours (Edis et al 1981). Unfortunately, absolute criteria for defining unresectability are not agreed but some guidelines have been established. Resection is clearly precluded if metastases are detected anywhere outside an area encompassed by an en bloc pancreatic resection. These include liver metastases, peritoneal implants, involvement of the omentum, mesentery and lymph nodes. Encasement of hepatic, splenic or superior mesenteric arteries or portal, splenic or superior mesenteric veins usually also indicates that resection is impossible (Fishman & Siegelman 1983, Ward et al 1983). The size of the primary tumour alone does not influence resectability.

Using these criteria, CT has been shown to be more accurate than angiography for assessing resectability based on vascular involvement (Freeny et al 1988).

The indeterminate mass

In general, the presence of a focal pancreatic mass indicates a neoplasm but an area of localized pancreatic enlargement is not an unusual manifestation of chronic pancreatitis, occurring in as many as 20% of cases (Ferrucci et al 1979). The mass remains indeterminate when secondary signs such as liver metastases, invasion of the peripancreatic tissues and adenopathy are absent. Pancreatic duct dilatation and pseudocyst formation occur both with inflammatory and neoplastic lesions and the pattern of duct dilatation is not generally helpful in distinguishing these entities. Intrahepatic bile duct dilatation is more likely to occur with carcinoma than chronic pancreatitis. Extensive calcification within a focal mass strongly suggests pancreatitis and occurs in 55% of cases but tiny foci of calcification may also be encountered in malignancy. Furthermore, in 6–10% of cases, carcinoma and pancreatitis may coexist (Fishman & Siegelman 1983). In practice, therefore, if any doubt exists as to the nature of the mass, a percutaneous biopsy should be performed.

The role of CT

Ultrasound remains the most readily available and least expensive of the imaging methods used in assessment of the pancreas. With modern equipment and careful technique the sensitivity and specificity of tumour detection may reach 90% (Campbell & Wilson 1988). However, in a relatively high number of patients, visualization of the whole pancreas remains unsatisfactory. In addition, ultrasound has a low sensitivity in identifying that disease is not resectable, mainly because vascular involvement is not detected (Freeny et al 1982). CT should be performed, therefore, in patients with a strong probability of pancreatic carcinoma and a normal or technically suboptimal ultrasound examination.

The remarkably high sensitivity and accuracy of CT in the diagnosis of pancreatic cancer must be seen in perspective as it is unlikely that diagnosis by CT significantly affects the mortality rate or prognosis of patients with pancreatic cancer. The accuracy of CT is now such that failure to show a pancreatic lesion reliably excludes pancreatic cancer in a patient with abdominal pain and weight loss.

Other forms of solid ductal neoplasms

These tumours are uncommon and include anaplastic carcinoma, mucinous adenocarcinoma, giant-cell carcinoma and solid and papillary epithelial neoplasms. The CT appearances may be sufficiently characteristic to suggest the definitive diagnosis.

Anaplastic carcinoma accounts for 5% of all pancreatic cancers and has an extremely poor prognosis. On CT the tumour tends to be a large, solid mass, otherwise similar to duct-cell adenocarcinoma.

Mucinous adenocarcinoma (colloid carcinoma) has an excess of mucin and can spread to the peritoneum, resulting in pseudomyxoma peritonei (Fig. 7.3). CT shows low-density areas consistent with mucin pools with or without calcification (Gustafson et al 1984).

Giant-cell carcinoma is composed of bizarre multinucleated giant cells. The tumour tends to be a large mass which undergoes haemorrhage and necrosis. The typical CT appearance is of a large, thick-walled cyst with ragged inner margins.

Solid and papillary epithelial neoplasms are uncommon tumours found mainly in young female patients (Choi et al 1988). They are of low-grade malignancy and metastases are rare. In most cases cure can be achieved following complete resection. CT shows a well-demarcated soft-tissue mass, usually in the tail of the pancreas. Cystic change due to haemorrhagic necrosis can occur within the mass. Calcification is infrequent.

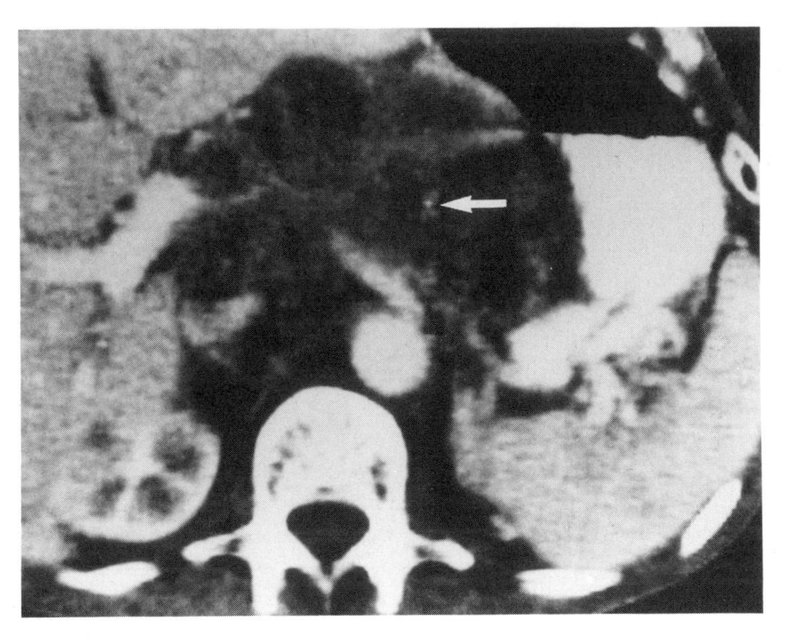

Fig. 7.3 Mucinous adenocarcinoma. Contrast-enhanced scan shows a large, low-density mass replacing the pancreas. It is encasing the coeliac artery and the portal confluence. A fleck of calcium is seen within the lesion (arrowed).

PRIMARY CYSTIC NEOPLASMS OF DUCT-CELL ORIGIN

Microcystic adenoma

The vast majority of these benign tumours occur in females over the age of 60 years. The tumour occurs in the head, body or tail but occasionally occupies the entire gland. Almost all the cysts are less than 2 cm in diameter and the CT appearance is usually of a water density mass which sometimes contains solid elements. Individual cysts are too small to be identified on CT. Calcification occurs more frequently than in any other pancreatic tumour. It is dystrophic within a central fibrotic scar and may have a stellate appearance on CT. The tumour does not have a well-developed capsule and is poorly demarcated from the normal gland. Contrast enhancement may be seen due to a rich network of capillaries within the tumour.

Mucinous cystic neoplasm

Like microcystic adenoma, this tumour occurs predominantly in females but unlike microcystic adenoma has a malignant potential, developing into a low-grade, mucinous adenocarcinoma. On CT, the mass is a well-demarcated, round or oval thick-walled cyst. The mass is generally > 5 cm in diameter and solid-enhancing excrescences can occasionally be seen in the wall, particularly if the tumour is malignant. Dystrophic peripheral calcification is seen in about 15% of cases. The main differential diagnosis is a pancreatic pseudocyst but a thick, irregular wall suggests the diagnosis of mucinous cystic neoplasm (Friedman et al 1983).

ISLET-CELL TUMOURS

The diagnosis of a functional islet-cell tumour is made by serum hormone assay and the role of the radiologist is to localize the tumour and judge the extent of its dissemination. About 20% of islet-cell tumours are non-functioning and these frequently remain silent until they are large enough to cause symptoms due to mass effect. Functioning tumours are generally quite small at the time of diagnosis.

Islet-cell tumours can produce clinical syndromes resulting from an excess of insulin, gastrin (Zollinger–Ellison), glucagon, somatostatin and vasoactive intestinal polypeptide (VIP). Other hormones, such as ACTH and melanocyte-stimulating hormone can also be secreted in excess.

Islet-cell tumours occur with equal frequency in the head, body and tail of the pancreas. The incidence of malignancy varies, e.g. gastrinomas and somatostatinomas are malignant in about 60% of cases, insulinomas in only about 10%.

Localization

There are a number of methods available for functioning islet-cell tumour localization and opinions vary as to which is the best technique. Pancreatic venous sampling, the most invasive, is reported to detect lesions with an accuracy of > 95% (Clark et al 1985). Its greatest value is in the detection of small insulinomas which are difficult to localize by other means.

The success rate of angiography varies in different series and with the type of islet-cell tumour being investigated. At best, angiography will detect about 80% of insulinomas but only about 15% of gastrinomas (Dunnick et al 1980). With modern CT equipment the accuracy rate for detecting islet-cell tumours is 70–80% (Stark et al 1984, Rossi et al 1985). Ultrasound is less accurate than CT and angiography and the most encouraging results to date show that ultrasound detected 60% of insulinomas (Galiber et al 1988).

CT is a useful initial investigation for the detection of islet-cell tumours because it has a relatively high accuracy and is non-invasive. A further major advantage of the technique is the ability to diagnose disseminated disease.

Insulinomas

Insulinomas are the most common islet-cell tumours of which 10% are

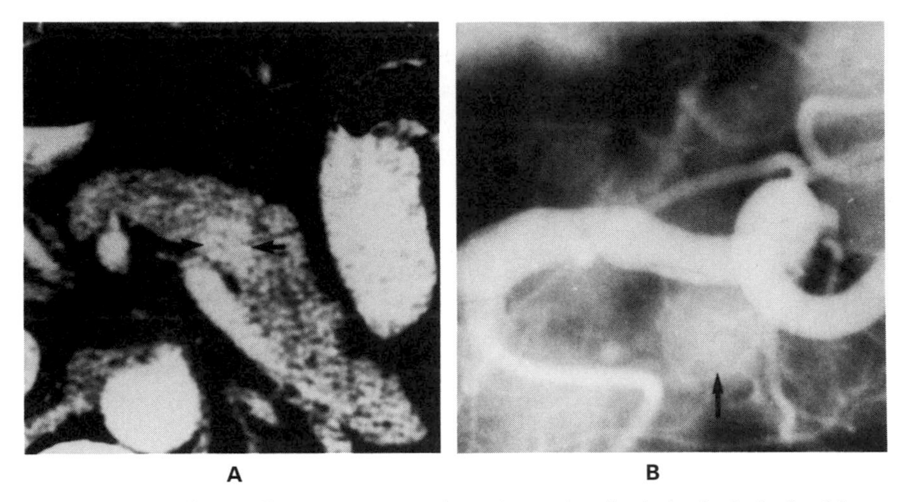

Fig. 7.4 **A** Insulinoma. Post-contrast scan shows 1 cm enhancing lesion in the body of the pancreas (arrowed) which is not distorting the pancreatic outline. **B** Coeliac arteriogram in the same patient shows the vascular blush corresponding to the small insulinoma (arrowed).

multiple and 10% malignant. They are generally the smallest, 80% being < 2 cm in diameter at the time of presentation (Fig. 7.4). For this reason they are more difficult to identify on CT than other islet-cell tumours and only about 60% of them will be detected. Insulinomas are only rarely ectopic, e.g. insulin-producing hepatomas or retroperitoneal sarcomas.

Large tumours produce sufficient distortion of the pancreatic contour to be seen on enhanced scans but may be isodense with the normal pancreas after bolus injection of contrast medium. Small lesions are not visible on pre-contrast scans because they have similar attenuation values to normal pancreatic tissue. They are only identified as a hyperdense 'blush' following bolus injection of contrast medium. Malignant insulinomas tend to be larger than benign lesions and calcification is more likely.

Gastrinomas

Gastrinomas are the second most common islet-cell tumour and account for the majority of cases of Zollinger–Ellison syndrome. Multiple lesions are seen in one-third of cases and in about 20% the entire gland is involved. In about 60% of patients with Zollinger–Ellison syndrome the tumour is malignant, in 30% the tumour a benign adenoma and in 10% the syndrome is due to hyperplasia. Multiple adenomas are particularly common in patients with multiple endocrine neoplasia Type I (see below). As with insulinomas, gastrinomas show an angiographic 'blush' on dynamic CT. Malignant lesions tend to be larger and may be calcified. The value of CT is not limited to detection of the pancreatic tumour since evidence of disseminated malignancy may be shown. Recently, the accuracy of CT in localizing gastrinomas has been reported as > 75% (Stark et al 1984) and it is particularly valuable in assessing resectability. In some patients stomach wall thickening due to mucosal hypertrophy can also be identified.

Other islet-cell tumours

Only a few examples of the CT appearances of glucagonomas, vipomas and somatostatinomas have been described. Their characteristics are similar to insulinomas except that they all tend to be larger than insulinomas at the time of presentation. Glucagonomas vary in size from 2.5 to 25 cm (Dodds et al 1985) and vipomas from 5 to 10 cm at presentation. As 90% of glucagonomas and 60% of vipomas are malignant, evidence of tumour spread is usually seen.

Multiple endocrine neoplasms – Type I (MEN I)

Type I MEN consists of tumours or hyperplasia of the pituitary gland, parathyroid gland and pancreatic islet cells (Dodds et al 1985). Less commonly, it may be associated with carcinoid tumours, thyroid disease, lipomas and nodular adrenocortical hyperplasia. Hyperparathyroidism is the most common manifestation of the syndrome (89%) and islet-cell tumours the second most common (81%).

Nearly all patients with MEN I syndrome eventually develop a neoplasm or hyperplasia of the pancreatic islet cells but the clinical signs of the islet-cell abnormality frequently do not arise until 5–10 years after the patient shows evidence of hyperparathyroidism. Gastrinoma is by far the most common islet-cell tumour, insulinoma being a much less common second. Occasionally the tumour produces both gastrin and insulin. About 20–40% of patients with Zollinger–Ellison syndrome have MEN I. MEN I is inherited as an autosomal dominant with high penetrance, thus, 50% of offspring are affected. However, imaging including CT is only justified if biochemical tests are positive. In the absence of symptoms or signs of a specific endocrinopathy, serum calcium and radioimmunoassay for serum gastrin are adequate to detect asymptomatic adult family members who have inherited the MEN I trait.

Non-functioning islet-cell tumours

Of islet-cell tumours 15–20% are non-functioning and those that produce symptoms are usually malignant. Hepatic or nodal metastases are frequently seen. The clinical presentation is identical to that of adenocarcinoma of the pancreas.

On CT, non-functioning islet-cell tumours tend to be larger and more frequently calcified than functioning tumours and about 75% enhance after

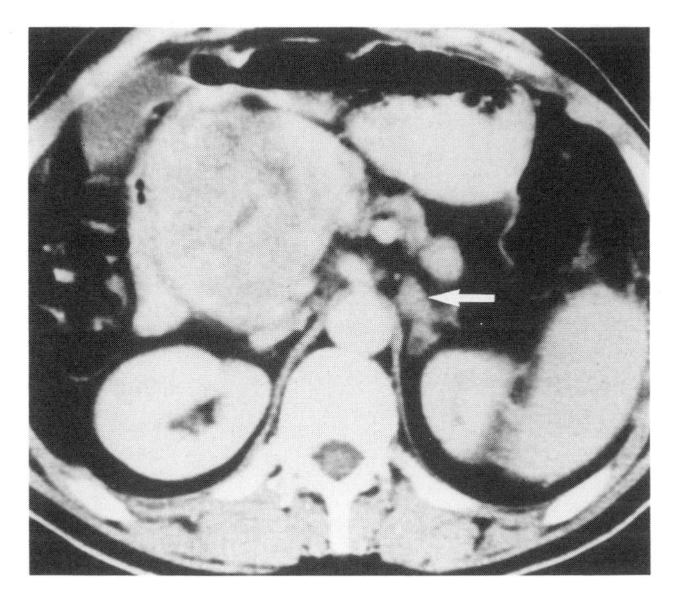

Fig. 7.5 Non-functioning islet-cell tumour. Post-contrast scan shows a large enhancing mass in the head of the pancreas with marked atrophy of the remainder of the pancreas. There is nodular hyperplasia of the left adrenal (arrowed) as the patient had MEN Type I syndrome.

injection of contrast medium (Fig. 7.5). Precise localization is important before surgery as complete resection can be achieved.

PANCREATIC LYMPHOMA AND METASTASES

Pancreatic involvement occurs in 1–2% of patients with intra-abdominal non-Hodgkin's lymphoma, almost invariably associated with massive retroperitoneal lymphadenopathy. Infrequently, isolated pancreatic involvement occurs and the CT appearances are indistinguishable from adenocarcinoma (Fig. 7.6). A mass of peripancreatic nodes, involved with lymphoma or with metastases from tumours of the breast, lung or from melanoma, may blend imperceptibly with the pancreas on CT and may be mistaken for an intrinsic pancreatic mass. Enhancement of the pancreas following the administration of intravenous contrast medium usually allows the pancreas to be identified separate from the nodes.

CONCLUSION

One of the most common reasons for referral for CT examination of the pancreas is for the detection of suspected carcinoma because CT is a highly effective method for demonstrating the presence and extent of the primary tumour as well as distant metastases. Although the information derived

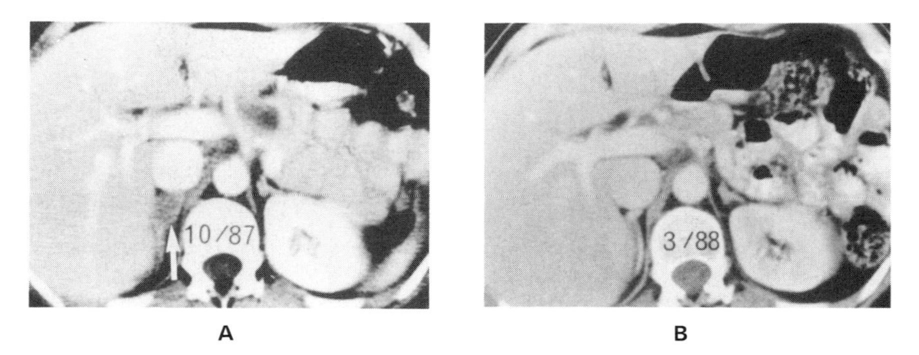

Fig. 7.6 **A** Pancreatic lymphoma. Post-contrast scan shows low attenuation mass in the body of the pancreas in a patient with non-Hodgkin's lymphoma. A mass lesion was also present in the right adrenal gland (arrow). **B** A scan five months later post-chemotherapy shows complete resolution of the lymphomatous masses in the pancreas and the right adrenal gland.

from CT is unlikely to benefit the individual patient it does enable the diagnosis to be made quickly and with little distress. Of perhaps equal importance is the confidence with which pancreatic carcinoma can be excluded.

With the advent of fast scanning techniques CT now plays a key role in the diagnosis of small functioning pancreatic tumours and as in pancreatic carcinoma has the advantage of demonstrating disseminated disease as well as the primary tumour.

REFERENCES

Campbell J P, Wilson S R 1988 Pancreatic neoplasms: how useful is evaluation with ultrasound. Radiology 167: 341–344

Choi B I, Kim K W, Han M C, Kim Y I, Kim C-W 1988 Solid and papillary epithelial neoplasms of the pancreas: CT findings. Radiology 166: 413–416

Clark L R, Jaffe M H, Choyke P L, Grant E G, Zeman R K 1985 Pancreatic imaging. Radiologic Clinics of North America 23: 489–502

Cubilla A L, Fitzgerald R J 1979 Classification of pancreatic cancer (non-endocrine). Mayo Clinic Proceedings 54: 449–458

Cubilla A L, Fitzgerald R J 1980 Cancer (non-endocrine) of the pancreas. A suggested classification. Monographs in Pathology 21: 82–100

Dodds W J, Wilson S D, Thorsen M K et al 1985 MEN I syndrome and islet-cell lesions of the pancreas. Seminars in Roentgenology 20: 57–64

Dunnick N R, Long J A, Krudy A et al 1980 Localizing insulinomas with combined radiography methods. American Journal of Roentgenology 135: 747–752

Edis A J, Kiernan P D, Taylor W F 1981 Attempted curative resection of ductal carcinoma of the pancreas: review of Mayo clinical experience 1951–1975. Mayo Clinic Proceedings 55: 531–536.

Ferrucci J T, Wittenberg J, Black E B et al 1979 Computed body tomography in chronic pancreatitis. Radiology 130: 175–182

Fishman E K, Siegelman S S 1983 CT of pancreatic carcinoma. In: Siegelman S S (ed) Computed Tomography of the Pancreas. Churchill Livingstone, New York, pp 123–156

Freeny P C, Marks W M, Ball T J 1982 Impact of high resolution computed tomography of

the pancreas on utilization of endoscopic retrograde cholangiopancreatography and angiography. Radiology 142: 35–39
Freeny P C, Marks W M, Ryan J A, Traverso L W 1988 Pancreatic ductal adenocarcinoma: diagnosis and staging with dynamic CT. Radiology 166: 125–133
Friedman A C, Lichtenstein J E, Dachman A H 1983 Cystic neoplasms of the pancreas: radiological-pathological correlation. Radiology 149: 45–50
Galiber A K, Reading C C, Charboneau J W et al 1988 Localization of pancreatic insulinoma: comparison of pre- and intraoperative ultrasound with CT and angiography. Radiology 166: 405–408
Gudjonsson B, Livstone E M, Spiro H 1978 Cancer of the pancreas. Diagnostic accuracy and survival statistics. Cancer 42: 2494–2506
Gustafson K D, Karnaze G C, Hattery R R, Scheithauer B W 1984 Pseudomyxoma peritonei associated with mucinous adenocarcinoma of the pancreas: CT findings and CT-guided biopsy. Journal of Computer Assisted Tomography 8: 335–338
Hosok T 1983 Dynamic CT of pancreatic tumours. American Journal of Roentgenology 140: 959–965
McMahon B, Yen S, Trichopoulos D, Warren K, Nardi G 1981 Coffee and cancer of the pancreas. New England Journal of Medicine 304: 630–633
Moosa A R, Levin B 1981 The diagnosis of 'early' pancreatic cancer: the University of Chicago experience. Cancer 47: 1688–1697
Robbins S C, Cotran S R 1979 Pathological Basis of Disease. W B Saunders, Philadelphia pp 1104–1107
Rossi P, Baert A, Marchal W, Tipaldi L, Wilms W, Pavone P 1982 Multiple bolus technique vs single bolus or infusion of contrast medium to obtain prolonged contrast enhancement of the pancreas. Radiology 144: 929–931
Rossi P, Baert A, Passariello R, Simonetti G, Pavone P, Tempesta P 1985 CT of functioning tumors of the pancreas. American Journal of Roentgenology 144: 57–60
Stark D D, Moss A A, Goldberg H I, Deveney C W 1984 CT of pancreatic islet-cell tumours. Radiology 150: 491–494
Ward E M, Stephens D H, Sheedy P F 1983 Computed tomographic characteristics of pancreatic carcinoma: an analysis of 100 cases. Radiographics 3: 547–565

8. Inflammatory disease of the pancreas

David H. Stephens

INTRODUCTION

Pancreatitis may be classified according to cause, duration, severity, structural alteration, functional impairment or by a combination of these and other criteria (Sarner & Cotton 1984, Singer et al 1985). The customary designation of pancreatitis as either acute or chronic is both convenient and clinically valid, as for the most part acute and chronic pancreatitis are separate and distinct conditions. This classification, however, does not entirely indicate the spectrum of disease encountered in practice. For example, there are relapsing forms of both acute and chronic pancreatitis. Furthermore, acute pancreatitis may enter a subacute phase, at which time some of the more important sequelae of the disease may occur. Rarely does acute pancreatitis progress into a chronic irreversible form of pancreatic inflammation (Magnuson & Stephens 1988).

ACUTE PANCREATITIS

Acute pancreatitis varies greatly in severity. The mild, self-limiting form is characterized by transient oedema of the gland, whereas severe cases may be complicated by necrosis, haemorrhage or suppuration. Between the extremes are cases of varying severity, many of which are associated with development of extrapancreatic fluid collections.

CT can serve a number of purposes in the evaluation of patients with acute pancreatitis. The technique can provide confirmatory evidence when the diagnosis is otherwise inconclusive but, perhaps more importantly, CT can be used to assess severity, detect complications and guide management of the disease. Although CT findings are generally accurate indicators of the severity of acute pancreatitis (Balthazar et al 1985, Vernacchia et al 1987), meaningful interpretation requires correlation with clinical information. Positive findings are present in the great majority of cases but the findings sometimes lack specificity. Since many of the manifestations are inconstant, sequential examinations may provide information that is not obvious on the initial study.

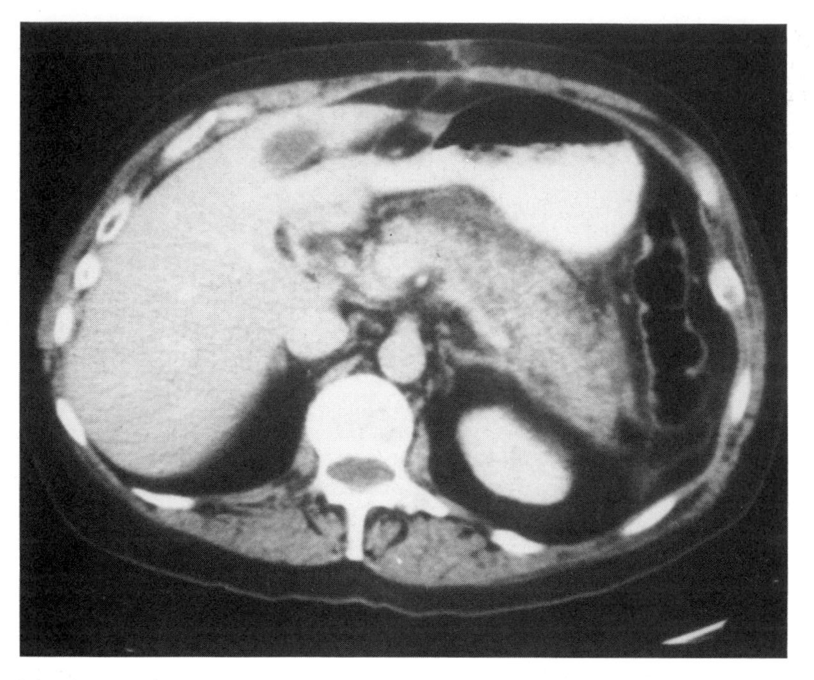

Fig. 8.1 Acute oedematous pancreatitis. The pancreas is swollen, its density is inhomogeneous and its margins are indistinct. The anterior layer of renal fascia on the left is thickened.

Oedematous pancreatitis

Although, in general, there is recognizable swelling of the gland in oedematous pancreatitis, CT evidence may be equivocal in uncomplicated cases. The margins of the pancreas may be indistinct and the density of the organ may be slightly diminished, usually in an inhomogeneous fashion (Fig. 8.1). Thickening of nearby retroperitoneal fascia is a very common but non-specific finding, most frequently involving the anterior layer of renal fascia on the left side (Parienty et al 1981) (Fig. 8.1). Although most cases of oedematous pancreatitis resolve without sequelae, we have observed generalized parenchymal atrophy and exocrine insufficiency appearing months after a single episode of oedematous pancreatitis (Magnuson & Stephens 1988).

Effusions

Peripancreatic effusions are common in acute pancreatitis, usually developing early in the course of the disease. When the acutely inflamed pancreas produces fluid in amounts greater than can be accommodated by ductal outflow, small pancreatic ducts and acini are subject to rupture.

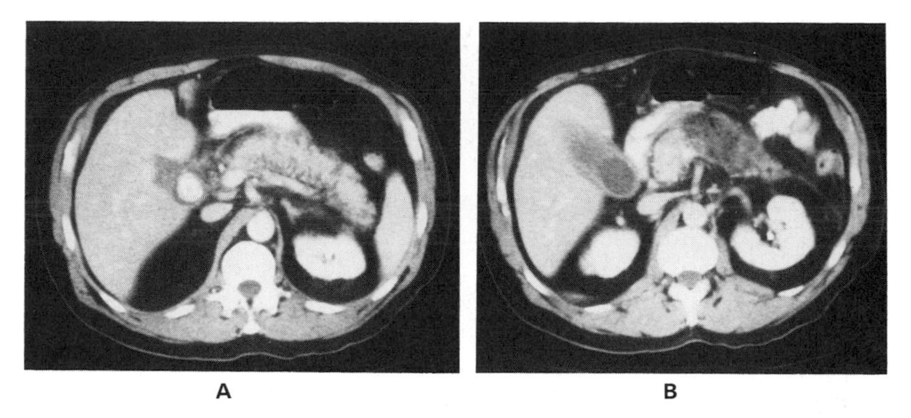

Fig. 8.2 Acute pancreatitis with peripancreatic effusion. Scans made at adjacent levels show a relatively normal pancreatic tail and body **A** and head **B** which have undergone appreciable intravenous contrast enhancement indicating adequate vascular perfusion. A fluid collection surrounds the pancreas, expanding the anterior pararenal space **B** below the level of the pancreatic tail and body. A calcified stone is present in the gallbladder **A**.

Fluid extravasated from the ductal system may collect within the pancreatic parenchyma, or it may migrate to the surface of the gland. The enzyme-rich effusion can escape beyond the confines of the gland by breaching the thin layer of fibrous tissue that serves ineffectively as a capsule for the pancreas (Siegelman et al 1980).

Extrapancreatic effusions first accumulate in the spaces that are the nearest to the pancreas: the anterior pararenal space (Fig. 8.2) and the lesser sac of the peritoneal cavity. Especially when the volume of extravasated fluid is large, effusions can also spread beyond the immediate vicinity of the pancreas. From the anterior pararenal space fluid may spread caudally into the iliac fossa. Sometimes a pancreatic effusion extends around or behind the kidney, usually without invading the perirenal space. In the greater peritoneal cavity fluid may spread along the transverse mesocolon or the leaves of small bowel mesentery, or it may accumulate as ascites. Fluid may enter the mediastinum by passing through the diaphragmatic hiatus. Since extrapancreatic fluid collections can be sources of serious complications of acute pancreatitis, it is important for the radiologist to understand the compartmental anatomy of the abdomen and routes of spread of fluid within the abdominal spaces (Love et al 1981, Dodds et al 1986, Raptopoulos 1986).

The outcome of acute pancreatitis with extrapancreatic effusion is variable. Spontaneous resolution of peripancreatic collections is common if pancreatic inflammation is brief, self-limiting and if the amount of extra-pancreatic fluid is not excessive. In fact, it has been suggested that the release of fluid from the pancreas may decompress the gland and thereby serve to lessen injury to the pancreatic parenchyma (Siegelman et al 1980). Fluid collections which do not resolve within a few weeks tend to become

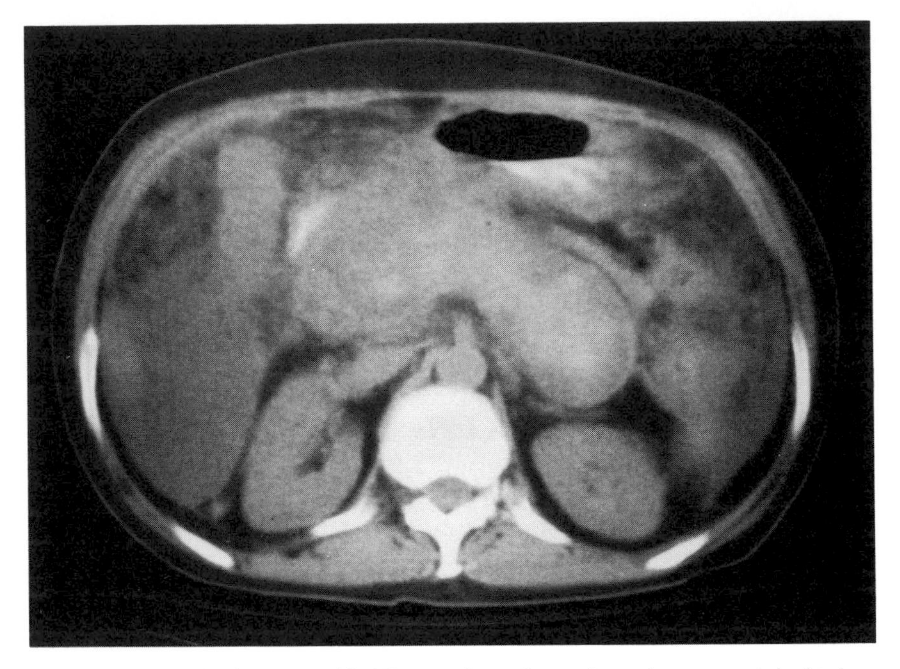

Fig. 8.3 Haemorrhagic pancreatitis. The unenhanced scan shows the pancreatic bed to be occupied by a saccular mass containing material of high-density (blood) as well as lower-density fluid. Ascites and mesenteric infiltration are also present. At autopsy the pancreas was found to have undergone liquefactive necrosis and haemorrhage.

encapsulated by fibrous connective tissue, thus becoming pseudocysts. A more serious complication is bacterial infection of a fluid collection with resultant abscess formation.

Necrosis

Tissue necrosis is an important determinant of the severity of acute pancreatitis (White et al 1986). Failure of pancreatic tissue to undergo normal or increased enhancement with intravenous contrast material indicates diminished vascular perfusion and thus the likelihood of necrosis (Kivisaari et al 1984). Extensive necrosis is associated with increased risk of haemorrhage (Fig. 8.3) and infection.

Haemorrhage

Haemorrhage, another potentially serious complication of acute pancreatitis, may be evident on CT because of the increased density of recently extravasated blood (Fig. 8.3). Haemorrhage may occur within the pancreas or at an extrapancreatic site of inflammation. Bleeding can occur into a pseudocyst, effusion or region of necrosis.

The clinical significance of haemorrhage associated with pancreatitis is variable. Not all patients with CT evidence of haemorrhage have clinically severe pancreatitis; some patients make uneventful recoveries with conservative management (Isikoff et al 1981). Haemorrhage, however, can be catastrophic and radiological evidence of this complication should be taken seriously.

Pseudocyst

The term pseudocyst should be reserved for a collection of pancreatic fluid encapsulated by fibrous tissue. Mature and uncomplicated pseudocysts typically appear as thin-walled, sharply circumscribed, round or oval masses that contain fluid of homogeneous water-like density (Williford et al 1983). Most pseudocysts occur within or adjacent to the pancreas (Fig. 8.4), but some are found at remote sites of extrapancreatic effusion.

Pseudocysts are far less likely to undergo spontaneous resolution than encapsulated effusions. However, spontaneous rupture and decompression of a pseudocyst may occur, sometimes into an adjacent hollow organ of the gastro-intestinal tract. Pseudocysts can also become infected, a compli-

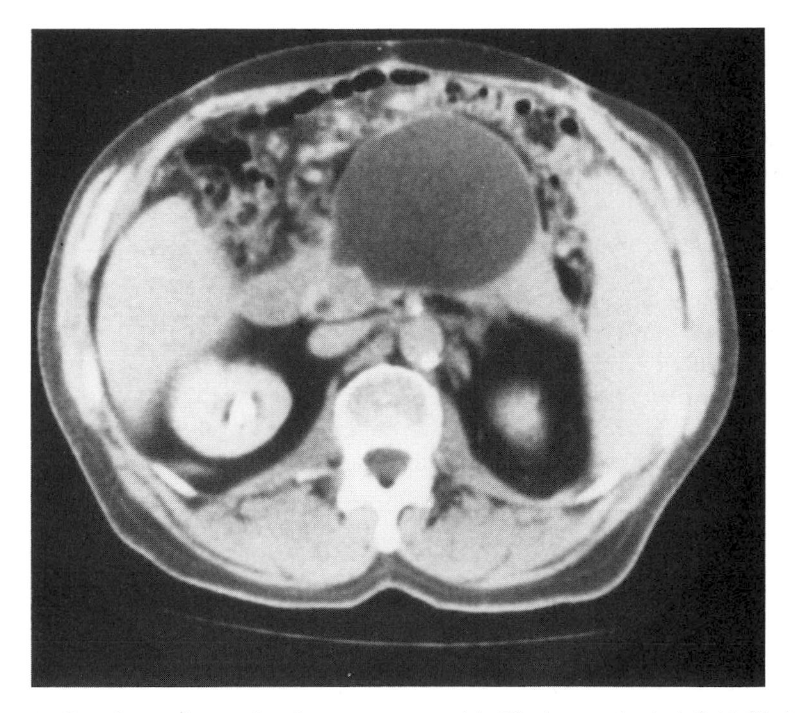

Fig. 8.4 Pseudocyst six months after acute pancreatitis. The large, spherical, fluid-filled mass has a thin but discernible capsular margin.

cation that may or may not result in the formation of gas within the cyst. Gas may also enter a pseudocyst from a communication with the gut.

Because relatively few mature pseudocysts disappear spontaneously, intervention is generally required to eliminate these masses. Surgical drainage has long been the standard treatment for pseudocysts but successful results are also being achieved by drainage under radiological guidance (Torres et al 1986).

Phlegmon

The term pancreatic phlegmon, introduced in the 1970s (Warshaw 1974), refers to a solid mass of indurated pancreas and adjacent retroperitoneal tissues which is characterized by oedema, infiltration of inflammatory cells and tissue necrosis (Sostre et al 1985). Since the introduction of sectional imaging, a variety of pancreatic and peripancreatic inflammatory lesions have been designated as phlegmons, although not all of these masses fit the description of the lesion originally given that name. While precise classification of inflammatory pancreatic masses is not always possible by radiological imaging, it is probably best to limit the term phlegmon to more or less solid-appearing inflammatory masses involving the pancreas and adjacent tissues.

Phlegmons usually develop after the initial attack of pancreatitis and may persist beyond the time of clinical recovery. Since phlegmons have necrotic components they may become infected. As it may not be possible to distinguish an uninfected phlegmon from an abscess on the basis of the radiological appearance, percutaneous diagnostic aspiration is often indicated when there is reason to suspect infection.

Abscess

Abscesses are life-threatening complications of acute pancreatitis. They have a variety of appearances on CT scans (Federle et al 1981, Freeny & Lawson 1982). In some cases they are indistinguishable from uninfected necrotizing pancreatitis or from sterile phlegmons or fluid collections. Like other fluid collections, abscesses may be confined to the pancreatic bed or they may extend beyond the immediate vicinity of the organ. For that reason, a CT examination for suspected pancreatic abscess should encompass the entire abdomen and the pelvis. Pancreatic abscesses may be unilocular or multilocular, solitary or multifocal. They may consist of liquid pus or they may be composed of semi-solid material or partially digested tissue.

The most impressive sign of an abscess is gas within an inflammatory mass (Mendez & Isikoff 1979, Federle et al 1981) (Fig. 8.5). However, despite its diagnostic value, the presence of gas within a pancreatic lesion does not constitute absolute evidence of a pyogenic abscess. For example,

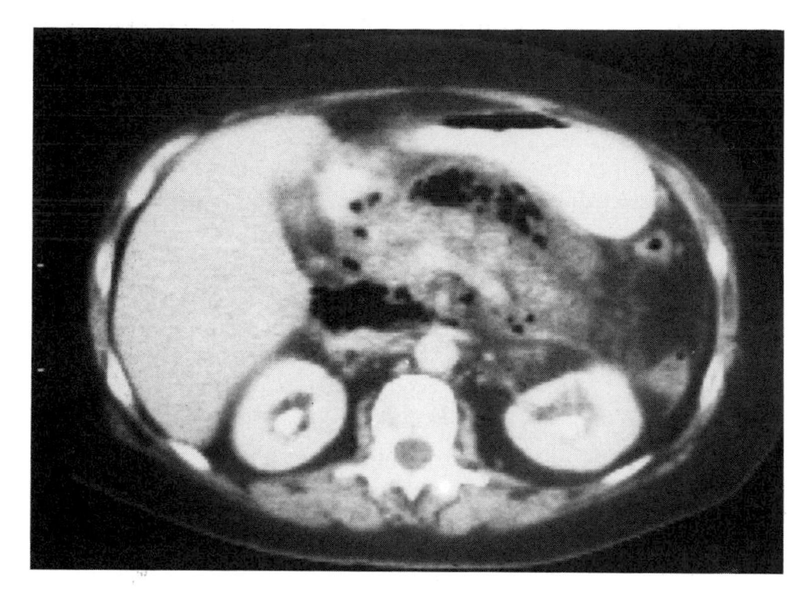

Fig. 8.5 Abscess. Collections of gas are present in the peripancreatic region. The pancreas itself appears relatively normal.

gas may be found in an uninfected pseudocyst that communicates with the gastrointestinal lumen and rarely gas has been observed in apparently sterile foci of pancreatic necrosis (Torres et al 1981). Furthermore, a substantial proportion of pancreatic abscesses, probably the majority, do not contain gas.

It is often impossible to determine whether or not an inflammatory mass or fluid collection is infected on the basis of the CT appearances alone and for this reason correlation with clinical information is imperative. When an abscess is a likely possibility, percutaneous aspiration of material for microscopic analysis and culture is usually indicated. Appropriate therapeutic intervention, which may include percutaneous drainage under CT guidance, can then be carried out (Karlson et al 1982, Hill et al 1983, van Sonnenberg et al 1985, Freeny et al 1988).

CHRONIC PANCREATITIS

The diagnosis of chronic pancreatitis is usually established before an imaging procedure is obtained but occasionally CT provides the first indication of the disease. Chronic pancreatitis is a common cause of pancreatic exocrine insufficiency (Schuman et al 1986) but recurrent or persistent abdominal pain may be the major clinical feature. Most of the pathological anatomy associated with pancreatitis is depicted well by CT (Leutmer et al 1988).

Alterations in pancreatic morphology

Parenchyma and ducts

Typically the pancreatic parenchyma atrophies in chronic pancreatitis although the overall thickness of the gland may be maintained as a result of concomitant ductal dilatation. Pancreatic ductal dilatation is a very common feature, best displayed on contrast-enhanced scans. The main pancreatic duct may be dilated diffusely or in a non-uniform fashion. Dilated side branches may also be visible.

Occasionally there is enlargement of the gland as a result of inflammatory infiltration or proliferation of fibrotic connective tissue. Usually the enlargement is focal and may be associated with atrophy of the remainder of the organ. In the absence of other evidence of chronic pancreatitis, a solid focal inflammatory mass may be impossible to distinguish from neoplasm on the basis of the CT appearances (Fishman et al 1983, Neff et al 1984, Leutmer et al 1988). Frequently, however, there are other features which indicate chronic inflammation. For example, dilated ductal branches or intraductal calculi distributed throughout such a mass points to the likelihood of chronic pancreatitis rather than a solid tumour.

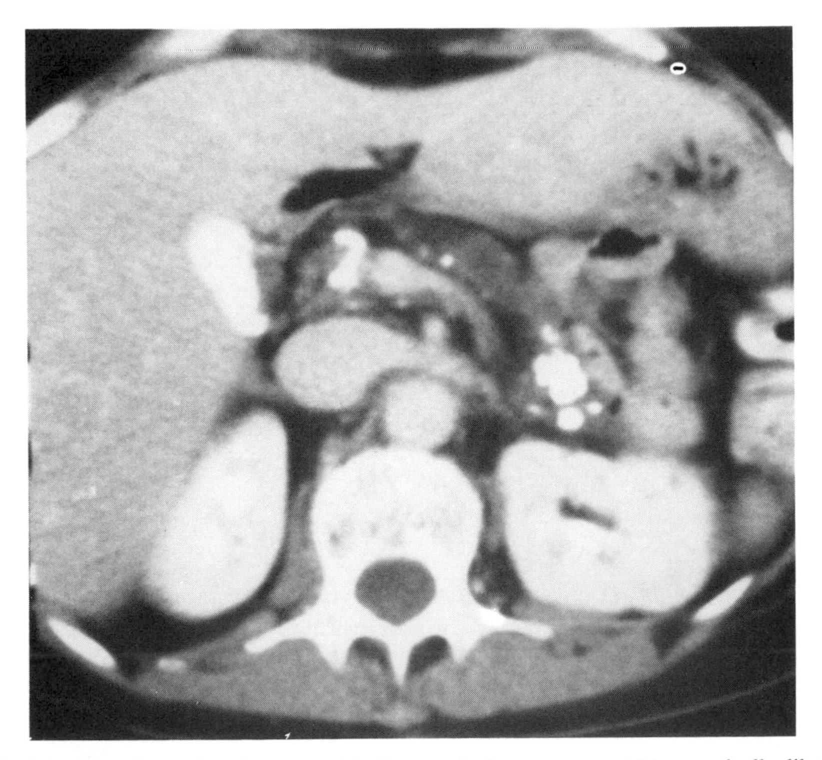

Fig. 8.6 Hereditary chronic pancreatitis. Large calculi are present within a markedly dilated main pancreatic duct. Pancreatic parenchyma is thinned.

Pancreatic calculi

CT is the most accurate method of detecting pancreatic calculi, a finding which is common in chronic pancreatitis and is practically diagnostic of this condition. The intraductal location of these calculi can often be recognized. In hereditary pancreatitis calculi tend to occur early in the disease; they are usually large and are often arranged in a linear pattern within the dilated main pancreatic duct (Fig. 8.6).

Fluid collections

Pseudocysts discovered in chronic pancreatitis are usually mature and relatively stable. They may be located in the vicinity of the pancreas or at some distance from the gland. Most are unilocular but some contain visible internal septa. The presence of unencapsulated peripancreatic fluid in chronic pancreatitis usually indicates superimposed acute inflammation.

Pseudoaneurysms

These lesions develop as a result of enzymatic disruption of arterial walls and most frequently occur in association with a pseudocyst. The commonest vessels involved are the splenic, gastroduodenal, pancreatico-duodenal and hepatic arteries. On CT, a pseudoaneurysm appears as a structure that undergoes dynamic contrast enhancement in the same fashion as neighbouring arteries. Often pseudoaneurysms are seen to lie within an unenhancing pseudocyst (Burke et al 1986). Recognition of this relatively uncommon complication is of considerable importance, as pseudoaneurysms can undergo massive haemorrhage.

CONCLUSION

The wide range of morphological changes seen in the spectrum of acute pancreatic inflammation are elegantly displayed on CT. For this reason, CT plays an integral role in the diagnosis, assessment of severity and in the detection of life-threatening complications of acute pancreatitis. In chronic pancreatitis the role of CT is more limited because the diagnosis is usually established before referral for CT examination. However, in those cases in which a conclusive diagnosis has not been reached the CT findings may be characteristic.

REFERENCES

Balthazar E J, Ranson J H C, Naidich D D et al 1985 Acute pancreatitis: prognostic value of CT. Radiology 156: 767–772

Burke J W, Erickson S J, Kellum C D et al 1986 Pseudoaneurysms complicating pancreatitis: detection by CT. Radiology 161: 447–450

Dodds W J, Darweesh R M A, Lawson T L et al 1986 The retroperitoneal spaces revisited. American Journal of Roentgenology 147: 1155–1161

Federle M P, Jeffrey R B, Crass R A, Van Dalsem V 1981 Computed tomography of pancreatic abscess. American Journal of Roentgenology 136: 878–882
Fishman E K, Jones B, Siegelman S S 1983 The indeterminate pancreatic mass: carcinoma versus focal pancreatitis. In: Siegelman S S (ed) Computed tomography of the pancreas. Vol 1. Contemporary issues in computed tomography. Churchill Livingstone, Edinburgh, pp 157–177
Freeny P C, Lawson T L 1982 Radiology of the pancreas. Springer-Verlag, New York
Freeny P C, Lewis G P, Traverso L W, Ryan J A 1988 Infected pancreatic fluid collections: percutaneous catheter drainage. Radiology 167: 435–441
Hill H C, Dach J L, Barkin J, Isikoff, M G, Morse B 1983 The role of percutaneous aspiration in the diagnosis of pancreatic abscess. American Journal of Roentgenology 141: 1035–1038
Isikoff M B, Hill M C, Silverstein W, Barkin J 1981 The clinical significance of acute pancreatic haemorrhage. American Journal of Roentgenology 136: 679–684
Karlson K B, Martin E C, Fankichen E I et al 1982 Percutaneous drainage of pancreatic pseudocysts and abscesses. Radiology 142: 619–624
Kivisaari L, Somer K, Strandertskjold-Nordenstam C G et al 1984 A new method for the diagnosis of acute haemorrhagic-necrotizing pancreatitis using contrast enhanced CT. Gastrointestinal Radiology 9: 27–30
Leutmer P H, Stephens D H, Ward E M 1988 Chronic pancreatitis: reassessment by current CT. Radiology (in press)
Love L, Meyers M A, Churchill R J et al 1981 Computed tomography of extraperitoneal spaces. American Journal of Roentgenology 136: 781–789
Magnuson J E, Stephens D H 1988 CT demonstration of pancreatic atrophy following acute pancreatitis. Journal of Computer Assisted Tomography 12: 1050–1053
Mendez G Jr, Isikoff M B 1979 Significance of intrapancreatic gas demonstrated by CT: a review of nine cases. American Journal of Roentgenology 132: 59–62
Neff C C, Simeone J F, Wittenberg J, Mueller P R, Ferrucci J T Jr 1984 Inflammatory pancreatic masses. Radiology 150: 35–38
Parienty R A, Pradel J, Pickard J-D et al 1981 Visibility and thickening of the renal fascia on computed tomograms. Radiology 139: 119–124
Raptopoulos V, Kleinman P K, Marks S Jr, Snyder M, Silverman P M 1986 Renal fascial pathways: posterior extension of pancreatic effusion within the anterior pararenal space. Radiology 158: 367–374
Sarner M, Cotton P B 1984 Classification of pancreatitis. Gut 25: 756–759
Schuman W P, Carter S J, Montana M A, Mack L A, Moss A A 1986 Pancreatic insufficiency: role of CT evaluation. Radiology 158: 625–627
Siegelman S S, Copeland B E, Saba G P, Camerson J L, Sanders R C, Zerhouni E A 1980 CT of fluid collections associated with pancreatitis. American Journal of Roentgenology 134: 1121–1132
Singer M, Gyr K, Sarles H 1985 Revised classification of pancreatitis. Gastroenterology 89: 683–690
Sostre C F, Flournoy J G, Bova J G, Goldstein H M, Schenker S 1985 Pancreatic phlegmon: clinical features and course. Digestive Disease Science 30: 918–927
Torres W E, Clements J L Jr, Sones P J, Knopf D R 1981 Gas in the pancreatic bed without abscess. American Journal of Roentgenology 137: 1131–1133
Torres W E, Evert M B, Baumgarter B R, Bernardino M E 1986 Percutaneous aspiration and drainage of pancreatic pseudocysts. American Journal of Roentgenology 147: 1007–1009
Van Sonnenberg E, Wittich G R, Casola G et al 1985 Complicated pancreatic inflammatory disease: diagnostic and therapeutic role of interventional radiology. Radiology 155: 335–340
Vernacchia F S, Jeffrey R B Jr, Federle M P et al 1987 Pancreatic abscess: predictive value of early abdominal CT. Radiology 162: 435–438
Warshaw A L 1974 Inflammatory masses following acute pancreatitis. Surgical Clinics of North America 54: 621–636
White E M, Wittenberg J, Mueller P R et al 1986 Pancreatic necrosis: CT manifestations. Radiology 158: 343–346
Williford M E, Foster W L Jr, Halvorsen R A, Thompson W M 1983 Pancreatic pseudocyst: comparative evaluation by sonography and computed tomography. American Journal of Roentgenology 140: 53–57

9. Detection of liver metastases

Jay P. Heiken

INTRODUCTION

Assessment of the liver for metastases is a critical part of the clinical evaluation of cancer patients, since the liver is second only to regional lymph nodes as a site of metastatic disease (Gilbert & Kagan 1976). Recently, imaging evaluation of the liver has taken on even greater importance with the increasing use of aggressive therapeutic regimens for metastatic disease, such as hepatic artery chemotherapy infusion, tumour embolization and surgical resection. It is, therefore, becoming increasingly important not only to identify patients who have hepatic metastases but to determine the exact number of lesions present and to define precisely their location within the hepatic parenchyma.

IMAGING TECHNIQUES

A variety of imaging techniques for evaluating the liver are currently available. For many years, radionuclide scintigraphy was the standard method for detecting hepatic abnormalities. Although its reported accuracy is reasonably high (80–95%) (Snow et al 1979, Knopf et al 1982, Alderson et al 1983), it has a number of limitations including inferior spatial resolution and inability to detect small (<2 cm) lesions located deep within the liver parenchyma. Despite the introduction of single photon emission computed tomography (SPECT) which should improve the ability of scintigraphy to detect deeply seated lesions, several other shortcomings are apparent:

1. Scintigraphy is unable to detect abnormalities outside the liver.
2. Lesions that are detected cannot be accurately localized because vascular anatomy is not visualized on hepatic scintigrams.
3. Liver lesions are difficult to detect in patients with hepatic dysfunction because activity is shifted to the spleen.
4. Scintigraphy is unable to differentiate between benign and malignant masses.
5. Variations in hepatic anatomy cause false positive diagnoses.

Although scintigraphy has the advantage of relatively low cost, additional studies are often required to confirm, further characterize or localize a suspected hepatic mass.

Ultrasonography provides higher spatial resolution for detecting hepatic lesions and is able to differentiate between cysts and solid masses. In addition, it allows accurate localization of lesions and provides information about structures outside the liver. However, the quality of an ultrasound examination is dependent on the technical skill of the ultrasonographer and on the patient's body habitus. Ultrasound evaluation of the liver is frequently suboptimal in obese patients and may be impaired by extensive bowel gas or by surgical scars or dressing. In addition, comparative studies have shown that ultrasound has a lower sensitivity and specificity for detecting hepatic metastases than CT (Snow et al 1979, Alderson et al 1983).

Like ultrasound, CT allows precise localization of lesions and provides information about structures outside the liver but it has the advantage of being more reproducible (not operator dependent). In addition, CT image quality is not impaired by obesity, bowel gas, surgical scars or appliances on the patient's body. Furthermore, CT is better able to differentiate between malignant neoplasms and benign cavernous haemangiomas.

Interpretation of studies comparing the accuracy of hepatic scintigraphy, ultrasonography and CT for detecting hepatic metastases (Snow et al 1979, Knopf et al 1982, Alderson et al 1983) is problematic for several reasons. During the years over which the studies were being performed, significant technological advances took place which improved the capabilities of all three imaging techniques. In the studies that included CT, a variety of imaging techniques were used, ranging from no use of intravenous contrast material to contrast-enhanced scanning achieved by drip infusion, bolus injection or bolus injection followed by drip infusion; the timing of scanning after administration of the intravenous contrast material varied from study to study (partly due to varying capabilities of the CT scanning equipment).

Although scintigraphy, ultrasonography and CT each have their proponents, the cumulative data support CT as the best overall screening test for hepatic metastases (Snow et al 1979, Knofp et al 1982, Alderson et al 1983). In a prospective, controlled multi-institutional study comparing hepatic scintigraphy, ultrasound and CT in patients with colon and breast carcinoma, Alderson et al (1983) concluded that CT provided the most accurate means for detecting liver metastases from both primary lesions.

COMPUTED TOMOGRAPHY

On non-contrast-enhanced CT scans, metastases are generally lower in attenuation than the liver parenchyma. An exception to this general rule occurs in patients with fatty infiltration of the liver in whom metastases may appear isodense or hyperdense due to the overall decrease in density of the liver. Calcified metastases also may occasionally appear isodense or hyperdense.

The objective of intravenous contrast material enhancement is to increase the difference in attenuation between the liver parenchyma and the lesions. Studies have shown that to maximize this effect, the contrast material should be administered as a bolus rather than as a drip infusion and the liver should be completely imaged within 3–4 minutes after the injection is started (Burgener & Hamlin 1983, Foley et al 1983). These data are based on the observation that the peak attenuation of the liver occurs between 1 and 4 minutes after the start of the bolus (Foley et al 1983). The initiation of scanning can be delayed 30–45 seconds after the start of the bolus to allow time for the hepatic parenchymal enhancement to approach its peak.

Approximately 50% of metastases show some degree of enhancement (peripheral, central or mixed) after administration of intravenous contrast material (Freeny & Marks 1986a). However, all but very vascular metastases increase in attenuation to a lesser degree than the normal hepatic parenchyma, thus increasing the difference in attenuation between metastases and normal liver. This differential enhancement occurs because the metastases are fed by branches of the hepatic artery, whereas the liver parenchyma receives approximately 75% of its blood supply from the portal vein which contributes no blood supply to the metastases. After intravenous injection, the contrast material rapidly moves from the intravascular to the interstitial space and within 3–4 minutes an equilibrium is reached. During the equilibrium phase metastases may become isodense with the liver parenchyma due to the interstitial accumulation of contrast material within the lesions at the same time that the intravascular concentration within the liver parenchyma is decreasing (Burgener & Hamlin 1983).

Before the availability of CT scanners that could image the liver completely within four minutes, investigators advocated the use of both pre-contrast and post-contrast-enhanced examinations in all patients to avoid missing lesions that became isodense with the liver parenchyma during the equilibrium phase (Berland et al 1982, Burgener & Hamlin 1983). However, because most CT scanners are now capable of imaging the entire liver before the equilibrium phase is reached, the usefulness of pre-contrast scans is limited. Nevertheless, non-contrast-enhanced scans may be helpful for detecting liver metastases from hypervascular tumours, such as carcinoids, pancreatic islet-cell tumours, renal-cell carcinomas and phaeochromocytomas.

CT screening techniques

The following contrast-enhancement techniques are used for detecting hepatic metastases.

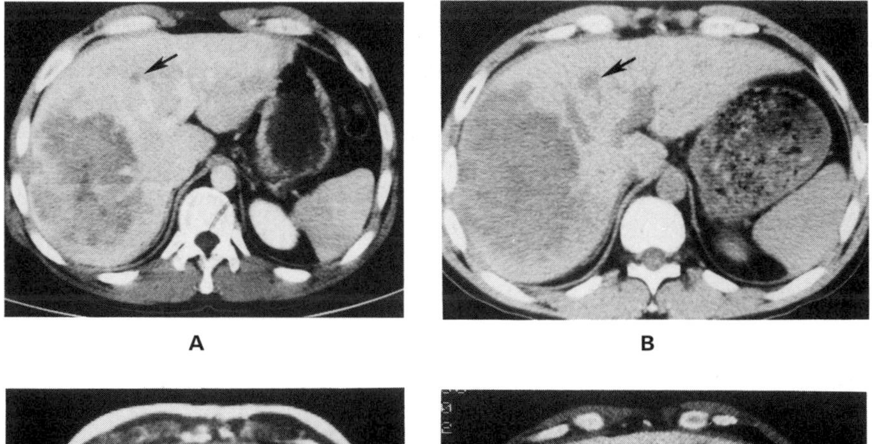

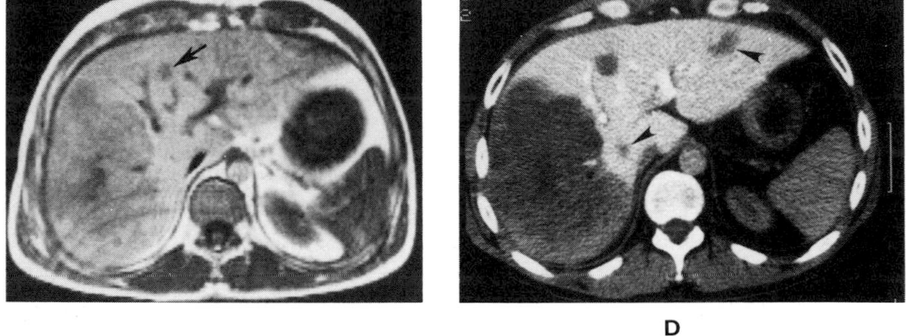

Fig. 9.1 Hepatoma with satellite metastases. **A** Dynamic intravenous contrast-enhanced CT image. **B** Delayed iodine CT (DICT) image. **C** T1 weighted spin echo MR image (TR 300 ms/TE 15 ms). All three studies show a small mass (arrow) in the medial segment of the left lobe in addition to a large mass in the right lobe. Note that both masses appear smaller on the dynamic intravenous contrast-enhanced scan (**A**) due to peripheral enhancement. **D** CT scan at the same level as **A**, **B** and **C** during arterial portography demonstrates two additional masses (arrowheads) not shown on the other studies.

Incremental dynamic contrast-enhanced CT

Fifty to 150 ml of 60% iodinated contrast material is injected as a bolus. After a 30–45 second delay, rapid incremental scanning is performed using contiguous 1-cm sections (Fig. 9.1a). The entire liver should be scanned within 3–4 minutes. This is the most useful routine method of hepatic screening by CT.

Delayed high-dose iodine CT (DICT)

The liver is scanned 4–6 hours after the administration of 60 grams of intravenous or intra-arterial iodine (Bernardino et al 1986). This type of imaging is based on the fact that the liver normally excretes 1–2% of the iodine load. This process produces a 20 HU increase in the attenuation of the normal hepatic parenchyma. Hepatic tumours appear as low-density defects because they do not excrete any iodine (Fig. 9.1b). DICT provides a more accurate assessment of tumour size than incremental dynamic contrast-enhanced CT, because with the delayed technique, there is no enhancement of the periphery of the neoplasm (Fig. 9.1a, b).

Two potential limitations of DICT are that small lesions may be difficult to differentiate from hepatic vessels and benign cavernous haemangiomas cannot be differentiated from malignant lesions. Review of the DICT scans in conjunction with the corresponding dynamic contrast-enhanced CT scans helps to avoid these potential pitfalls.

Hepatic specific contrast-enhanced CT

A number of liver-specific contrast agents including liposomes, iodinated starch particles and oily emulsions have been studied. These agents are either phagocytosed by the reticulo-endothelial system or taken up by the hepatocytes. They increase the density of the liver because they contain iodine. Consequently, focal hepatic masses appear as low-density defects since they do not accumulate the contrast material. The most widely studied liver-specific contrast agent is EOE-13 (ethiodized oil emulsion 13) which is an iodinated ester of poppyseed oil in an emulsified form (Miller et al 1984, Sugarbaker et al 1984). After intravenous injection of EOE-13, attenuation of the liver increases by a mean of 32.5 HU and the spleen by 52.3 HU, whereas tumours show a negligible increase in attenuation (Miller et al 1984).

CT using EOE-13 is highly sensitive for the detection of hepatic metastases (Sugarbaker et al 1984). However, because of the high incidence of side effects, such as fever and chills, after its use (Miller et al 1984), EOE-13 has remained an experimental agent.

Computed tomographic arteriography (CTA)

Computed tomographic arteriography is usually performed after coeliac and/or superior mesenteric artery (SMA) angiography has been performed. With the angiographic catheter secured in the hepatic artery, coeliac axis or SMA, the patient is transferred to the CT scanner. Iodinated contrast material is infused slowly through the catheter during rapid incremental CT scanning of the liver (Freeny & Marks 1983, Matsui et al 1983).

When CTA is performed with the catheter in the hepatic artery or coeliac axis, 30% contrast material is infused at a rate of 0.5–1.0 ml/second. Alternatively, the same effect can be achieved by hand injection of 10–12 ml of contrast material during each scan. The less dense (30%) contrast material is preferred to avoid beam-hardening artefacts that can occur when 60% iodinated contrast material is used. On CTA images obtained with this technique, hepatic metastases appear as peripherally-enhancing

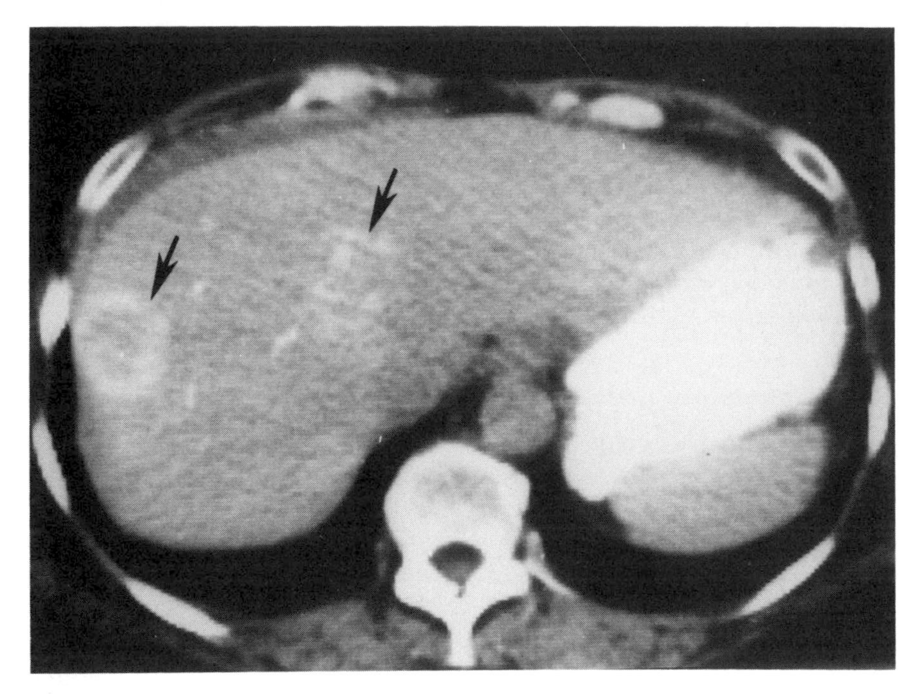

Fig. 9.2 Metastatic carcinoid tumour. A CTA image obtained during slow infusion of 30% iodinated contrast material through the hepatic artery demonstrates two peripherally-enhancing lesions (arrows).

hyperdense masses compared to the normal hepatic parenchyma (Fig. 9.2). This technique has been shown to be significantly more sensitive for detecting liver metastases than CT performed with intravenous injection of contrast material (Freeny & Marks 1983). A potential pitfall of this method is that homogeneous enhancement of the normal hepatic parenchyma is obtained in only about two-thirds of patients due to a variety of causes including replaced hepatic arteries and altered hepatic haemodynamics (Freeny & Marks 1986b).

Computed tomographic arterial portography (CTAP)

Computed tomographic arterial portography performed during infusion of contrast material through a catheter in the superior mesenteric artery (SMA), more consistently produces homogeneous enhancement of the normal hepatic parenchyma (Matsui et al 1983, Heiken et al in press). However, perfusion abnormalities can also occur with this technique and may be responsible for false positive diagnoses (Miller et al 1987). For CTAP approximately 100 ml of 60% iodinated contrast material is infused through the SMA catheter at a rate of 0.5 ml/second. CT scans are initiated

20 seconds after the start of the infusion and obtained in a rapid incremental fashion.

On CTAP images, hepatic metastases appear as low attenuation masses because they have an arterial blood supply, whereas the normal hepatic parenchyma is supplied predominantly by the portal venous system (Fig. 9.1d). After the dynamic phase scans have been obtained, rescanning the

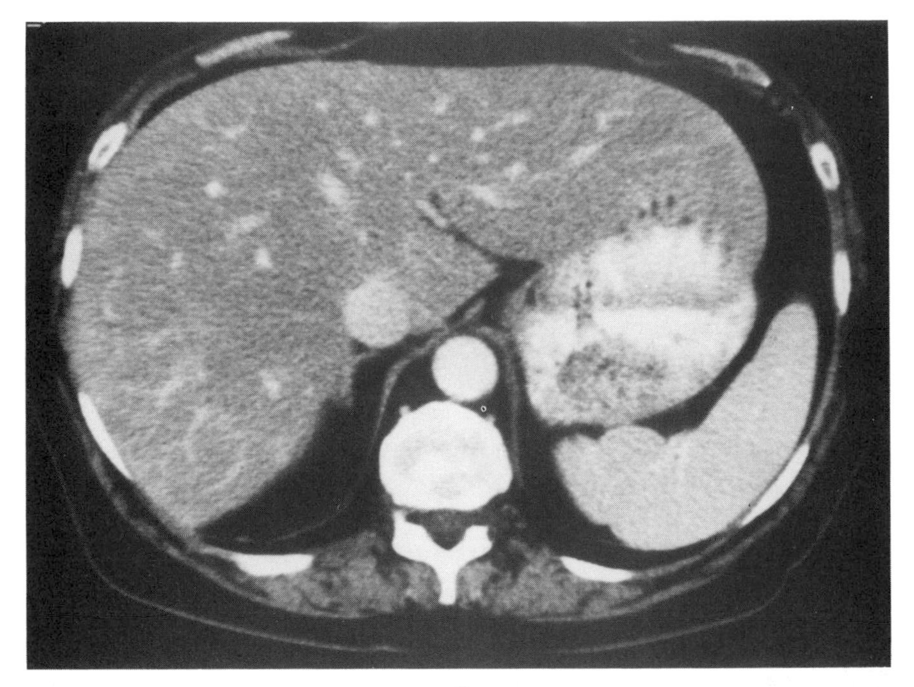

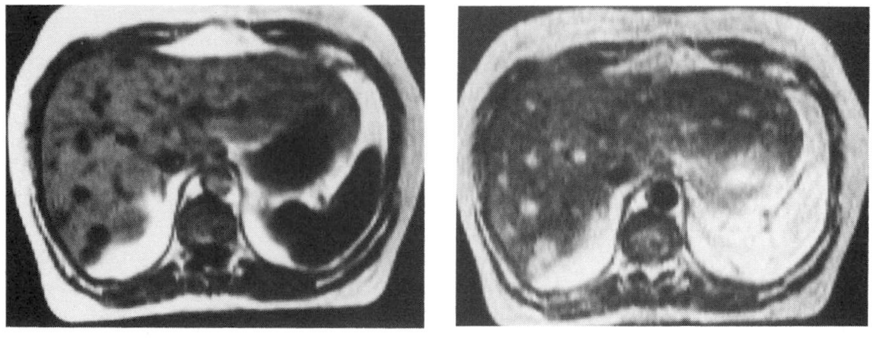
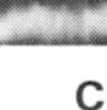

Fig. 9.3 Metastatic small-cell carcinoma of the lung. **A** A dynamic intravenous contrast-enhanced CT scan shows minimal inhomogeneity of the hepatic parenchyma but no discrete metastatic lesions. **B** T1 weighted spin echo MR image (TR 300 ms/TE 15 ms). **C** T2 weighted spin echo MR image (TR 3000 ms/TE 90 ms). The MR images demonstrate multiple discrete hepatic metastases.

liver during the equilibrium phase of contrast enhancement helps to avoid misdiagnoses caused by abnormalities of hepatic perfusion. CTAP, like CTA with hepatic artery infusion, is a highly sensitive technique for detecting liver metastases. It is markedly superior to CT obtained after intravenous contrast material administration for detecting lesions >2 cm (Matsui et al 1987, Heiken et al in press). However, since CTA is an invasive procedure it is not used as a routine hepatic screening examination. Nevertheless, it is an excellent technique for the preoperative evaluation of selected patients with liver metastases who are being considered for hepatic resection.

MAGNETIC RESONANCE (MR) IMAGING

MR imaging combines the advantages of CT, such as high spatial resolution and ability to precisely localize lesions, with superior intrinsic tissue contrast. In two recent comparative studies, MR imaging at intermediate field strength (0.3–0.6 Tesla) was found to be superior to contrast-enhanced CT for detecting hepatic metastases (95.4% versus 87.1%) (Reinig et al 1987) and 64% versus 51% (Stark et al 1987). In a third study, MR imaging and CT were reported to be equivalent with MR imaging having a sensitivity of 96% and CT 93% (Chezmar et al 1988). Despite the fact that another study reported MR imaging to be less useful than CT (Glazer et al 1986), it appears that state-of-the-art MR imaging is at least as sensitive and probably slightly more sensitive than intravenous contrast-enhanced CT for the detection of hepatic metastases (Fig. 9.3). However, MR imaging is not as sensitive as CT for detecting extrahepatic disease (Stark et al 1987, Chezmar et al 1988). Thus, CT remains a better overall screening examination of cancer patients.

CONCLUSION

Ultrasound and CT are the most frequently used screening techniques for the detection of liver metastases and of these contrast-enhanced CT is the most sensitive. Currently, the role of MR imaging versus CT in screening for hepatic metastases remains controversial. Relative cost, availability of equipment and examination time are important determinants of which test is used. Prospective comparative studies and additional clinical experience will be necessary to determine the ultimate place of MR imaging as a screening test for hepatic metastases. Intravenous contrast-enhancing agents for MR imaging, such as superparamagnetic iron oxide, show substantial potential for increasing even further the already high sensitivity of MR imaging (Stark et al 1988).

REFERENCES

Alderson P O, Adams D F, McNeil B J et al 1983 Computed tomography, ultrasound and scintigraphy of the liver in patients with colon or breast carcinoma: a prospective comparison. Radiology 149: 225–230

Berland L L, Lawson T L, Foley W D, Melrose B L, Chintapilli K N, Taylor A J 1982 Comparison of pre- and post-contrast CT in hepatic masses. American Journal of Roentgenology 138: 853–858

Bernardino M E, Erwin B C, Steinberg H V, Baumgartner B R, Torres W E, Gedgaudas-McClees R K 1986 Delayed hepatic CT scanning: increased confidence and improved detection of hepatic metastases. Radiology 159: 71–74

Burgener F A, Hamlin D J 1983 Contrast enhancement of hepatic tumours in CT: comparison between bolus and infusion techniques. American Journal of Roentgenology 140: 291–295

Chezmar J L, Rumancik W M, Megibow A J, Hulnick D H, Nelson R C, Bernardino M E 1988 Liver and abdominal screening in patients with cancer: CT versus MR imaging. Radiology 168: 43–47

Foley W D, Berland L L, Lawson T L, Smith D F, Thorsen M K 1983 Contrast enhancement technique for dynamic hepatic computed tomographic scanning. Radiology 147: 797–803

Freeny P C, Marks W M 1983 Computed tomographic arteriography of the liver. Radiology 148: 193–197

Freeny P C, Marks W M 1986a Patterns of contrast enhancement of benign and malignant hepatic neoplasms during bolus dynamic and delayed CT. Radiology 160: 613–618

Freeny P C, Marks W M 1986b Hepatic perfusion abnormalities during CT angiography: detection and interpretation. Radiology 159: 685–691

Gilbert H A, Kagan A R 1976 Metastases: incidence, detection and evaluation. In: Weiss L (ed) Fundamental aspects of metastases. Elsevier, New York

Glazer G M, Aisen A M, Francis I R, Gross B H, Gyves J W, Ensminger W D 1986 Evaluation of focal hepatic masses: a comparative study of MRI and CT. Gastrointestinal Radiology 11: 263–268

Heiken J P, Weyman P J, Lee J K T et al (in press) Detection of focal hepatic masses: prospective evaluation using CT, delayed CT, CT during arterial portography and MR. Radiology (in press)

Knopf D R, Torres W E, Fajman W J, Sones P J Jr 1982 Liver lesions: comparative accuracy of scintigraphy and computed tomography. American Journal of Roentgenology 138: 623–627

Matsui O, Kadoya M, Suzuki M et al 1983 Work in progress: dynamic sequential computed tomography during arterial portography in the detection of hepatic neoplasms. Radiology 146: 721–727

Matsui O, Takashima T, Kodoya M et al 1987 Liver metastases from colorectal cancers: detection with CT during arterial portography. Radiology 165: 65–69

Miller D L, Vermess M, Doppman J L et al 1984 CT of the liver and spleen with EOE-13: review of 225 examinations. American Journal of Roentgenology 143: 235–243

Miller D L, Simmons J T, Chang R et al 1987 Hepatic metastasis detection: comparison of three CT contrast enhancement methods. Radiology 165: 785-790

Reinig J W, Dwyer A J, Miller D L et al 1987 Liver metastasis detection: comparative sensitivities of MR imaging and CT scanning. Radiology 164: 43–47

Snow J H, Goldstein H M, Wallace S 1979 Comparison of scintigraphy, sonography and computed tomography in the evaluation of hepatic neoplasms. American Journal of Roentgenology 132: 915–918

Stark D D, Wittenberg J, Butch R J, Ferrucci J T Jr 1987 Hepatic metastases: randomised, controlled comparison of detection with MR imaging and CT. Radiology 165: 399–406

Stark D D, Weissleder R, Elizondo G et al 1988 Superparamagnetic iron oxide: clinical application as a contrast agent for MR imaging of the liver. Radiology 168: 297

Sugarbaker P H, Vermess M, Doppman J L, Miller D L, Simon R 1984 Improved detection of focal lesions with computerized tomographic examination of the liver using ethiodized oil emulsion (EOE-13) liver contrast. Cancer 54: 1489–1495

10. Focal benign liver disease*

David H. Stephens

INTRODUCTION

Benign, focal lesions of the liver comprise a diverse group of abnormalities. The vast majority of these abnormalities produce no ill effects but some benign hepatic lesions cause significant clinical disturbances and a small proportion lead to life-threatening complications. For the radiologist, the challenge is not only to distinguish potentially troublesome benign tumours from insignificant ones but also to differentiate malignant neoplasms from benign lesions.

FOCAL FATTY INFILTRATION

The excessive accumulation of fat in a focal or regional distribution within the liver has only recently been described (Brawer et al 1980) and the widespread use of abdominal CT is mainly responsible for the current awareness of the condition.

Focal fatty infiltration occurs in a variety of configurations, many of which are characteristic. Frequently the low density zones seen on CT extend to the surface of the liver and they are often fan-shaped or have an irregular 'geographic' configuration (Halversen et al 1982, Clain et al 1984) (Fig. 10.1). Occasionally fatty infiltration has a segmental or lobar distribution (Fig. 10.1). Unlike most space-occupying lesions of the liver, fatty infiltration usually does not disturb the vessels that pass through the zone of involvement.

Occasionally, the CT appearances are indistinguishable from those of a neoplasm. This is especially true when the process occurs in a nodular form (Yates & Streight 1986). In some cases percutaneous biopsy is the best approach but if a precise diagnosis is not of immediate consequence, a follow-up CT examination may be worthwhile, as fatty infiltration often undergoes rapid resolution or redistribution, especially when the

* Based on Stephens D H Benign masses of the Liver. In: Silverman P, Zeman R (eds) Computed Tomography and Magnetic Resonance Imaging of the Liver and Biliary System. Contemporary Issues in Computed Tomography. Churchill Livingstone, New York (in press).

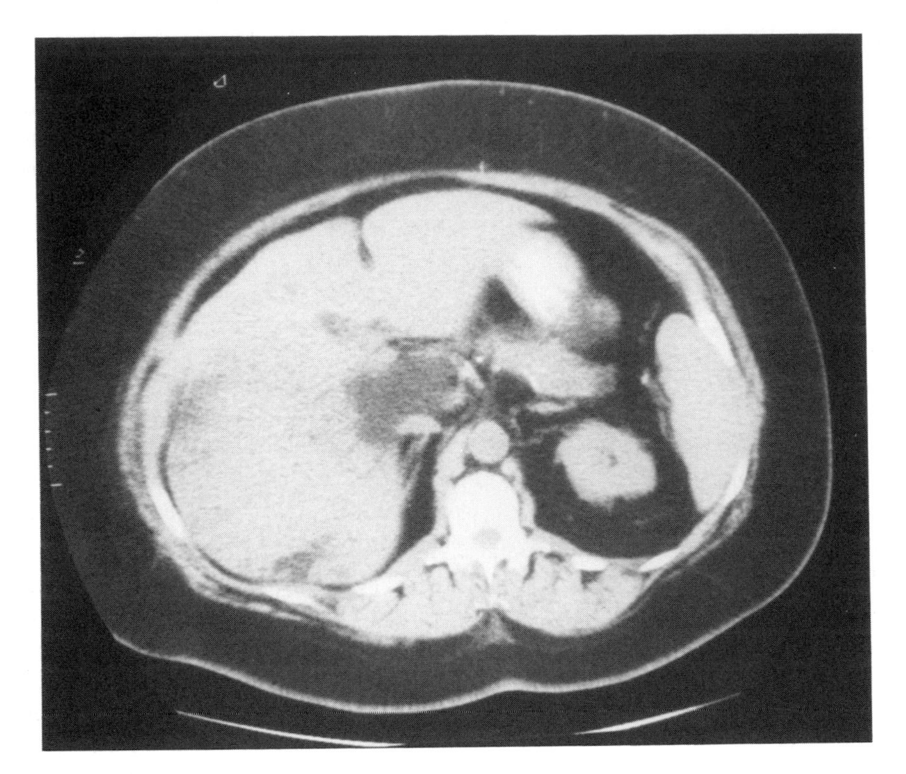

Fig. 10.1 Focal fatty infiltration in a diabetic patient. The involved zones are non-spherical and extend to the surface of the liver. The largest region of fatty infiltration involves the caudate lobe.

underlying metabolic disturbance is brought under control (Clain et al 1984).

CYSTS

Epithelial-lined simple cysts of the liver are thought to be congenital, probably of biliary derivation. They may occur as isolated lesions or, far less commonly, as components of polycystic disease.

CT features of individual cysts

The CT appearance of uncomplicated benign hepatic cysts is usually characteristic enough to permit a correct diagnosis without further investigation. The typical features of sharp definition, smooth margination, spherical shape and homogeneous composition, are accurately depicted and the density of fluid within a simple cyst is usually similar to that of water. The wall of a cyst is not seen unless the lesion abuts the capsule of the liver or the wall of another cyst. Cysts do not enhance with intravenous contrast medium.

Haemorrhage into a cyst can alter the CT density of the contents (Swensen et al 1984). If blood is distributed evenly within the cyst, the density of the lesion may be elevated uniformly but as a thrombus forms the density of a haemorrhagic cyst becomes heterogeneous, the clotted component having a higher density than the surrounding fluid.

A variety of cavitating lesions can mimic benign hepatic cysts but properly performed contrast-enhanced CT usually permits distinction. These lesions include cavitating malignant tumours, hydatid cysts and amoebic or pyogenic abscess.

Polycystic disease

Autosomal dominant polycystic disease is an inherited disorder that most often affects the kidneys but also frequently involves the liver and sometimes affects the pancreas. The cysts in a polycystic liver are subject to the same kinds of complications that affect solitary hepatic cysts and because there are more of them, these complications are more likely to occur (Levine et al 1985). Polycystic liver disease is almost always easy to recognize on CT. Typically, there are innumerable cysts of varied sizes distributed throughout the liver but sometimes only a portion of the liver is involved and, in some cases, the number of cysts is not so great. The coexistence of polycystic renal disease helps to establish the polycystic nature of hepatic cysts when liver involvement is not typical.

Cavernous haemangioma

Among the mixed benefits to result from the widespread application of sectional imaging of the liver is a vastly improved rate of detection of cavernous haemangiomas.

The imaging features that characterize a cavernous haemangioma are based on the distinctive structural morphology and haemodynamics of the lesion. Cavernous haemangiomas are composed mainly of enlarged blood-filled vascular spaces (sinusoids). Blood circulates slowly through the vascular spaces, tending to flow from the sinusoids at the periphery of the mass towards those at the centre. Although not encapsulated, cavernous haemangiomas are sharply defined and there are no reactive changes in the adjacent normal hepatic parenchyma. They may be single or multiple and vary greatly in size.

Many cavernous haemangiomas also contain non-vascular elements, usually in the form of fibrotic scar-like tissue. Foci of haemorrhage, thrombosis or calcification are less frequent components (Ros et al 1987). Awareness that a heterogeneous composition is not inconsistent with the diagnosis of cavernous haemangioma should clarify any misunderstanding regarding the criteria for diagnosis of this tumour (Ros et al 1987, Scatarige et al 1987).

A CT examination that is performed primarily to determine whether a lesion that is known to exist is a cavernous haemangioma should begin with a series of unenhanced scans at contiguous levels through the entire liver. Unenhanced scans not only indicate the best level or levels at which to conduct the contrast-enhanced examination but may also provide important clues as to the nature of the mass. The vascular components of cavernous haemangiomas on unenhanced scans are uniformly hypodense relative to normal liver because their attenuation values are comparable with those of normal blood vessels or the spleen, which is also of blood-vessel density on unenhanced scans. Since the density of hepatic parenchyma is usually greater than the density of intravascular blood, haemangiomas are usually hypodense relative to normal liver (Fig. 10.2a). However, if the density of hepatic parenchyma is at the lower limit of normal and therefore isodense with normal blood vessels, a cavernous haemangioma is also likely to be isodense with hepatic parenchyma. When fatty infiltration causes the density of the liver to be lower than the density of flowing blood, a cavernous haemangioma will appear hyperdense on unenhanced scans.

The fibrotic elements that are frequently present within cavernous haemangiomas are usually of lower density than the blood-filled portions of these tumours and appear as sharply defined hypodense structures within the tumours (Fig. 10.2a). These components may have nodular, linear, angular or stellate configurations. Calcification is rarely seen.

The most distinctive CT features of cavernous haemangiomas are depicted by the pattern of sequential opacification following a rapid bolus injection of intravenous contrast material. A series of scans at one or more predetermined levels of interest is obtained and our usual dose of contrast material is 150 ml of a 60% iodinated agent (42 g iodine). Timing of the scans after injection may be influenced by the size of the lesion, as complete enhancement usually occurs earlier in smaller tumours than in larger ones. Since circulation within cavernous haemangiomas is slow, scans made at intervals of 20–30 seconds are usually adequate early in the series. After the initial few scans, intervals can be determined according to the findings as they appear on the monitor.

Iodinated blood can often be seen in peripheral vascular spaces shortly after contrast material is delivered but sometimes there is a delay of a minute or more before opacification of the tumour is observed. Initial enhancement usually takes place at the outer margin of the tumour but always within its perimeter. The first clusters of sinusoids to become opacified may have the appearance of individual vascular lakes or puddles (Fig. 10.2b). As more spaces become filled with iodinated blood, the zones of opacification enlarge and coalesce. Opacification usually progresses in a centripetal fashion but sometimes it spreads from one side of the mass to the

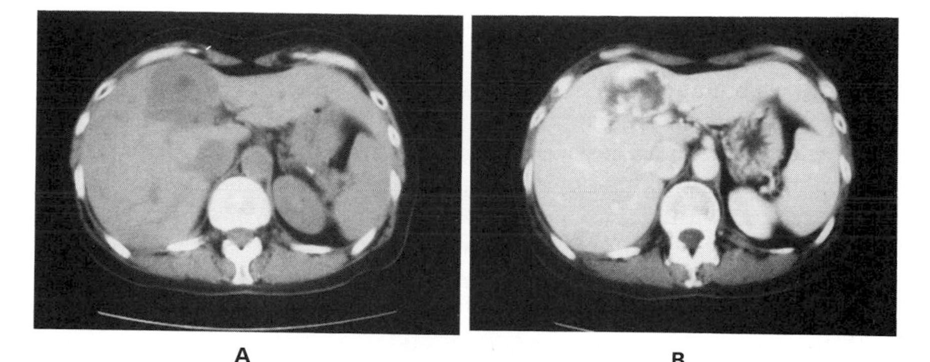

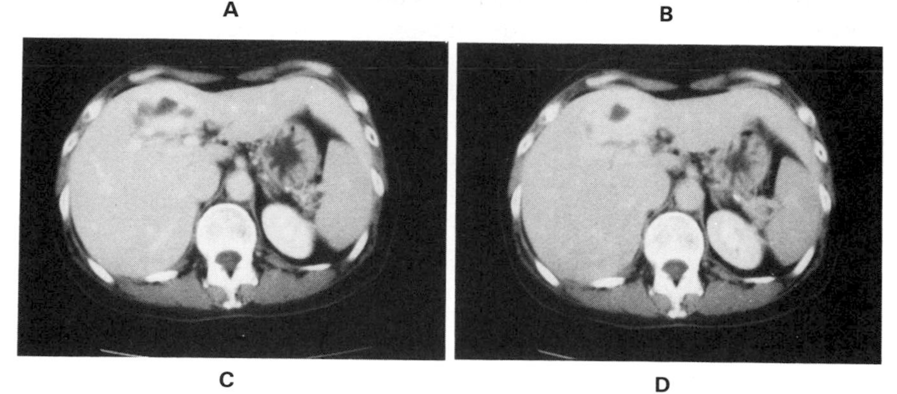

Fig. 10.2 Cavernous haemangioma. **A** Unenhanced scan showing a mass in the medial segment of the left hepatic lobe. Except for a small central hypodense component, the tumour is of the same density as normal blood vessels. **B, C** and **D** Scans taken after contrast enhancement show progressive opacification of the tumour with enhanced portions of the mass of similar density to normal blood vessels on the same scan. The central fibrous component remains unenhanced even on the final scan **D**. Slight biliary ductal dilatations along the posterior margin of the haemangioma are due to partial ductal obstruction at the porta hepatis.

other, and occasionally opacification is displayed first within the interior of the lesion. Eventually all of the vascular spaces become filled with iodinated blood. Even in small tumours this process usually requires at least three minutes (Ashida et al 1987).

The intensity of opacification that occurs within vascular spaces of a cavernous haemangioma varies according to the concentration of iodine within the blood stream. On any scan in the series, the density of the enhanced vascular spaces approximates to the density of the normal vessels on the same scan (Fig. 10.2b, c and d). Although complete enhancement has been suggested as a necessary criterion for the diagnosis of cavernous haemangiomas by CT (Freeney & Marks 1986), the presence of one or more well-defined, low-density, homogeneous, unenhancing components should not preclude the diagnosis because they represent fibrotic components.

Other types of well-vascularized tumours, especially hypervascular metastases, can become hyperdense during early phases of contrast enhancement. However, unlike haemangiomas, these metastases become hyperdense suddenly during the arterial phase of enhancement but their density fades more rapidly than the density of normal vessels during subsequent phases. Occasionally, malignant tumours may undergo a spreading type of enhancement similar to that of haemangiomas but not with the same degree of density as that which typifies a cavernous haemangioma. One feature of some enhancing neoplasms that is not seen with cavernous haemangiomas is a circumferential hypodense zone outside the perimeter of the tumour.

There remains a small but significant minority of tumours that cannot be classified with confidence as either haemangiomatous or non-haemangiomatous by CT. A technically adequate scan is not always possible, for example, when the use of intravenous contrast material may be inadvisable. Very small tumours may be difficult to scan repeatedly because of inconsistencies in depth of respiration. Multiplicity of lesions can also present a problem, although it is usually possible to obtain an adequate study of more than one tumour by scanning at alternative levels after injection of contrast material. There are also cases in which the tumours themselves do not have features sufficiently characteristic to permit a confident diagnosis of cavernous haemangioma. Occasionally so much of the tumour is occupied by fibrotic tissue that the vascular portion is not conspicuous. In other cases the circulatory characteristics of a cavernous haemangioma may be atypical, in which case the pattern of progressive enhancement will also be atypical (Mikulis et al 1985).

FOCAL NODULAR HYPERPLASIA

Focal nodular hyperplasia is an uncommon tumour of the liver. It occurs most often in young women but is not restricted to people of that age group or sex. According to prevailing opinion, any relationship between the use of oral contraceptives and the development of focal nodular hyperplasia is probably coincidental rather than causal (Kerlin et al 1983).

Focal nodular hyperplasia usually produces no symptoms, though larger masses occasionally cause discomfort as a result of space-occupying effects. Most tumours discovered during life are found incidentally by hepatic imaging or at laparotomy. If left undisturbed, focal nodular hyperplasia practically never causes serious trouble, has no malignant potential and there have been no documented deaths associated with its natural history.

Focal nodular hyperplasia usually occurs as a solitary mass but multiple tumours are present in about 20% of cases (Wanless et al 1985). The condition can occur anywhere in the liver but there is a predilection for subcapsular locations. Tumours arising near the surface of the liver often bulge the contour of the organ and some even become pedunculated. Internally, focal nodular hyperplasia is usually divided into lobules by

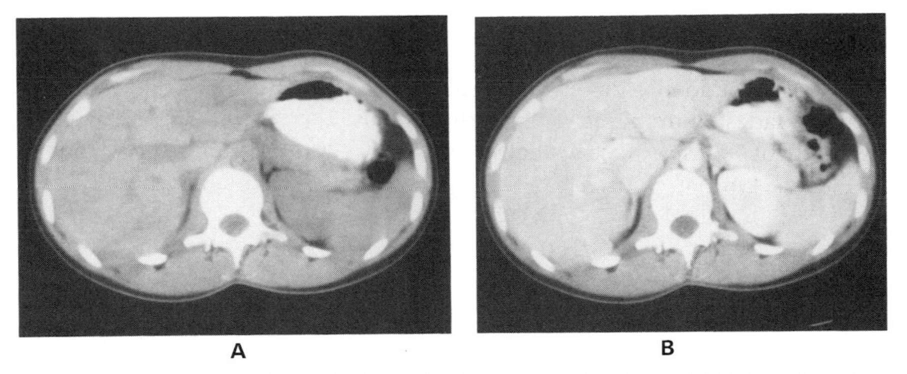

Fig. 10.3 Focal nodular hyperplasia. **A** Unenhanced scan showing a slightly hypodense mass in the left hepatic lobe. Centrally there is a low density scar. **B** With contrast enhancement the tumour, except for the central fibrous scar, becomes uniformly hyperdense. Unlike the cavernous haemangioma in Figure 2, the enhanced focal nodular hyperplasia is not quite as dense as the normal portal veins on the enhanced scan and the enhancement did not occur in a gradual, progressive fashion.

fibrous bands that often radiate in 'spoke-like' fashion from a central or eccentric fibrous scar. Within the fibrous scar and septa there are vascular channels and proliferating bile ducts. The parenchymal lobules contain normal constituents of the liver: hepatocytes, Kupffer cells, blood vessels and bile ducts. The architectural arrangement of these elements, however, is notably abnormal (Wanless et al 1985).

CT findings in focal nodular hyperplasia often lack specificity but in many cases they are characteristic enough to provide a strong indication of the tumour's histological type (Mathieu et al 1986). Except for their fibrous tissue components, these solid masses are of homogeneous soft-tissue density, usually slightly less than that of normal liver on unenhanced scans (Fig. 10.3a). Tumours that project beyond the normal contour of the liver may be evident as protuberant masses even when they are isodense with normal parenchyma. Fibrous bands, and more often a central scar, may be recognized as structures of relatively low density within some of these tumours (Fig. 10.3a). The central scar typically has a stellate configuration. It is not a consistent CT finding in focal nodular hyperplasia but its presence in a solid-appearing hepatic tumour should indicate the likelihood of that diagnosis.

Since focal nodular hyperplasia is well vascularized, it often undergoes an appreciable degree of enhancement with intravenous contrast material. Enhancement is greatest on scans made during the early phases and at this time a hypervascular tumour may become hyperdense relative to normal liver (Fig. 10.3b). Subsequently such a tumour may become isodense with normal liver and later hypodense. A tumour that is not so highly vascularized may remain hypodense relative to normal parenchyma at all stages of enhancement. The internal fibrotic components usually undergo less enhancement than the parenchymal lobules of the tumour (Fig. 10.3b).

Even though sectional imaging or angiography may provide findings highly indicative of focal nodular hyperplasia, many of these features overlap those occasionally found in hepatic neoplasms, such as a fibrolamellar type of hepatocellular carcinoma. This type of hepatocellular carcinoma often contains stellate collagenous scars (Freidman et al 1985). Hepatic-cell adenoma is another lesion which may be difficult to distinguish from focal nodular hyperplasia.

Focal nodular hyperplasia is perhaps the only type of hepatic tumour in which ^{99m}Tc-sulphur colloid scintigraphy can often provide definite diagnostic information. Unlike other space-occupying lesions of the liver, focal nodular hyperplasia often contains functioning Kupffer cells in sufficient concentration to exhibit normal or increased uptake on sulphur colloid scans. When a zone of normal to increased radionuclide activity correlates in location with that of a demonstrated hepatic mass, the finding is virtually diagnostic of focal nodular hyperplasia (Sandler et al 1980, Welch et al 1985).

HEPATIC-CELL ADENOMAS

Hepatic-cell adenomas are also relatively uncommon. They occur mainly but not exclusively in women of child-bearing age. Most women who develop hepatic adenomas have used contraceptive hormones, and there is strong evidence to implicate oral contraceptives as a major cause of these tumours (Klatskin et al 1977, Kerlin et al 1983). Anabolic steroids have also been implicated and a significant proportion of men who develop hepatic adenomas have received these hormones. Hepatic adenomas may also be associated with glycogen storage disease, in which case the tumours are often multiple and frequently occur in childhood (Doppman et al 1984).

The principal clinical significance of hepatic-cell adenomas is related to their tendency to haemorrhage. For this reason, hepatic-cell adenomas are generally regarded as tumours which should be resected. The rare existence of hepatocellular carcinoma within an adenoma suggests that malignant transformation is also possible (Kerlin et al 1983).

Hepatic-cell adenomas are well circumscribed, often encapsulated and usually solitary. Uncomplicated adenomas consist mostly of normal or slightly atypical hepatocytes (Kerlin et al 1983). They also contain blood vessels, Kupffer cells and internal deposits of fat may be present (Mathieu et al 1986, Lubbers et al 1987). Bile ducts are notably absent. The composition of these tumours is frequently altered by haemorrhage, in which case haematoma or clot may be a major component.

The appearance of an adenoma of the liver is influenced mainly by whether or not haemorrhage has occurred. On CT, solid adenomas usually have a density slightly less than that of normal liver (Welch et al 1985, Mathieu et al 1986) (Fig. 10.4a). Since the composition of an uncomplicated adenoma is similar to that of normal hepatic parenchyma,

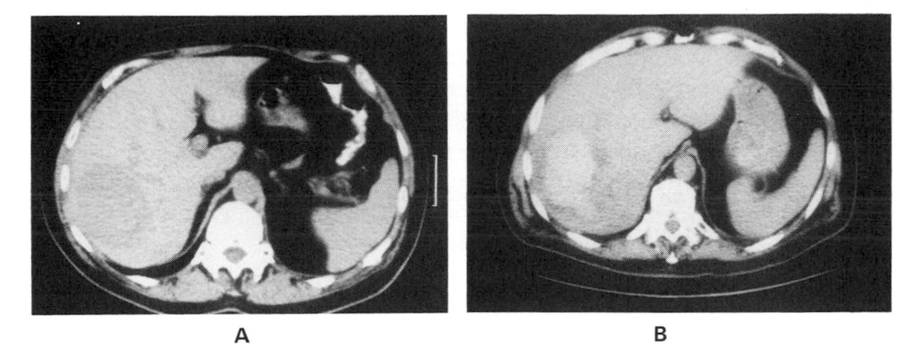

Fig. 10.4 Hepatic-cell adenoma before and after haemorrhage. **A** Scan taken before haemorrhage shows a solid-appearing hypodense mass. **B** Unenhanced scan taken at a later date after onset of acute upper abdominal pain, shows material of increased density occupying most of the mass. At resection the adenoma was largely occupied by haematoma. (Reproduced by kind permission of Churchill Livingstone, New York.)

some of these tumours are nearly isodense with adjacent parenchyma. Adenomas occurring in patients with glycogen storage disease may appear relatively hyperdense if the hepatic parenchyma is diffusely infiltrated with fat. If a deposit of fat is present in the tumour, the CT image of an adenoma may contain a corresponding radiolucent focus (Mathieu et al 1986). Rarely, an adenoma may have a central necrotic region that could resemble the fibrous scar sometimes seen in focal nodular hyperplasia or hepatocellular carcinoma. The response of a solid adenoma to intravenously administered contrast material is variable and generally non-specific. In a well-vascularized adenoma there may be transient hyperdensity or isodensity during the early phase of vascular enhancement. In other cases the tumours remain hypodense relative to normal liver at all stages of enhancement.

The presence of extravasated blood within an adenoma significantly alters the CT appearance of the lesion. A scan taken during or shortly after haemorrhage will typically show an area of homogeneously increased density within the mass (Fig. 10.4b). After the haematoma begins to organize, however, a scan will usually show the tumour to be of heterogeneous density with a hyperdense component that represents coagulating blood surrounded by hypodense components representing serous fluid or tumour tissue. Much later, a residual chronic haematoma or seroma may resemble a cyst.

BILIARY CYSTADENOMAS

Cystadenomas may arise from either intrahepatic or extrahepatic bile ducts but most of these rare cystic tumours are situated within the liver. Most biliary cystadenomas reported to date have been in women over the age of thirty but their occurrence is not limited to that age group or sex (Stanley et al 1983, Korobkin et al 1988). Upper abdominal pain, abdominal swelling and a palpable mass are among the common clinical presentations. Malignant transformation resulting in the development of a biliary cystadenocarcinoma is considered to be the major potential complication of these tumours. For that reason and because it is usually impossible to distinguish a benign cystadenoma from a cystadenocarcinoma on the basis of macroscopic features (Stanley et al 1983), complete surgical excision is the treatment of choice (Korobkin et al 1988).

The typical CT appearance of a biliary cystadenoma is that of a large, sharply-defined, fluid-filled mass with or without visible internal septations, mural nodules or papillary projections (Stanley et al 1983, Korobkin et al 1988). Calcification has been observed uncommonly in the walls or septa. The internal architecture is sometimes displayed better by ultrasound than by CT.

Differential diagnostic considerations include other types of cystic hepatic masses, especially simple cysts, echinococcal cysts and amoebic or pyogenic abscesses. The appearance of the lesion together with relevant clinical and laboratory information, can usually reduce the number of likely diagnostic possibilities.

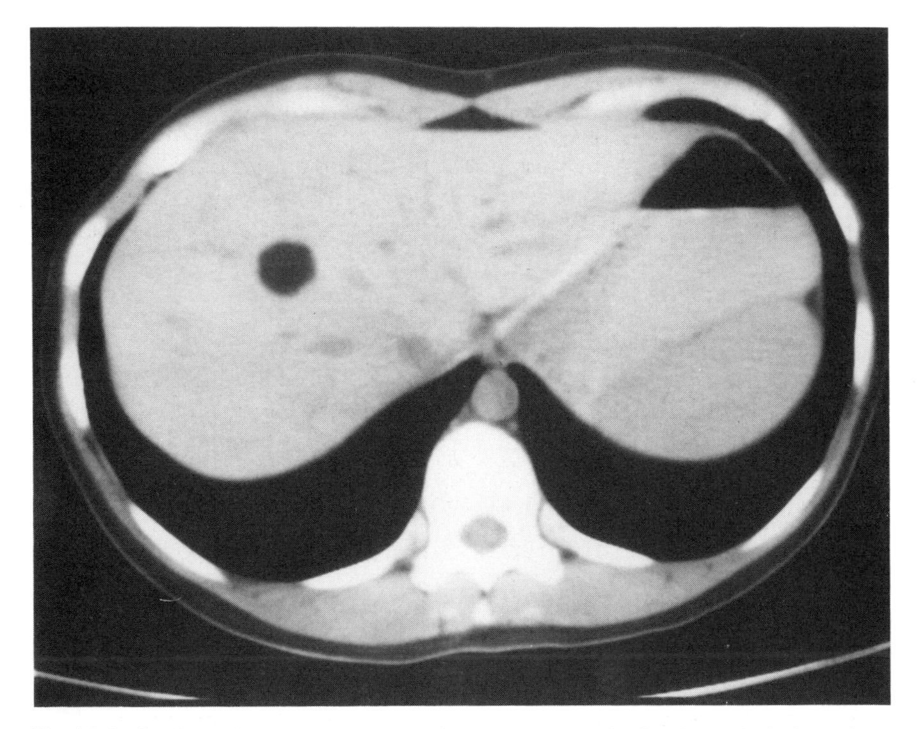

Fig. 10.5 Angiomyolipoma in a patient with tuberous sclerosis. CT shows the lesion to have the radiolucency of fat.
(Reproduced by kind permission of Churchill Livingstone, New York.)

LIPOMA AND ANGIOMYOLIPOMA

Benign lipomatous tumours of the liver occur either as pure lipomas or as angiomyolipomas. Either type of tumour may occur in the liver as an isolated lesion but angiomyolipomas may also be found in patients who have tuberous sclerosis (Roberts et al 1986).

Benign lipomatous tumours are distinctly uncommon in the liver. Of the small number reported thus far, all but a very few have been little asymptomatic lesions discovered incidentally by ultrasound or CT (Roberts et al 1986, Brunneton et al 1987). They are discrete lesions, typically round or oval in shape. Most angiomyolipomas have similar features (Fig. 10.5). Despite the rarity of these tumours in the liver, there is hardly any other isolated lesion that could have the same CT appearance. Hepatocellular carcinomas (Itai et al 1987) and hepatic adenomas (Mathieu et al 1986) have been reported to contain foci of fat but in these tumours non-fatty components of the masses should predominate. A tiny lipoma could easily be mistaken for a simple cyst on CT if volume averaging caused the density of the mass to appear falsely high, but such a misdiagnosis would have no ill effects on the patient.

CONCLUSION

Benign space-occupying lesions of the liver, once considered rare, are encountered frequently in modern diagnostic radiology. A small proportion of these masses are potentially harmful. Many more of them are troublesome to those who strive to determine their nature but a thorough knowledge of the natural history of these lesions and their characteristic appearances on CT should be of considerable help in making the correct diagnosis.

REFERENCES

Ashida C, Fishman E K, Zerhouni E A, Herlong F H, Siegelman S 1987 Computed tomography of hepatic cavernous haemangiomas. Journal of Computer Assisted Tomography 11: 455–460

Brawer M K, Austin G E, Lewin K J 1980 Focal fatty change of the liver a hitherto poorly recognised entity. Gastroenterology 78: 247–252

Brunneton J-N, Kerbou P, Drouillard J et al 1987 Hepatic lipomas: ultrasound and computed tomographic findings. Gastrointestinal Radiology 12: 299–303

Clain J E, Stephens D H, Charboneau J W 1984 Ultrasonography and computed tomography in focal fatty liver: report of two cases with special emphasis on changing appearances over time. Gastroenterology 87: 948–952

Doppman J L, Cornblath M, Dwyer A J et al 1984 Computed tomography of the liver and kidneys in the glycogen storage disease. Journal of Computer Assisted Tomography 8: 46

Freeny P C, Marks W M 1986 Hepatic haemangioma: dynamic bolus CT. American Journal of Roentgenology 147: 711–719

Freidman A C, Lichtenstein J E, Goodman Z et al 1985 Fibrolamellar hepatocellular carcinoma. Radiology 157: 583–587

Halversen R A, Korobkin M, Ram P C, Thompson W M 1982 CT appearance of focal fatty infiltration of the liver. American Journal of Roentgenology 139: 277–281

Itai Y, Ohtomo K, Kokubo T et al 1987 CT and MR imaging of fatty tumours of the liver. Journal of Computer Assisted Tomography 11: 253–257
Kerlin P, Davis G L, McGill D B et al 1983 Hepatic adenoma and focal nodular hyperplasia: clinical, pathological and radiologic features. Gastroenterology 84: 994–1002
Klatskin G 1987 Hepatic tumours: possible relationship to use of oral contraceptives. Gastroenterology 73: 386–397
Korobkin M, Stephens D H, Fishman E K et al Biliary cystadenoma and cystadeno-carcinoma: CT and sonographic findings in 11 patients. Radiology (in press)
Levine E, Cook L T, Grantham J J 1985 Liver cysts in autosomal dominant polycystic kidney disease: clinical and computed tomographic study. American Journal of Roentgenology 145: 229–233
Lubbers P R, Ros P R, Goodman Z D, Ishak K G 1987 Accumulating of technetium-99m sulfur colloid by hepatocellular adenoma: scintigraphic-pathologic correlation. American Journal of Roentgenology 148: 1105–1108
Mathieu D, Bruneton J-N, Drouillard J, Pointreau C C, Vasile N 1986 Hepatic adenomas and focal nodular hyperplasia: dynamic CT study. Radiology 160: 53–58
Mikulis D J, Costello P, Clouse M E 1985 Hepatic hemangioma: atypical appearance. American Journal of Roentgenology 145: 77–78
Roberts J R, Fishman E K, Hartman D S et al 1986 Lipomatous tumours of the liver: evaluation with CT and ultrasound. Radiology 158: 613–617
Ros P R, Lubbers P R, Olmsted W W, Morillo G 1987 Hemangioma of the liver: heterogeneous appearance on T2-weighted images. American Journal of Roentgenology 149: 1167–1170
Sandler M A, Petrocelli R D, Marks D S, Lopez R 1980 Ultrasonic features and radionuclide correlation in liver cell adenoma and focal nodular hyperplasia. Radiology 135: 393–397
Scatarige J C, Kenny J M, Fishman E K, Herlong F H, Seigelman S S 1987 CT of giant cavernous haemangioma. American Journal of Roentgenology 149: 83–85
Stanley J, Vujic I, Schabel S I, Gobien R P, Reines H D 1983 Evaluation of biliary cystadenoma and cystadenocarcinoma. Gastrointestinal Radiology 8: 245–248
Swensen S J, McLeod R A, Stephens D H 1984 CT of extracranial hemorrhage and hematomas. American Journal of Roentgenology 143: 907–912
Wanless I R, Mawdsley C, Adams R 1985 On the pathogenesis of focal nodular hyperplasia of the liver. Hepatology 5: 1194–1200
Welch T J, Sheedy P F II, Johnson C M et al 1985 Focal nodular hyperplasia and hepatic adenoma. Comparison of angiography, CT, ultrasound and scintigraphy. Radiology 156: 593–595
Yates C K, Streight R A 1986 Focal fatty infiltration of the liver simulating metastatic disease. Radiology 159: 83–84

11. Evaluation of colonic disease

Jay P. Heiken

INTRODUCTION

The barium enema examination has long served as the primary imaging technique for evaluating the colon and remains the technique of choice for detecting colonic mucosal abnormalities. However, the contrast enema examination provides limited information about the extramucosal extent of colonic disease processes. CT is capable of providing this important additional information and serves as a valuable complementary study. CT is useful for:

1. Characterizing and determining the extent of a known colonic abnormality.
2. Staging selected known colonic neoplasms.
3. Detecting recurrent neoplasms.
4. Demonstrating the presence of a colonic abnormality when colonic pathology is unsuspected.

TECHNIQUE

Routine CT examination of the abdomen and pelvis requires the administration of at least 500 ml of oral contrast material (dilute 2–5% barium or iodine) approximately one hour prior to scanning. Although this technique generally provides adequate opacification of distal small bowel loops, it results in inconsistent opacification of the colon. In addition, incomplete distension of the colon may give the appearance of colonic wall thickening and faeces may obscure or simulate a colonic neoplasm. For adequate opacification of the colon, administration of 600–1000 ml of oral contrast material 12–24 hours prior to the examination is generally recommended (Mitchell et al 1985). CT evaluation of the colon is significantly improved if the colon is distended by rectally administered positive contrast material (dilute barium or iodine) or by insufflation of air through a rectal tube (Megibow et al 1984). Intravenous administration of glucagon (0.5–1 mg) may help the patient retain the colonic contrast material or air without discomfort. When a colonic lesion is known or suspected prior to CT scanning, the colon should be prepared with a standard barium enema preparation to provide optimal visualization of the colonic wall and lumen. Occasionally, re-scanning the patient in the prone or lateral decubitus position can help for demonstrating or confirming a suspected lesion. In addition, when a small intraluminal mass is suspected, the use of wider than standard window widths (1000–2000 HU) and lower window levels (−200 to −500 HU) can be useful for demonstrating the lesion (Balthazar 1986).

NORMAL APPEARANCES

The thickness of the wall of the normal colon depends on the degree of colonic distension. When the colon is well distended the wall should not exceed 3 mm in thickness, whereas a wall thickness of 5 mm is within normal limits for a collapsed colon (Fisher 1982). The normal colonic wall should be symmetric, should have homogeneous soft-tissue attenuation, should be sharply defined and surrounded by normal-appearing mesenteric fat.

INFLAMMATORY DISEASES

Ulcerative colitis

In early ulcerative colitis when disease is limited to the mucosa, the colon usually has a normal appearance on CT (Gore et al 1984). In patients with chronic ulcerative colitis, the colonic wall is usually thickened and often has an inhomogeneous attenuation with regions of fat density (Gore et al 1984). The mural thickening is related to infiltration of the lamina propria by round cells in patients with active disease and to hypertrophy of the muscularis mucosa and fatty infiltration of the submucosa in patients with longstanding disease (Gore et al 1984). Fat deposition within the submucosa is not specific for ulcerative colitis and has been seen in granulomatous colitis as well (Jones et al 1986).

The rectum of patients with chronic ulcerative colitis often has a 'target-like' appearance due to submucosal fat deposition. This target pattern consists of a thickened rectal wall with an inner ring of soft-tissue density (mucosa, oedematous infiltrated lamina propria and hypertrophied muscularis mucosae), surrounded by a ring of lower attenuation (fatty infiltration of the submucosa), which in turn is surrounded by a second ring of soft-tissue density (muscularis propria) (Gore 1987). In addition, the rectal lumen is usually narrowed and the presacral space widened, primarily due to proliferation of perirectal fat. Characteristically, the perirectal fat is higher in attenuation than normal extraperitoneal fat and contains an increased number of streaky soft-tissue densities.

Granulomatous (Crohn's) colitis

Mural thickening is a characteristic finding in granulomatous colitis

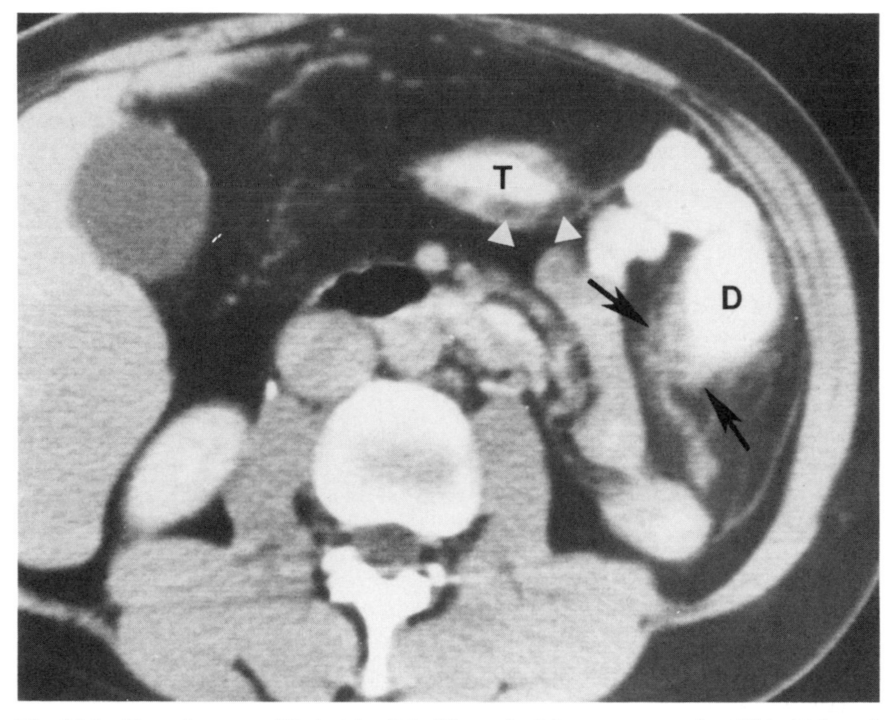

Fig. 11.1 Granulomatous (Crohn's) colitis. The wall of the transverse colon (T) is thickened and contains areas of fat density (arrowheads) indicative of submucosal fat accumulation. The medial wall (arrows) of the descending colon (D) is thick and ill defined. Strands of soft-tissue density extending into the adjacent fat represent pericolic mesenteric inflammation.

because pathologically the disease involves all layers of the bowel wall. The thickening is secondary to oedema, fibrosis, inflammation and lymphangiectasis (Sommers 1978). The bowel wall is usually homogeneous in attenuation but may be inhomogeneous in patients with longstanding disease due to submucosal fat deposition (Gore et al 1984, Jones et al 1986) (Fig. 11.1). Although there is significant overlap, the bowel wall in patients with granulomatous colitis tends to be thicker (mean 13 mm) than in patients with ulcerative colitis (mean 7.8 mm) (Gore et al 1984). The CT scan may be normal in patients with early disease.

The major benefit of CT scanning in patients with granulomatous colitis is to identify and characterize the extramucosal abnormalities that cause separation of bowel loops on barium studies (Goldberg et al 1983). Most importantly, CT is helpful for differentiating mesenteric abscess from fibrofatty proliferation or diffuse inflammatory reaction of the mesentery. Fibrofatty mesenteric proliferation, the most common cause of bowel loop separation, is characterized by increased density of the fat between the separated loops (−70 to −90 HU) and lack of a soft-tissue mass or fluid collection in the affected region (Goldberg et al 1983). An abscess can be confidently diagnosed when a well-marginated, near-water density mass is

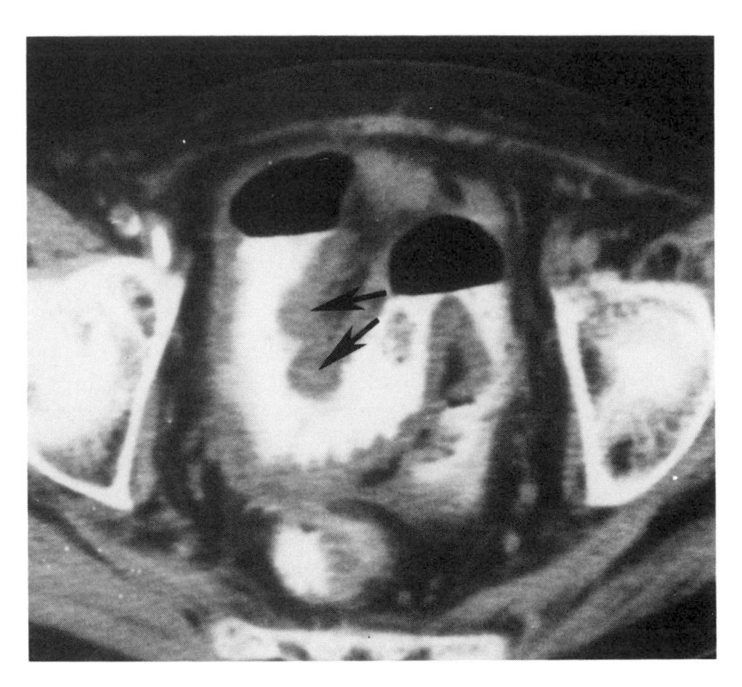

Fig. 11.2 Ischaemic colitis. The wall of the sigmoid colon is diffusely thickened. Areas of 'thumb-printing' (arrows) can be identified.

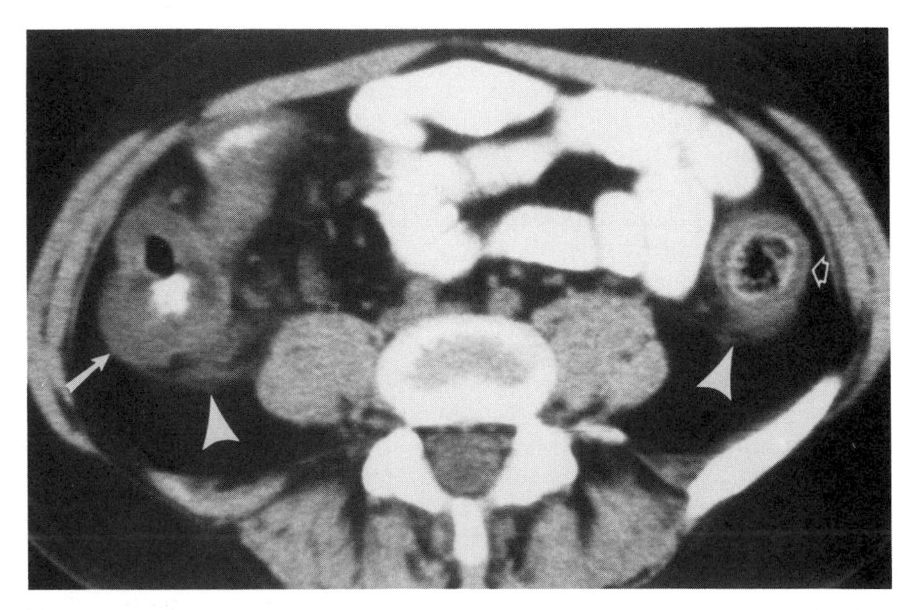

Fig. 11.3 Pseudomembranous colitis. Wall thickening is seen in the ascending (solid arrow) and descending (open arrow) colon. Ill-defined soft-tissue densities extending into the pericolic fat (arrowheads) represent inflammatory changes.

identified. Occasionally, the mass may contain air and oral contrast material indicating communication with bowel (Goldberg et al 1983, Kerber et al 1984). CT can also be helpful for identifying and defining the extent of sinus tracts and fistulae. In cases in which a mesenteric mass has an attenuation value near that of soft tissue, it may be difficult to differentiate an abscess from an inflammatory mass (Kerber et al 1984). CT is also capable of demonstrating many of the extra-intestinal complications of Crohn's disease, such as sclerosing cholangitis, gallstones, renal calculi, osteomyelitis, aseptic necrosis and sacro-ileitis (Kerber et al 1984).

Other inflammatory bowel diseases

Thickening of the colon wall associated with abnormalities in the pericolic fat is not limited to patients with ulcerative or granulomatous colitis. It may be seen in patients with ischaemia (Fig. 11.2), infectious, pseudomembranous (Fig. 11.3) or radiation colitis as well as in patients with graft versus host disease. More localized areas of bowel wall thickening are seen in patients with diverticulitis and appendicitis.

Diverticulitis

The most common CT findings in patients with diverticulitis include inflammation of the pericolic fat (98%), colonic diverticula (84%) and colon wall thickening (70%) (Hulnick et al 1984) (Fig. 11.4). The relative role of CT versus the traditional contrast enema examination in patients with suspected diverticulitis is controversial. In a study by Hulnick et al (1984), CT demonstrated the extracolonic extent and complications of diverticulitis more accurately than contrast enema examinations in 41% of cases. However, Johnson et al (1987) found that patient management was altered in only 1 of 28 patients as a result of the additional information provided by CT. Although CT and contrast enema examination are approximately equally sensitive for diagnosing diverticulitis, CT is preferable if a diverticular abscess is strongly suspected (Fig. 11.5). In addition, because CT images the whole abdomen, it is useful for demonstrating complications of diverticulitis such as bladder involvement, ureteral obstruction and distant abscesses (Hulnick et al 1984). CT also serves as an excellent method for guiding the percutaneous drainage of diverticular abscesses. Percutaneous diverticular abscess drainage can convert complex two or three-stage surgical procedures to safer one-stage colonic resections.

It is important to keep in mind that an extensive or perforated carcinoma of the colon may have an appearance indistinguishable from that of diverticulitis. A discrete mass or thickening of the colon wall out of proportion to the infiltrative changes in the pericolic fat should suggest a carcinoma. In addition, diverticulitis of the right colon may be mistaken for appendicitis (Balthazar et al 1987).

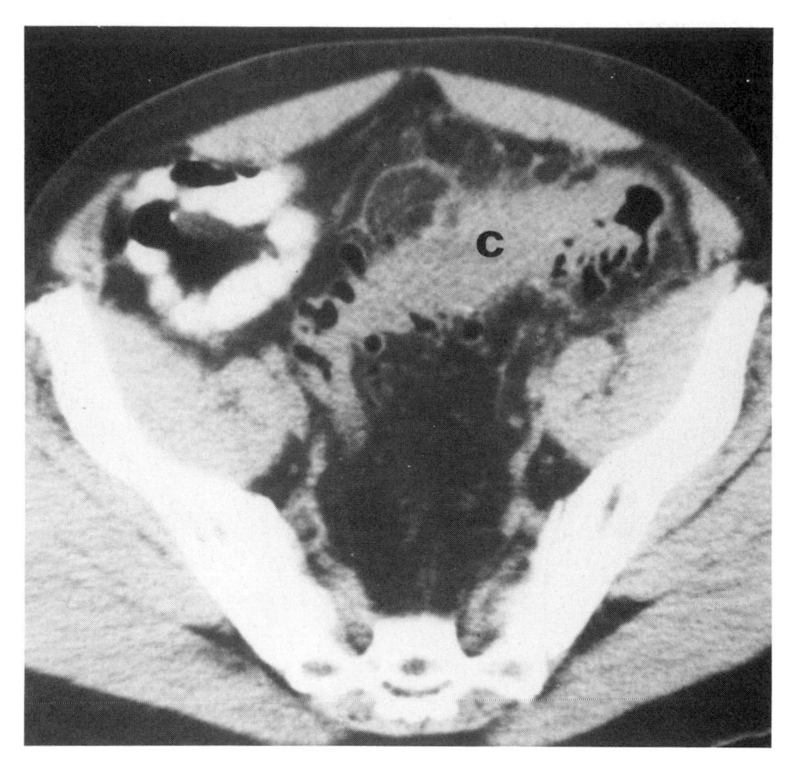

Fig. 11.4 Diverticulitis. The wall of the sigmoid colon (C) is thickened and strands of soft-tissue density extend into the adjacent mesenteric fat. Multiple air-filled diverticula can be identified along the wall of the colon.

Appendicitis

CT is a valuable adjunct to conventional barium studies for evaluating patients with suspected appendicitis and may be particularly useful in patients with an atypical clinical presentation (Jones et al 1983). The most common CT finding is pericaecal inflammation which consists of linear and streaky densities in the adjacent mesenteric or pelvic fat (Balthazar et al 1986). An associated pericaecal soft-tissue mass is usually indicative of a phlegmon, whereas an appendiceal abscess appears as a right lower quadrant or pericaecal fluid collection (Fig. 11.6a). CT is an excellent method for guiding percutaneous drainage of such abscesses which, in some cases, eliminates the need for surgery (van Sonnenberg et al 1987). An appendicolith can be identified in up to 25% of cases (Balthazar et al 1986) (Fig. 11.6b). A less frequently seen but specific sign of appendicitis is circumferential, symmetric thickening of the appendix.

The sensitivity of CT for detecting appendicitis is similar to that of the barium enema examination. A normal CT scan does not exclude appendicitis since mild forms without periappendiceal disease may escape detection (Balthazar et al 1986).

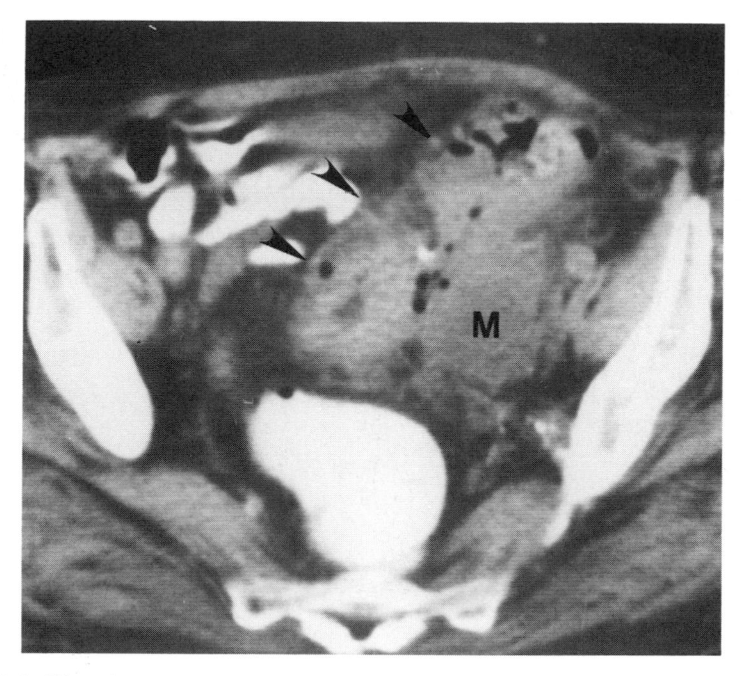

Fig. 11.5 Diverticulitis with a pericolonic abscess. An ill-defined near-water density mass (M) abuts the thickened sigmoid colon (arrowheads).

ADENOCARCINOMA

Although CT is capable of demonstrating 65–100% of known colorectal carcinomas (Freeny et al 1986) and of occasionally identifying colonic neoplasms that are unsuspected, it is not the primary imaging technique for detecting colorectal carcinoma. The barium examination remains the most

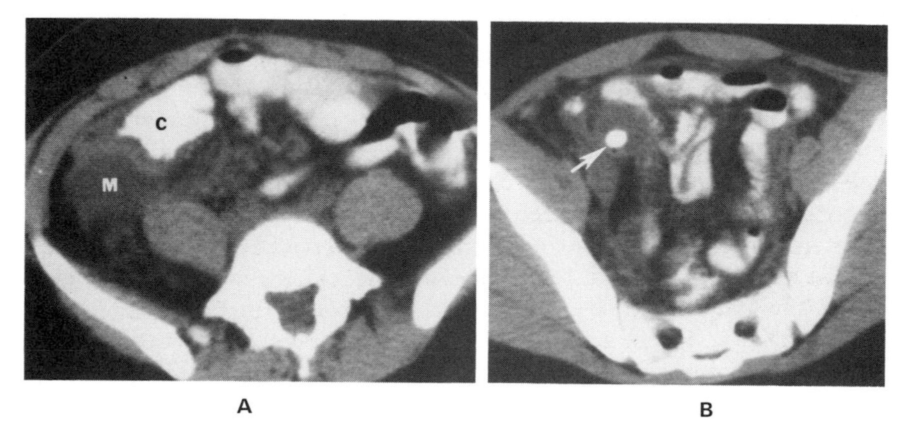

Fig. 11.6 Appendiceal abscess. **A** A near-water attenuation mass (M) abuts the caecum (C). **B** At a slightly more caudal level an appendicolith (arrow) is identified within the mass.

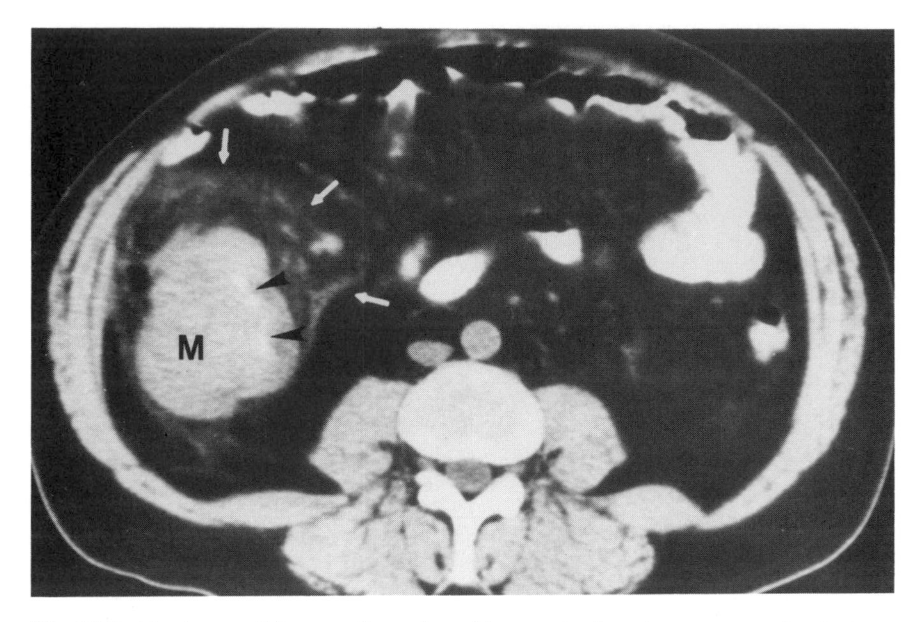

Fig. 11.7 Carcinoma of the ascending colon with extension into the mesentery. A soft-tissue mass (M) compresses the contrast material-containing lumen (arrowheads) of the ascending colon. Strands of soft-tissue density within the surrounding fat (arrows) represent infiltration of tumour into the mesentery.

sensitive radiological method for colorectal carcinoma detection. The strength of CT lies in its ability to image colonic masses directly, thereby showing extension to adjacent tissues and demonstrating distant metastases.

On CT, colon carcinoma has a varied appearance including focal asymmetric colonic wall thickening (> 5 mm), semicircular or circumferential wall thickening or a discrete mass (Fig. 11.7). The tumour is usually homogeneous in attenuation although large masses may have central areas of decreased attenuation due to necrosis. A mild degree of contrast enhancement (10–30 HU increase) is usually seen after bolus injection of intravenous contrast material (Balthazar 1986).

The differential diagnosis of colorectal adenocarcinoma on CT includes other primary malignant neoplasms, such as lymphoma and leiomyosarcoma, from which adenocarcinoma may be indistinguishable based on the CT scan appearances alone. Marked colonic wall thickening in association with extensive mesenteric and retroperitoneal adenopathy should suggest lymphoma. Colonic lipomas are easily differentiated from carcinomas due to their fat density (Heiken et al 1982). Localized inflammatory processes, such as diverticulitis or appendicitis, may be difficult to distinguish from a colonic carcinoma that has perforated or has extended beyond the bowel wall to infiltrate the pericolic fat.

Table 11.1 Dukes' (1938) classification of carcinoma of the rectum

A	Tumour limited to the wall of the rectum
B	Spread by direct extension through extrarectal tissues
C	Involvement of regional lymph-nodes

Preoperative staging of colorectal carcinoma

In 1938, Dukes devised a classification for staging rectal carcinoma (Table 11.1). Over the years the Dukes' system has undergone multiple modifications to include the presence or absence of lymph-node involvement and a fourth category (D) has been added to include peritoneal seeding of tumour or distant metastases to liver, lung or bone (Kirklin et al 1949, Astler & Coller 1954, Turnbull et al 1967). Although the Dukes' classification remains a useful standard for assessing prognosis and determining appropriate treatment it is a pathological staging system. Since CT cannot accurately determine the depth of tumour in the bowel wall and is inaccurate in assessing pelvic lymph-node metastases, the Dukes' classification is not useful for the staging of colorectal cancers by CT and for these reasons Thoeni et al (1981) have proposed an alternative system for the CT staging of rectal and rectosigmoid tumours (Table 11.2).

A number of investigators have used CT preoperatively to stage patients with colorectal cancer. Although the early reports indicated that CT was an accurate preoperative staging method (Thoeni et al 1981), more recent studies have found CT to be of limited value in this regard (Freeny et al 1986, Thompson et al 1986). Possible reasons for these discrepancies include the large numbers of patients with advanced disease and the lack of assessment of lymph-node involvement in some of the early studies (Thoeni et al 1981, van Waes et al 1983). More recent CT studies have found accuracy rates for detecting invasion of perirectal fat of 55–79% with sensitivities for detection of lymph-node metastases of only 22–73% (Freeny et al 1986, Thompson et al 1986, Balthazar et al 1988). Using modifications of the Dukes' classification, Freeny et al (1986), Thompson et al (1986) and Balthazar et al (1988) correctly staged only 38 of 80 patients (47.5%), 15 of 25 patients (60%) and 31 of 76 patients (41%) respectively. The vast majority of the incorrectly staged patients were understaged due to inability to detect lymph-node metastases and inability to determine extension of tumour into the perirectal fat.

Table 11.2 Staging of primary rectal and rectosigmoid tumours by CT (Thoeni et al 1981)

Stage I	Intraluminal polypoid mass without thickening of the bowel wall
Stage II	Thickening of the bowel wall (> 0.5 cm) without invasion of surrounding tissue
Stage IIIA	Invasion of surrounding tissue but no extension to the pelvic side walls
Stage IV	Pelvic tumour and distant metastases

Thus, CT is not an accurate method for the pre-operative local staging of primary colorectal carcinoma. However, it is useful for identifying patients with advanced (Dukes' Stage D) disease, which may lead to changes in surgical planning or preoperative management (Thompson et al 1986, Balthazar et al 1988). CT may also be useful for evaluating patients with a suspected complication of the tumour, such as a perforation (Thompson et al 1986).

Recurrent colorectal carcinoma

Tumour recurrence after resection of rectosigmoid carcinoma occurs in 30–50% of patients (Welch & Donaldson 1978). Up to one-third of recurrences are detected within the first six months after surgery and more than 80% occur within two years (Welch & Donaldson 1978). Of patients with recurrent carcinoma, one-third to one-half have local recurrence only (Olson et al 1980) and 45–72% of patients who die of colorectal cancer following attempted curative surgery do so as a direct result of locally recurrent disease (Gunderson & Sosin 1974). The importance of early detection of pelvic recurrence cannot be overstated.

CT is currently the imaging test of choice for detecting and assessing the overall extent of recurrent disease. It is particularly valuable in patients who have been treated with abdominoperineal (AP) resection, sincc

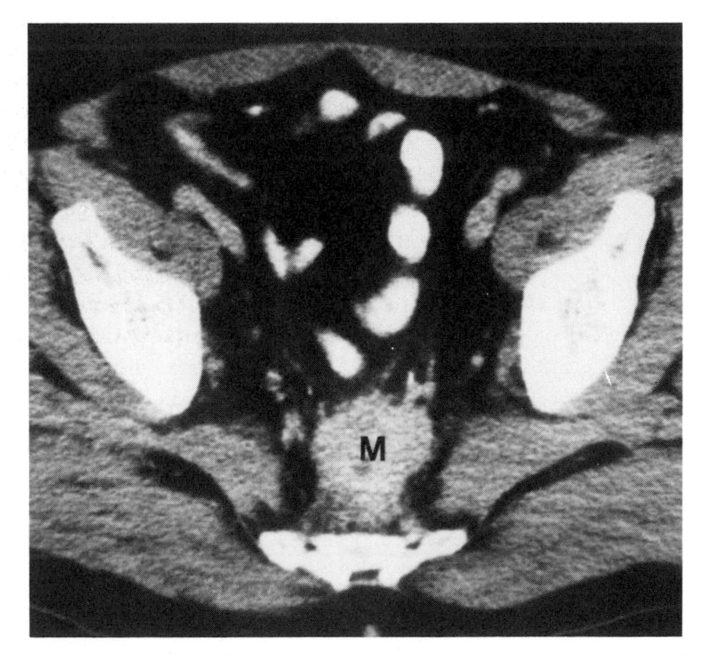

Fig. 11.8 Recurrent rectal carcinoma after abdominoperineal resection. A mass (M) showing contrast enhancement is present in the presacral space.

absence of the rectum precludes evaluation by barium enema or endoscopy. The value of CT in detecting recurrent rectosigmoid carcinoma has been documented in a number of studies with overall accuracy ranging from 87 to 95% (Moss et al 1981, Grabbe et al 1983, Freeny et al 1986, Thompson et al 1986). Lesions as small as 1–2 cm have been detected (Heiken & Lee 1985).

After AP resection, the most frequent site of recurrence is the presacral (precoccygeal) space. Tumour recurrence usually appears as a globular soft-tissue mass (Fig. 11.8). Several authors have described the difficulty in differentiating recurrent carcinoma from postoperative changes, such as fibrosis, haematoma, abscess and normal pelvic structures (Lee et al 1981, Kelvin et al 1983). After AP resection, the urinary bladder falls posteriorly to occupy the presacral space. The seminal vesicles in men and the uterus in women also move posteriorly with the bladder, whereas the prostate in men remains fixed in its normal retropubic position. In addition, small bowel loops occupy a significant portion of the rectal fossa. CT examinations performed within the first month after AP resection may show an amorphous soft-tissue density mass in the pelvis with obliteration of normal fascial planes due to postoperative oedema. In the majority of cases, presacral masses due to postoperative fibrosis diminish in size, elongate and become better defined between 4 and 9 months after surgery (Kelvin et al 1983). In many cases, these early postoperative changes resolve significantly within the first 4 months, after which postoperative fibrotic changes appear as minimal streaky soft-tissue densities in the presacral and precoccygeal space (Lee et al 1981). However, some benign postoperative presacral masses show no change with time (Kelvin et al 1983). Masses due to recurrent tumour and postoperative fibrosis can usually be differentiated on serial CT examinations; it may be difficult to make this distinction on a single study. CT-guided needle biopsy is, therefore, often necessary to make a diagnosis. It is recommended that after AP resection a baseline CT examination be performed 2–4 months after surgery, followed by repeat examinations at 6-monthly intervals for at least the first 2 years (Heiken & Lee 1985). Any new or enlarging presacral mass should be biopsied under CT guidance. Since at least half of patients with recurrence develop distant metastases (Olson et al 1980), the upper abdomen including the liver should always be included as part of the postoperative CT examination.

In patients who have undergone resection of rectosigmoid carcinoma with primary colonic reanastomosis, tumour often recurs in the anterior portion of the anastomosis (Moss et al 1981). Barium enema examination and CT are complementary procedures for the postoperative evaluation of these patients. The barium enema examination is more sensitive than CT for detecting metachronous colonic neoplasms and recurrent carcinoma at the anastomosis, whereas CT better evaluates recurrences or metastases remote from the anastomotic site (Chen et al 1987).

Magnetic resonance (MR) imaging is potentially useful for differentiating postoperative fibrosis or radiation fibrosis from recurrent tumour because fibrosis has a low signal intensity on T2 weighted images, whereas recurrent tumour has a medium to high intensity due to its long T2 values. However, oedema and inflammation also show a high signal intensity on T2 weighted images and further investigation is necessary to determine the reliability of MR imaging for distinguishing fibrosis from tumour recurrence.

CONCLUSION

CT is a useful complementary examination to barium studies in patients with benign and malignant colonic disease because the extent of extramucosal pathology can be defined. In benign conditions CT can identify abscess formation, fluid collections, sinus tracts and fistulae. In malignancy CT is helpful for delineating the extent of direct tumour spread beyond the colonic wall as well as the presence of distant metastases. In patients with suspected recurrence, CT is highly accurate for detecting tumour recurrence but on occasion tumour may be indistinguishable from fibrosis.

REFERENCES

Astler V B, Coller F A 1954 The prognostic significance of direct extension of carcinoma of the colon and rectum. Annals of Surgery 139: 846

Balthazar E J 1986 Colon. In: Megibow A J, Balthazar E J (eds) Computed tomography of the gastrointestinal tract. C V Mosby, St Louis

Balthazar E J, Megibow A J, Hulnick D H, Gordon R P, Naidich D P, Beranbaum E R 1986 CT of appendicitis. American Journal of Roentgenology 147: 705–710

Balthazar E J, Megibow A J, Gordon R B, Hulnick D 1987 Cecal diverticulitis: evaluation with CT. Radiology 162: 79–81

Balthazar E J, Megibow A J, Hulnick D, Naidich D P 1988 Carcinoma of the colon: detection and preoperative staging by CT. American Journal of Roentgenology 150: 301–306

Chen Y M, Ott D J, Wolfman N T, Gelfand D W, Karstaedt N, Bechtold R E 1987 Recurrent colorectal carcinoma: evaluation with barium enema examination and CT. Radiology 163: 307–310

Fisher J K 1982 Normal colon wall thickness on CT. Radiology 145: 415–418

Freeny P C, Marks W M, Ryan J A, Bolen J W 1986 Colorectal carcinoma evaluation with CT: preoperative staging and detection of postoperative recurrence. Radiology 158: 347–353

Goldberg H I, Gore R M, Margulis A R, Moss A A, Baker E L 1983 Computed tomography in the evaluation of Crohn's disease. American Journal of Roentgenology 140: 227–228

Gore R M 1987 Cross-sectional imaging of inflammatory bowel disease. Radiologic Clinics of North America 25: 115–131

Gore R M, Marn C S, Kirby D F, Vogelzang R L, Neiman H L 1984 CT findings in ulcerative, granulomatous and indeterminate colitis. American Journal of Roentgenology 143: 279–284

Grabbe E, Lierse W, Winkler R 1983 The perirectal fascia morphology and use in staging of rectal carcinoma. Radiology 149: 241–246

Gunderson L L, Sosin H 1974 Areas of failure found at reoperation (second or symptomatic look) following 'curative surgery' for adenocarcinoma of the rectum. Cancer 34: 1278–1292

Heiken J P, Forde K A, Gold R P 1982 Computed tomography as a definitive method for diagnosing gastrointestinal lipoma. Radiology 142: 409–414

Heiken J P, Lee J K T 1985 Recurrent pelvic malignancy. In: Walsh J W (ed) Computed tomography of the pelvis. Churchill Livingstone, New York, pp 185–209
Hulnick D H, Megibow A J, Balthazar E J, Naidich D P, Bosniak M A 1984 Computed tomography in the evaluation of diverticulitis. Radiology 152: 491–495
Johnson C D, Baker M E, Rice R P, Silverman P, Thompson W M 1987 Diagnosis of acute colonic diverticulitis: comparison of barium enema and CT. American Journal of Roentgenology 148: 541–546
Jones B, Fishman E K, Hamilton S R et al 1986 Submucosal accumulation of fat in inflammatory bowel disease: CT/pathologic correlation. Journal of Computer Assisted Tomography 10: 759–763
Jones B, Fishman E K, Siegelman S S 1983 Computed tomography and appendiceal abscess: special applicability in the elderly. Journal of Computer Assisted Tomography 7: 434–438
Kelvin F M, Korobkin M, Heaston D K, Grant J P, Akwari O 1983 The pelvis after surgery for rectal carcinoma: serial CT observations with emphasis on non-neoplastic features. American Journal of Roentgenology 141: 959–964
Kerber G W, Greenberg M, Rubin J M 1984 Computed tomography evaluation of local and extraintestinal complications of Crohn's disease. Gastrointestinal Radiology 9: 43–48
Kirklin J W, Docherty M D, Waugh J M 1949 The role of the peritoneal reflection in the prognosis of carcinoma of the rectum and sigmoid colon. Surgery, Gynecology, Obstetrics 88: 326
Lee J K T, Stanley R J, Sagel S S, Levitt R G, McClennan B L 1981 CT appearance of the pelvis after abdominoperineal resection for rectal carcinoma. Radiology 141: 737–741
Megibow A J, Zerhouni E A, Hulnick D H, Beranbaum E R, Balthazar E J 1984 Air insufflation of the colon in CT of the pelvis. Journal of Computer Assisted Tomography 8: 797–800
Mitchell D G, Bjorgvinsson E, terMeulen D, Lane P, Greberman M, Friedman A C 1985 Gastrografin versus dilute barium for colonic CT examination: a blind randomized study. Journal of Computer Assisted Tomography 9: 451–453
Moss A, Thoeni R F, Schnyder P, Margulis A R 1981 Value of computed tomography in the detection and staging of recurrent rectal carcinoma. Journal of Computer Assisted Tomography 5: 870–874
Olson R M, Parencevich N P, Malcolm A W et al 1980 Patterns of recurrence following curative resection of adenocarcinoma of the colon and rectum. Cancer 45: 2969–2974
Sommers S C 1978 Ulcerative and granulomatous colitis. American Journal of Roentgenology 130: 817–823
Thoeni R F, Moss A A, Schnyder P, Margulis A R 1981 Detection and staging of primary rectal and rectosigmoid cancer by computed tomography. Radiology 141: 135–138
Thompson W M, Halvorsen R A, Foster W L Jr, Roberts L, Gibbons R 1986 Preoperative and postoperative CT staging of rectosigmoid carcinoma. American Journal of Roentgenology 146: 703–710
Turnbull R B, Kyle K, Watson F R, Spratt J 1967 Cancer of the colon: the influence of the no-touch isolation technique on survival rates. Annals of Surgery 160: 420–427
van Sonnenberg E, Wittich G R, Casola G et al 1987 Periappendiceal abscess: percutaneous drainage. Radiology 163: 23–26
van Waes P F G, Koehler P R, Feldberg M A M 1983 Management of rectal carcinoma: impact of computed tomography. American Journal of Roentgenology 140: 1137–1142
Welch J P, Donaldson G A 1978 Detection and treatment of recurrent cancer of the colon and rectum. American Journal of Surgery 135: 505–511

12. Renal cystic disease

N. Reed Dunnick

INTRODUCTION

Renal cysts, cystic disease and cystic masses are among the most common abnormalities encountered in uroradiology. In some cases the renal cysts are part of a systemic process which also involves the liver. In most patients, however, one or several cystic masses are detected and the question is whether the lesion is benign or malignant. In the vast majority of cases, the radiographic findings are sufficiently characteristic that surgery is not required. However, a variety of radiographic modalities may be needed before a confident diagnosis can be reached.

BENIGN CORTICAL CYSTS

The CT appearances of a simple cyst are the same as those found on excretory urography. A cyst is round, well-defined, has a smooth margin and a sharp interface with the normal renal cortex. The density of the cyst fluid should be close to that of water. A density greater than 15 Hounsfield units (HU) is suspicious for a complicated cyst or even a solid mass lesion (Bosniak 1986). There should be no contrast enhancement of a simple cyst. However, small increases (2–5 HU) in density are normally seen after intravenous contrast injection. Renal cysts may be detected as an incidental finding during a contrast-enhanced CT examination of the abdomen and in this situation there is no opportunity to test for contrast enhancement. However, if the density of the cyst fluid is less than 15 HU and other criteria of a single cyst are present, the lesion is almost certainly benign.

The wall of a benign cortical cyst is too thin to be seen on CT. However, when evaluating wall thickness it is important to look at a portion of the cyst that extends well away from the parenchyma. If the cyst is completely intrarenal, wall thickness cannot be assessed.

The accuracy of the radiographic diagnosis of a renal cyst depends upon how well it is seen by each modality. When all the criteria of a benign simple cyst are present, it is highly unlikely to be anything else and further evaluation is not warranted. However, cysts are often not visualized well enough by excretory urography to make this determination. Due to cost considerations, ultrasound is the most efficient method of confirming the presence of a simple cyst which is poorly seen during urography.

CT is currently the gold standard for the evaluation of renal mass lesions, but it is a more expensive examination than ultrasound and requires intravenous contrast material. It is indicated when the ultrasound examination is indeterminate or technically inadequate due to obesity or overlying gas. It is also appropriate to proceed directly to CT if the urogram indicates that the mass is complex or likely to be solid.

COMPLICATED CYSTS

Those cystic masses which do not satisfy the criteria of a benign simple cyst must be further evaluated to exclude malignancy (Friedland 1987, Papanicolaou et al 1986). A variety of abnormalities are now recognized which exclude the diagnosis of a simple cyst. As experience accumulates, especially with CT and ultrasound, the likelihood of these abnormalities representing malignancy can be better judged.

Septations

Thin internal septations can be detected by ultrasound but their presence alone does not suggest malignancy (Rosenberg et al 1985). Many of these thin septations are not seen during either urography or CT, and it is likely that they will be classified as typical simple cysts.

Other septations may be thick enough to be seen on CT examination. If the septa are thin, smooth and do not have localized areas of thickening or irregularity, a benign diagnosis can be made. However, if there is an associated solid mass, the lesion must be considered to be malignant.

Calcification

The presence of calcification is also a non-specific finding. When evaluation of the kidney depended primarily on urography, the presence of calcification, especially central calcification, was an ominous sign. However, CT has made the presence or absence of calcification almost irrelevant, as wall thickening and soft-tissue masses can easily be detected. Thin calcification in the wall of a cyst or in a septation does not, in itself, warrant surgical exploration (Fig. 12.1).

Thick wall

A thick wall is incompatible with a simple cyst (Fig. 12.2). It indicates either that the lesion is another type of cystic mass, or that the cyst has become complicated by a process such as infection or haemorrhage. In addition, the lesion may be a cystic renal adenocarcinoma. Thick-walled

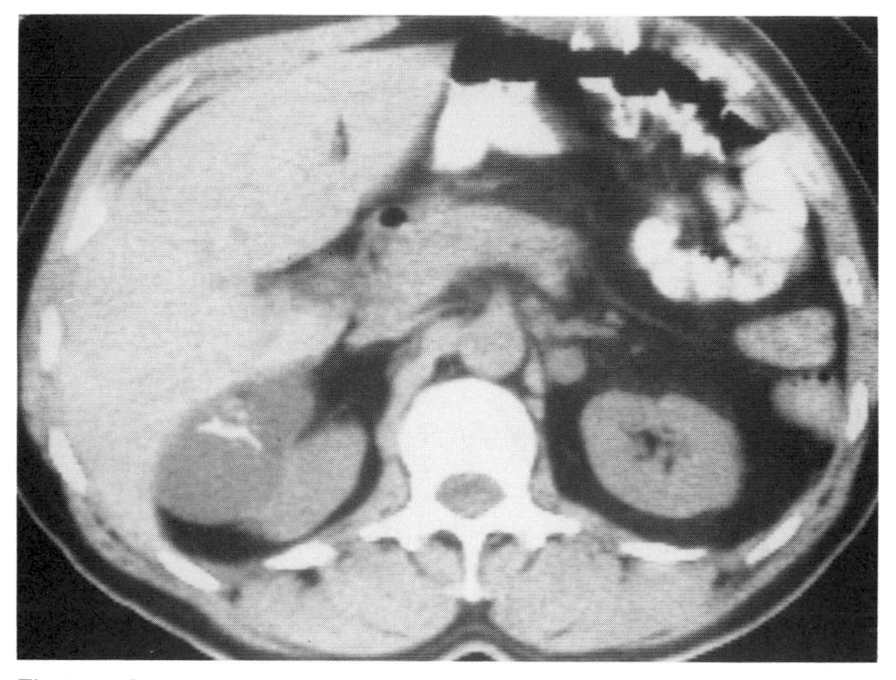

Fig. 12.1 CT scan showing calcific septations within a renal cyst. However, no soft-tissue mass is seen to suggest malignancy.

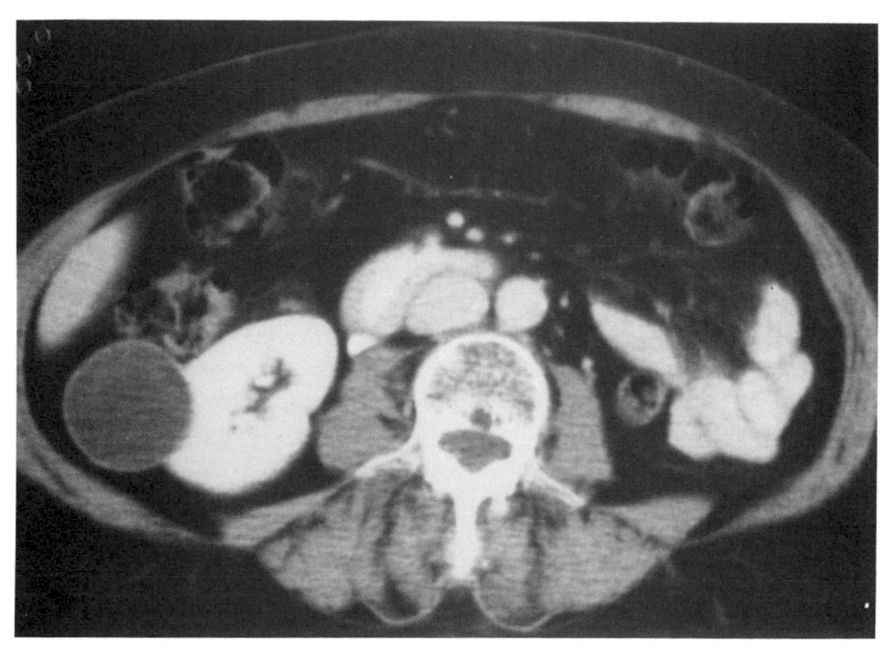

Fig. 12.2 CT scan showing a thickened wall which excludes a simple cyst and further evaluation is needed.

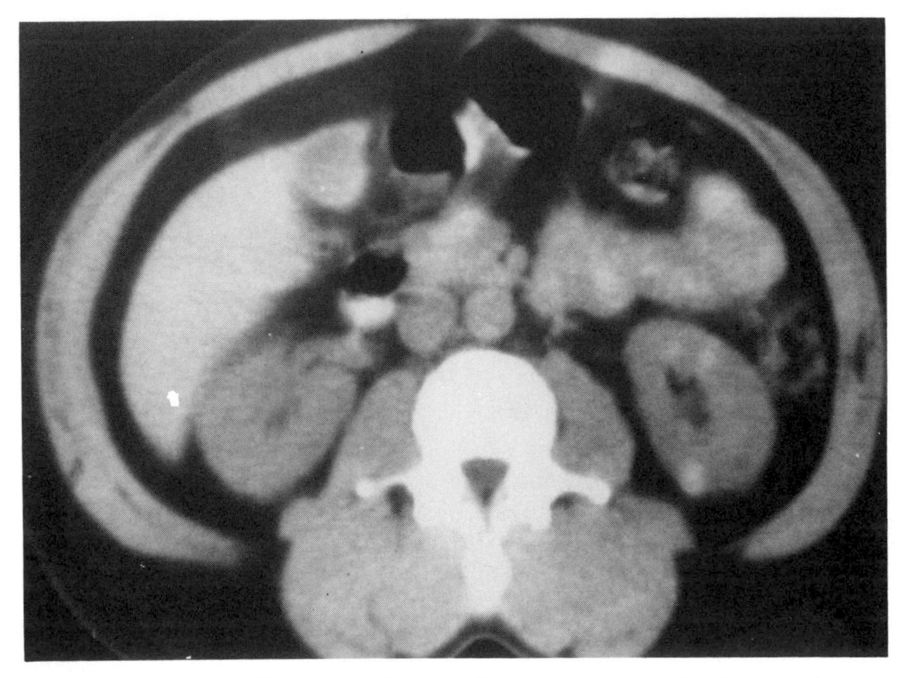

Fig. 12.3 Unenhanced CT scan showing several small, homogeneous but dense renal lesions. They are most likely haemorrhagic cysts.

lesions must be considered indeterminate and surgical exploration is indicated. The presence of an associated soft-tissue tumour mass is an even more serious finding and is highly suspicious of malignancy.

Hyperdense renal cysts

One category of atypical renal cysts which has been frequently described is the hyperdense cyst (Coleman et al 1984, Dunnick et al 1984a). These lesions look like typical simple cysts on CT examination in that they are rounded, well-defined, homogeneous masses that do not enhance with intravenous contrast injection (Fig. 12.3). They are usually small, peripheral lesions, measuring less than 3 cm in diameter. However, instead of displaying a density near to that of water their attenuation values are between 60 and 90 HU (Sussman et al 1984). They are easily recognized on unenhanced CT examination but are often masked on scans taken after injection of intravenous contrast medium because the densities of the cyst and enhanced renal parenchyma are similar. For these reasons, it is likely that hyperdense cysts are more common than are generally appreciated as abdominal CT scans are frequently performed after intravenous contrast material has been given.

There are several possible aetiologies for a hyperdense renal cyst. The most common are haemorrhage and a high protein content of the cyst fluid. However, the cyst may contain diffuse 'paste-like' calcified material. The vast majority of these hyperdense cysts are benign, but they must be carefully examined for other atypical features. CT examination prior to, and following, intravenous contrast injection is often helpful since a cyst does not enhance, whereas a solid tumour will show definite enhancement (Dunnick et al 1984b).

Ultrasound examination is a useful modality in the evaluation of the hyperdense renal mass. The distinction between a cystic and solid lesion can be made and blood elements can sometimes be seen floating within the cyst. However, if the lesion cannot be clearly evaluated, surgical exploration may still be needed.

PARAPELVIC CYSTS

These benign cysts lie in the region of the renal hilum and cause extrinsic compression of the collecting system. The CT appearance is that of a benign cyst which is located in the hilar area rather than the cortex of the kidney (Hidalgo et al 1982) (Fig. 12.4).

Parapelvic cysts may not be renal in origin, but could be lymphocytic or may arise from embryological remnants in the renal hilum. With increased

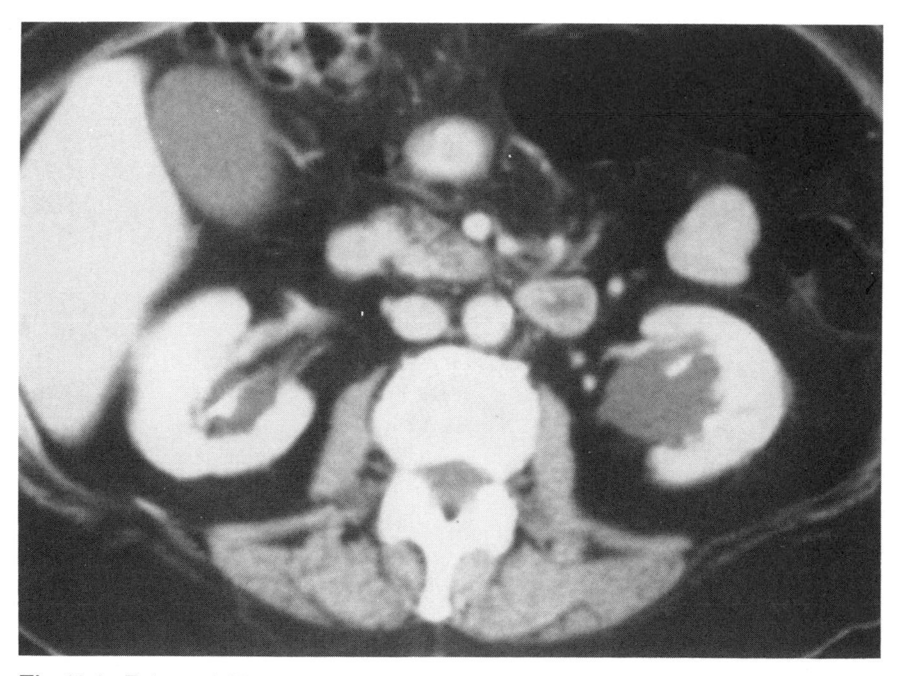

Fig. 12.4 Enhanced CT scan which shows bilateral parapelvic renal cysts which are easily recognized.

use of CT and ultrasound, they are frequently recognized and are often multiple and bilateral. Problems arise when they are confused with other entities.

Parapelvic cysts should not be confused with renal sinus fat (sinus lipomatosis) (Cronan et al 1982) as CT can easily separate these processes. The low density fat is clearly different from the water density cysts on CT examination.

ADULT POLYCYSTIC DISEASE

Adult polycystic disease is the most common form of cystic kidney disease and is transmitted by autosomal dominant inheritance. Although the aetiology is unknown, the cysts seem to arise from nephrons which initially were able to function normally.

Patients with adult polycystic disease present most commonly in the third or fourth decade. The initial complaint is usually pain which may be in the lumbar spine, groin or upper abdomen. Hypertension, which occurs in over half of the patients, is due to increased renin production by the kidneys. Almost half of the patients have cerebral (berry) aneurysms in the circle of Willis, and stroke from rupture of a berry aneurysm is a significant cause of morbidity and mortality.

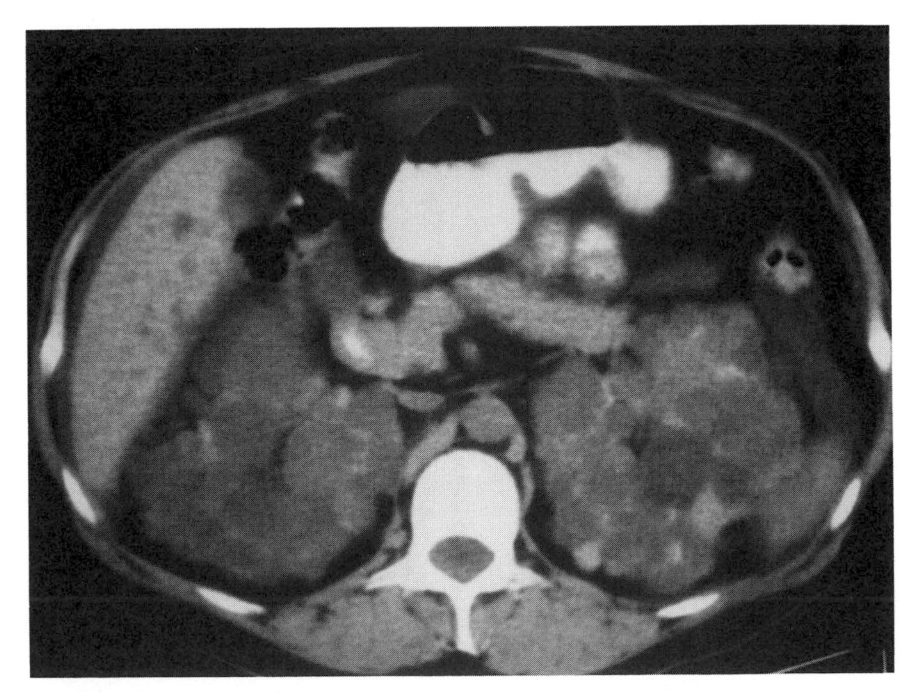

Fig. 12.5 Unenhanced CT scan showing polycystic renal disease. Note associated hepatic cysts as well as several hyperdense, presumably haemorrhagic, renal cysts.

Ultrasound and CT have replaced nephrotomography as the standard method of examination (Segal & Spataro 1982). Innumerable renal cysts are seen with either modality (Fig. 12.5). The kidneys are markedly enlarged but maintain their basic reniform shape (McCallum & Gildiner 1981).

CT has the advantage of clearly demonstrating the cysts and collecting systems of both kidneys. Pre-contrast scans are needed to demonstrate renal stones and facilitate the diagnosis of haemorrhagic cysts. Since the kidneys are typically riddled with innumerable cysts which abut each other, they are not round in shape but assume a variety of irregular contours.

CT is also useful for demonstrating hepatic cysts which are present in 57–74% of patients with adult polycystic disease (Levine et al 1985). These liver cysts develop from dilatation of aberrant bile ducts that embryologically failed to establish communication with the biliary tree. The cysts gradually accumulate fluid secreted by the lining cuboidal epithelial cells.

Bleeding into renal cysts is common and may be the source of acute flank pain. If the cyst ruptures into the renal pelvis, haematuria will occur. Cyst haemorrhage may be more common in adult polycystic disease because of the associated hypertension, the increased bleeding tendency of uraemia, or heparinization during dialysis. Haemorrhagic renal cysts may be seen in 70% of patients and perinephric haemorrhage has also been reported but is rare (Levine & Grantham 1985, Levine & Grantham 1987).

Although both kidneys are affected in adult polycystic disease, involvement may be asymmetric. Rare cases of unilateral disease are reported but these may represent manifestations which are too small for macroscopic imaging (Lee et al 1978).

Since ultrasound is a non-invasive technique, it is the method of choice for screening the children of affected families.

ACQUIRED CYSTIC DISEASE OF URAEMIA

With improvements in dialysis and renal transplantation, patients with end-stage renal disease are now living much longer. As a result, we are beginning to detect acquired cystic disease and an occasional renal adenocarcinoma in the native kidneys (Cho et al 1984).

Although the mechanism of cyst formation in these uraemic patients is unknown, it is postulated that dialysis incompletely removes toxins and their accumulation may induce these changes. The involution of the cysts after successful renal transplantation supports this hypothesis.

Cysts occur in approximately 45% of patients followed for three years or more (Levine et al 1984). Radiographic evaluation is needed, not for detection of renal cysts, but to identify carcinomas which occur in about 7% of patients. Ultrasound examination of native kidneys is difficult as they are often small, distorted and surrounded by highly echogenic fat. In addition, calcification frequently occurs, either in the cyst walls or in the

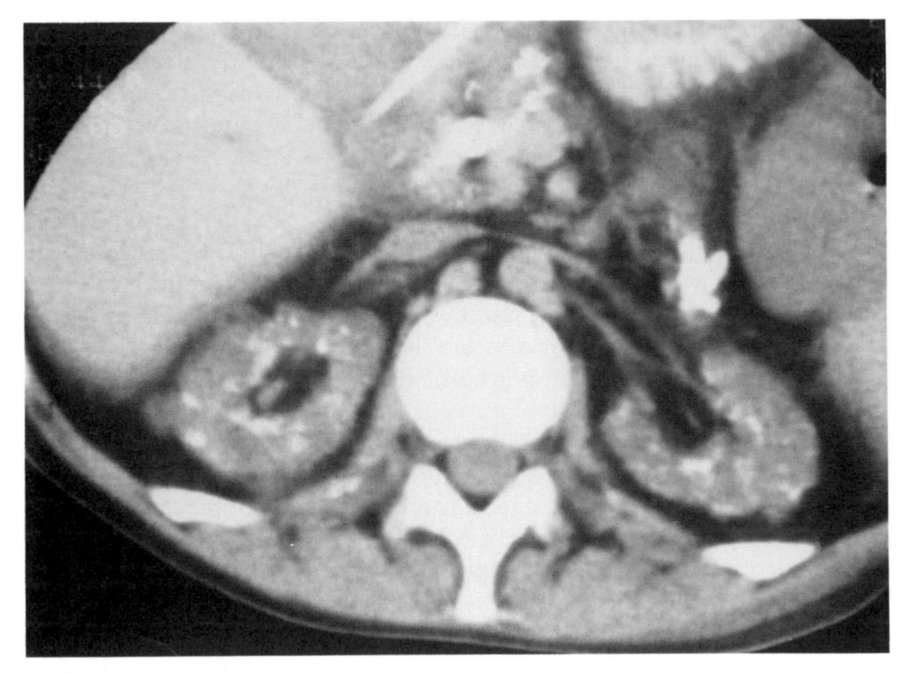

Fig. 12.6 CT scan showing multiple small cysts and dystrophic calcifications are present in this patient on chronic haemodialysis.

renal interstitium, which further hampers ultrasound examination. CT is, therefore, the method of choice for examining the native kidneys and has the advantage of a higher sensitivity than ultrasound for detecting small lesions (Fig. 12.6).

MULTICYSTIC DYSPLASTIC KIDNEY

A multicystic dysplastic kidney consists of a collection of irregularly sized cysts and fibrous tissue but no functioning renal parenchyma. The cysts do not communicate, the renal collecting system is small or absent and there are atretic ipsilateral renal vessels. The anomaly results from occlusion of the fetal ureters usually before 8–10 weeks.

A variant, the hydronephrotic type of multicystic dysplasia, may result from incomplete ureteral obstruction later in gestation. In such cases, the cysts communicate with the renal pelvis.

Most renal dysplasias are detected as an abdominal mass in infancy. Multicystic dysplastic kidney is the second most common cause of an abdominal mass in the neonate, following only hydronephrosis in frequency. Males are more commonly affected than females and there is a predilection for the left kidney.

Malformations including bilateral multicystic dysplastic kidney, pelvi-ureteric junction obstruction, hypoplasia of the opposite kidney and horseshoe kidney are commonly associated with multicystic dysplastic kidney. These occurred in 41% of fetuses examined by ultrasound by Kleiner et al (1986). Since some of these contralateral anomalies are fatal, less severe changes are more commonly seen and pelvi-ureteric junction obstruction is the most common malformation demonstrated in children or adults. If the multicystic dysplastic kidney is not detected in infancy it may remain asymptomatic and be detected as an incidental finding in an adult (Pedicelli et al 1986).

Abdominal radiographs may demonstrate a soft-tissue flank mass. In adults calcification is common, usually in the cyst walls. There is no functional renal parenchyma on the affected side, but excretory urography will demonstrate compensatory hypertrophy of the contralateral kidney. If retrograde pyelography is performed, an atretic ureter may be demonstrated. Extravasation is common because cannulation of the small ureteric opening may be difficult.

The multiple cysts with thick septa are well shown by CT. Mural calcifications can be demonstrated in the cyst walls, but there is no evidence of contrast excretion (Fig. 12.7).

Ultrasound is particularly valuable for assessing infants and demonstrates multiple cysts of varying sizes (Sanders & Hartman 1984). There is no connection between adjacent cysts, nor is there renal parenchyma

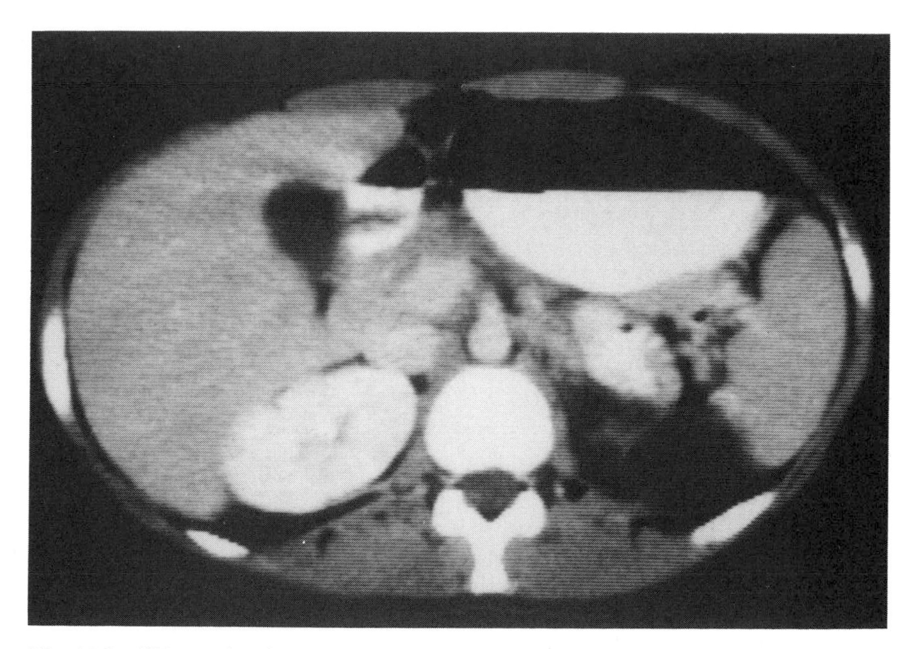

Fig. 12.7 CT scan showing a collection of cysts, but no functioning tissue, in this multicystic dysplastic kidney. The contralateral (right) kidney is normal.

surrounding the cysts. If angiography is performed, no ipsilateral renal artery will be identified.

Segmental multicystic renal dysplasia in an upper pole moiety may be seen in patients with obstruction from an ectopic ureterocoele. The dysplastic segment has the same features as the multicystic dysplastic kidney and causes compression of the normally functioning lower pole moiety.

MULTILOCULAR CYSTIC NEPHROMA

This uncommon lesion has been described by a variety of names including multilocular renal cyst, cystic adenoma, lymphangioma, segmental multicystic kidney, segmental polycystic kidney, cystic hamartoma, benign cystic nephroma and Perlman's tumour. It is a congenital renal lesion which is not genetically transmitted.

Multilocular cystic nephroma is a well-circumscribed lesion containing many cysts of variable size. The cystic mass is surrounded by a thick fibrous capsule which compresses adjacent renal parenchyma and often projects into the renal pelvis.

The presenting signs and symptoms depend upon the patient's age.

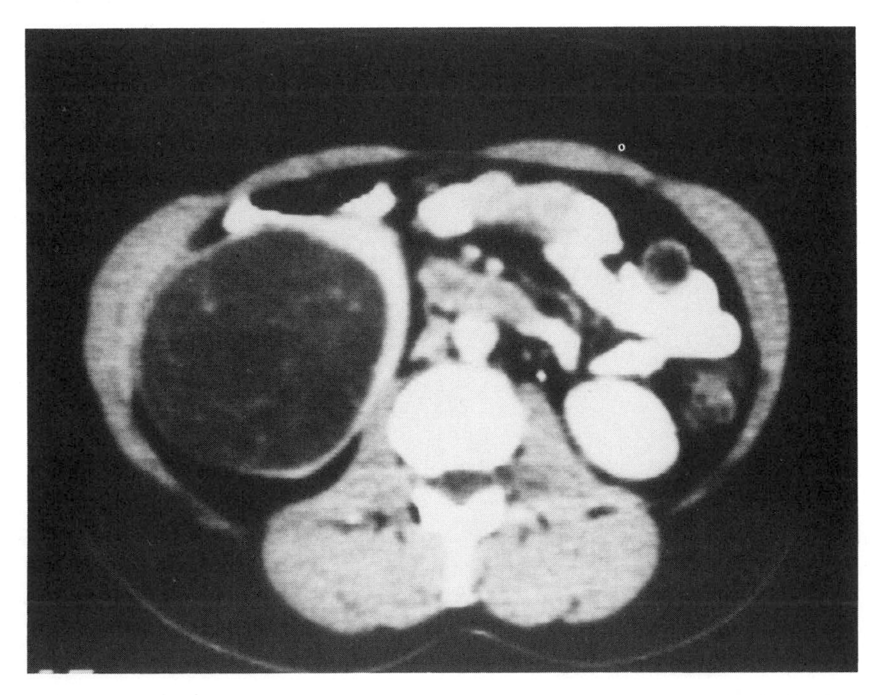

Fig. 12.8 CT scan showing a well-circumscribed multilocular cystic nephroma in the right kidney. Thin internal septations are identified on an enhanced CT examination.

Males are usually under 4 years of age and present with a palpable abdominal mass. Females typically present between the ages of 4 and 20 years or over 40 years. Among children presenting under 4 years of age, 73% are male; when the patient is over 4 years at presentation, 89% are female. In the adult, multilocular cystic nephroma may be found during examination for an unrelated complaint or during the investigation of pain, haematuria or urinary tract infection. Haematuria may result from herniation of the tumour into the renal pelvis which causes tissue necrosis of the overlying thin layer of transitional cell epithelium (de Wall et al 1986).

Calcification is uncommon, especially in the paediatric patient. However, radiographically detected calcifications were found in 7 of 12 adult patients reported by Banner et al (1981). Calcification is usually seen in the cyst walls or intervening stroma. The pattern of calcification is non-specific and may be central or peripheral. A large renal mass is seen on excretory urography. The cystic mass occurs with equal frequency on either side but is more common in the lower pole. Projection of the mass into the renal pelvis can often be demonstrated. The mass is hypovascular and mottled in appearance.

The multiple cystic spaces are best demonstrated with ultrasound. If the cysts are large, multiple locules separated by echogenic stroma suggest the diagnosis of multilocular cystic nephroma. If the cysts are small, they may not be defined by ultrasound and the echogenic stroma may suggest a complex or solid renal mass.

The CT appearances of multilocular cystic nephroma are usually characteristic. The masses are large, averaging about 10 cm in diameter and are sharply delineated from the normal renal parenchyma. They are hypovascular but the septations show enhancement after injection of intravenous contrast medium (Fig. 12.8). When large cysts are present the internal septations are well defined (Madewell et al 1983). If the cysts are small, the mass may have a pitted appearance (Parienty et al 1981).

Multilocular cystic nephroma must be differentiated from a cystic renal adenocarcinoma. Although adenocarcinoma arising in this condition has been reported, Madewell et al (1983) believe that these cases are multiloculated renal adenocarcinomas and the pathological features of multilocular cystic nephroma are not present.

Radiological imaging studies are not adequate to exclude malignancy and further evaluation is needed. Cyst aspiration is usually inadequate as the locules do not communicate and an excessive number of punctures would be required to evaluate all portions of the lesion. Thus, surgical excision is indicated.

Since multilocular cystic nephroma is a benign lesion and the diagnosis can often be suggested preoperatively, local excision may be appropriate. Frozen section should be obtained, however, to exclude malignancy. If malignant tissue is seen, a radical nephrectomy should be performed.

HYDATID DISEASE

Hydatid disease in man is usually due to *Echinococcus granulosus* but may also be caused by *Echinococcus multilocularis*.

Hydatid cysts are composed of three layers: an outer protective pericyst, an easily broken middle membrane and a thin inner germinal layer which produces the scolices. The organs most commonly involved are the liver (75%) and lung (15%). Other organs, such as the brain, bone and the kidneys are infected in less than 10% of cases.

Although most hydatid cysts are acquired in childhood, they usually remain undetected until adulthood. The symptoms of renal hydatid disease are non-specific and many patients are asymptomatic. Flank pain, haematuria or signs of urinary tract infection may be present (Lewall & McCorkell 1986). A serological test is available for patients suspected of having hydatid disease, either on the basis of contact or radiological findings.

Curvilinear calcifications in the wall of the hydatid cyst may be detected on plain radiographs. A hypovascular mass is detected with urography but the thick rim distinguishes the hydatid cyst from a simple cortical cyst.

Thick-walled cysts are also well demonstrated by either CT or ultrasound (Beggs 1985). If daughter cysts are present, they can be detected by ultrasound or CT as soft tissue components next to the clear water density of cyst fluid.

CONCLUSION

Renal cystic disease encompasses a wide range of congenital and acquired lesions that have been identified more frequently during recent years due to the increased use of non-invasive imaging. Although many of these cystic masses can be adequately categorized with ultrasound, CT is required for evaluation of those lesions in which the ultrasound diagnosis is not conclusive. Incidental renal cystic lesions are sometimes found on CT carried out for other purposes and knowledge of their CT characteristics is required for differential diagnosis. CT is the method of choice for assessing renal cystic disease in patients with longstanding renal failure.

REFERENCES

Banner M P, Pollack H M, Chatten J, Witzleben C 1981 Multilocular renal cysts: radiologic–pathologic correlation. American Journal of Roentgenology 136: 239–247
Beggs I 1985 The radiology of hydatid disease. American Journal of Roentgenology 145: 639–648
Bosniak M A 1986 The current radiological approach to renal cysts. Radiology 158: 1–10
Cho C, Friedland G W, Swenson R S 1984 Acquired renal cystic disease and renal neoplasms in hemodialysis patients. Urologic Radiology 6: 153–157
Coleman B G, Arger P H, Mintz M C, Pollack H M, Banner M P 1984 Hyperdense renal masses: a computed tomographic dilemma. American Journal of Roentgenology 143: 291–294

Cronan J J, Yoder I C, Amis E S Jr, Pfister R C 1982 The myth of anechoic renal sinus fat. Radiology 144: 149–152
de Wall J G, Schroder F H, Scholtmeijer R J 1986 Diagnostic workup and treatment of multilocular cystic kidney. Urology 28: 73–77
Dunnick N R, Korobkin M, Clark W M 1984b CT demonstration of hyperdense renal carcinoma. Journal of Computer Assisted Tomography 8: 1023–1024
Dunnick N R, Korobkin M, Silverman P M, Foster W L Jr 1984a Computed tomography of high density renal cysts. Journal of Computer Assisted Tomography 8: 458–461
Friedland G W 1987 Shrinking and disappearing renal cysts. Urologic Radiology 9: 21–25
Hidalgo H, Dunnick N R, Rosenberg E R, Ram P C, Korobkin M 1982 Parapelvic cysts: appearance on CT and sonography. American Journal of Roentgenology 138: 667–671
Kleiner B, Filly R A, Mack L, Callen P W 1986 Multicystic dysplastic kidney: observations of contralateral disease in the fetal population. Radiology 161: 27–29
Lee J K T, McClennan B L, Kissane J M 1978 Unilateral polycystic kidney disease. American Journal of Roentgenology 130: 1165–1167
Levine E, Cook L T, Grantham J J 1985 Liver cysts in autosomal-dominant polycystic kidney disease: clinical and computed tomographic study. American Journal of Roentgenology 145: 229–233
Levine E, Grantham J J 1985 High-density renal cysts in autosomal dominant polycystic kidney disease demonstrated by CT. Radiology 154: 477–482
Levine E, Grantham J J 1987 Perinephric hemorrhage in autosomal dominant polycystic kidney disease: CT and MR findings. Journal of Computer Assisted Tomography 11: 108–111
Levine E, Grantham J J, Slusher S L, Greathouse J L, Krohn B P 1984 CT of acquired cystic kidney disease and renal tumours in long-term dialysis patients. American Journal of Roentgenology 142: 125–131
Lewall D B, McCorkell S J 1986 Rupture of echinococcal cysts: diagnosis, classification and clinical implications. American Journal of Roentgenology 146: 391–394
Madewell J E, Goldman S M, Davis C J, Hartman D S, Feigin D S, Lichtenstein J E 1983 Multilocular cystic nephroma: a radiographic-pathologic correlation of 58 patients. Radiology 146: 309–321
McCallum R W, Gildiner M 1981 Diminished visualization of renal outlines in adult renal polycystic disease. Journal of the Canadian Association of Radiology 32: 13–16
Papanicolaou N, Pfister R C, Yoder I C 1986 Spontaneous and traumatic rupture of renal cysts: diagnosis and outcome. Radiology 160: 99–103
Parienty R A, Pradel J, Imbert M C, Picard J D, Savart P 1981 Computed tomography of multilocular cystic nephroma. Radiology 140: 135–139
Pedicelli G, Jequier S, Bowen A, Boisvert J 1986 Multicystic dysplastic kidneys: spontaneous regression demonstrated with US. Radiology 161: 23–26
Rosenberg E R, Korobkin M, Foster W, Silverman P M, Bowie J D, Dunnick N R 1985 The significance of septations in a renal cyst. American Journal of Roentgenology 144: 593–595
Sanders R, Hartman D 1984 The sonographic distinction between neonatal multicystic kidney and hydronephrosis. Radiology 151: 621–625
Segal A J, Spataro R F 1982 Computed tomography of adult polycystic disease. Journal of Computer Assisted Tomography 6: 777–780
Sussman S, Cochran S T, Pagani J J et al 1984 Hyperdense renal masses: a CT manifestation of hemorrhagic renal cysts. Radiology 150: 207–211

13. Solid renal masses

Rodney H. Reznek

INTRODUCTION

CT is a highly reliable technique for establishing the solid nature of a focal renal mass. Most masses considered indeterminate by ultrasound can be characterized using CT and this is the major reason for referral. With modern CT technology small incidental solid renal masses are also being detected with increasing frequency in patients undergoing abdominal CT examinations.

RENAL-CELL CARCINOMA

Once a renal mass is identified on intravenous urography, ultrasound is performed to determine whether the mass is cystic or solid. The kidneys are scanned with CT either if the mass is considered indeterminate on ultrasound or for staging if the mass is solid and presumed to be a renal carcinoma.

Bilateral tumours have been described in < 2% of patients with renal adenocarcinoma and half of them are bilateral at presentation (Bracken 1987).

CT appearances

On unenhanced scans a renal-cell carcinoma usually has a density equal to, or slightly less than, normal renal parenchyma and the interface between the tumour and normal tissue is generally ill-defined. The mass may appear inhomogeneous due to varying amounts of tumour haemorrhage or necrosis and central amorphous calcification is common. Large tumours alter the renal contour but small isodense and uncalcified tumours may not be visible on unenhanced scans. Most frequently the pattern of enhancement is patchy. However, occasionally the tumour may be avascular and therefore does not enhance or there may be uniform dense uptake of contrast medium. As on unenhanced scans the interface between the tumour and surrounding parenchyma is indistinct.

Cystic malignant neoplasms account for 5–7% of all renal cancers

(Parienty et al 1985). CT is undertaken when ultrasound shows an atypical cyst requiring further diagnostic evaluation. On CT, malignancy is suspected if the attenuation values of the contents of the cyst are higher than those of a simple cyst and if its wall is thick and irregular. The wall, which enhances to a lesser degree than normal parenchyma, should be actively sought, particularly when the cyst lies adjacent to normal renal tissue.

Small renal neoplasms

CT is far more sensitive than intravenous urography or ultrasound for identifying renal neoplasms smaller than 3 cm in diameter (Curry et al 1986). It has been suggested that almost as many renal cancers are detected incidentally as those identified in patients with symptoms (Bracken 1987, Amendola et al 1988).

The diagnosis of small renal tumours may pose problems for CT because partial volume averaging may falsely increase attenuation values, thus a cyst may be misinterpreted as a solid mass. To some extent this difficulty can be overcome by using thin slices (2–5 mm). Any evidence of enhancement indicates a solid vascular lesion.

Occasionally the first clinical manifestation of a tumour is a spontaneous haemorrhage into the subcapsular and perirenal spacc (Davidson 1985a). CT readily shows the haematoma as a high-density perirenal collection and usually identifies the underlying cortical tumour.

Staging of renal cancer

The most widely used staging scheme of Robson et al (1969) is shown in (Table 13.1).

Vascular invasion

Assessment of renal vein and inferior vena caval invasion is critical to planning the surgical approach. If the inferior vena cava is involved care must be taken to ensure that the upper extent of the tumour is delineated (Fig. 13.1). In particular, the relationship between the entrance of the

Table 13.1 Staging of renal cancer (Robson et al 1969)

Stage	Description
Stage I	Neoplasm confined within the renal capsule
Stage II	Tumour invasion of perinephric fat but confined by Gerota's fascia
Stage IIIA	Invasion of renal vein or inferior vena cava
Stage IIIB	Regional lymph-node involvement
Stage IVA	Invasion of adjacent organ (excluding adrenal gland)
Stage IVB	Distant metastases

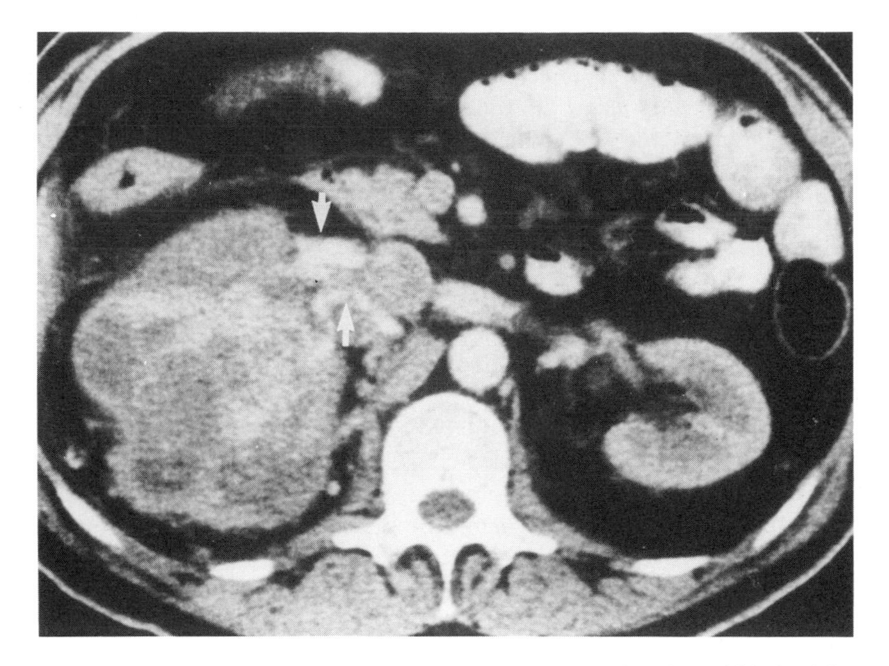

Fig. 13.1 Renal carcinoma of the right kidney showing tumour thrombus within the right renal vein and inferior vena cava. Multiple enhancing collateral vessels can also be seen (arrowed).

hepatic veins into the vena cava and the tumour within the cava must be ascertained. When the tumour is below this point, thrombectomy can be performed through an incision that allows control of the vena cava above and below the thrombus. Tumour extending to or above the hepatic veins, or into the heart is more safely resected with cardiopulmonary bypass.

Renal vein involvement should be assessed using careful dynamic scanning with bolus injection of intravenous contrast material. Intraluminal defects within the opacified veins are the only reliable evidence of tumour. Venous dilatation alone cannot be considered as diagnostic of renal vein invasion because highly vascular lesions may cause dilatation of the artery and vein. The right renal vein is frequently short and oblique and may be particularly difficult to visualize. Nevertheless, using thin collimation and dynamic CT, renal vein involvement can be detected in $> 95\%$ of cases (Zeman et al 1988).

Vena caval involvement is often easy to detect as a filling defect in the inferior vena cava. About 75% of tumours which involve the vena cava are right sided, presumably due to the short course of the right renal vein (Marshall 1984). Difficulty in interpretation may arise, particularly on the right side, because the tumour mass may compress the vena cava and be misinterpreted as tumour within the cava.

Laminar flow defects can also be misleading. Rapid injection of contrast medium may result in opacification of the renal veins before enhancement of the inferior vena cava. Opacified renal venous return surrounds the unopacified caval blood producing a ‘pseudothrombus’. If this occurs, delayed scans through the cava should resolve the problem.

Direct tumour extension

Extension of tumour into the perinephric fat should only be diagnosed when there is a mass of >1 cm in the perinephric space. Thickening of Gerota’s fascia and irregular perinephric soft tissue strands are not reliable criteria of tumour extension as these appearances may also be caused by a resolving haematoma, oedema or dilated collateral vessels.

CT is ideal for showing direct invasion of adjacent muscles (psoas, quadratus lumborum, erector spinae and the diaphragm), and adjacent organs. Enlargement and/or change in density of the muscle must be present before invasion is diagnosed, since loss of fat planes is not necessarily a sign of invasion. Tumour growth usually occurs by displacing adjacent structures and it is unusual for renal carcinoma to directly infiltrate organs (Bracken 1987).

Nodal involvement

At surgery about 20% of patients will have lymph-node involvement. Left-sided tumours spread via the lymphatics to periaortic lymph nodes. Right-sided tumours spread to hilar, perivenacaval and interaortico-caval lymph-nodes. Occasionally, iliac nodes are involved, probably due to lymphatic obstruction causing retrograde spread down the periureteral lymphatics (Marshall 1984).

Lymph nodes >2 cm in diameter almost always contain tumour. Tumour involvement of nodes reduces survival by half as compared with Stage I disease, even if radical resection with lymphadenectomy is performed (Zeman et al 1985).

Accuracy

CT has proved more accurate than angiography for assessing renal vein and vena cava involvement, perirenal extension and lymph node involvement (Weyman et al 1980). The overall accuracy of CT in staging renal carcinoma is currently at least 90–92% (Levine 1987, Zeman et al 1988).

In a recent study using dynamic scanning with thin slices, ipsilateral renal vein involvement was detected in 94% of patients (Zeman et al 1988). Ultrasound is also highly specific for diagnosing venous invasion but is less accurate for assessing perinephric invasion, adjacent muscle and nodal involvement (Webb et al 1987).

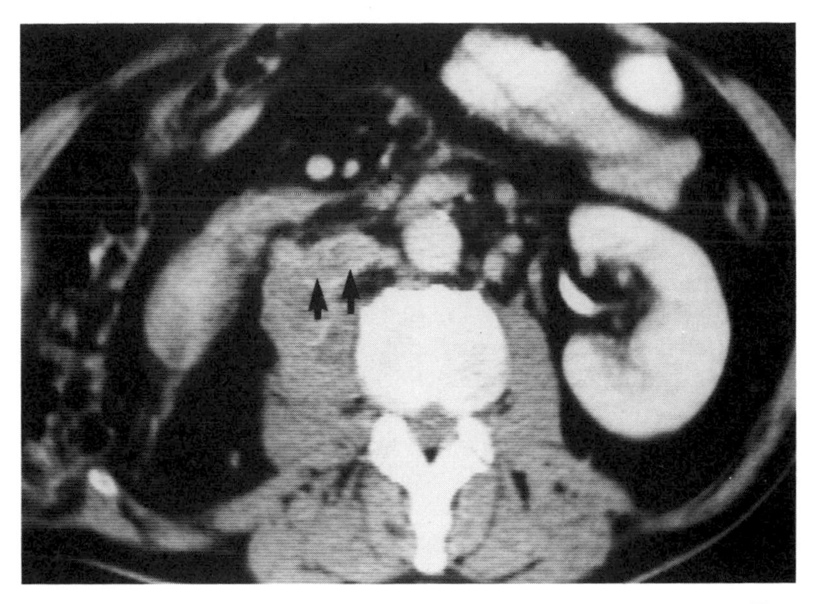

Fig. 13.2 Recurrence of tumour following right nephrectomy for renal carcinoma. Tumour thrombus within the inferior vena cava (arrows).

Postoperative assessment

Early detection of recurrence before it becomes clinically apparent may improve survival by permitting easy resection. CT is ideally suited to the follow-up of patients who have undergone nephrectomy. The use of ultrasound is limited by bowel loops which frequently fill the renal fossa. The tail of the pancreas and spleen may also occupy this area. The features which suggest recurrence on CT are a soft-tissue mass in the renal fossa, together with enlargement or irregularity of the contour of the ipsilateral psoas muscle (Fig. 13.2). Postoperative fibrosis or even an abscess can mimic recurrence.

OTHER MALIGNANT RENAL NEOPLASMS

Renal lymphoma, metastases, transitional-cell carcinomas and Wilms' tumours are the most common other forms of malignant renal neoplasms. Sarcomas account for only about 1% of renal malignancies and there are no specific features to distinguish them from other tumours unless they contain bone or fat (Pollack et al 1987).

Renal lymphoma

Renal involvement is much more frequent in non-Hodgkin's lymphoma than in Hodgkin's disease and may be identified in up to 33% of autopsies.

However, on CT, carried out for routine staging, it is only detected in up to 6% of patients. Renal lymphoma rarely causes impairment of renal function and it is unlikely to be the first manifestation of disease.

CT appearances

The most common CT appearances (30–40% of cases) are multiple, discrete renal masses which have similar features to renal-cell carcinomas. They may be unilateral or bilateral and vary in size from 1 to 5 cm (Pollack et al 1987, Reznek et al 1988). In 15–20% of patients the mass is solitary. In about 10% of patients global enlargement of one or both kidneys is seen. The majority of patients with intrinsic renal lymphoma do not have evidence of retroperitoneal lymph-node enlargement, irrespective of whether renal involvement is diagnosed at the time of presentation or recurrence (Reznek et al 1988). Direct invasion of one or both kidneys by adjacent retroperitoneal masses accounts for about 25% of cases. In most cases lymphomatous tissue infiltrates directly into the renal parenchyma but occasionally the perinephric space or renal sinus may be invaded without evidence of renal parenchymal involvement.

Renal metastases

At post-mortem the most common malignant renal neoplasm is a metastasis. They usually occur late in the course of the disease and few cause symptoms.

The majority of tumours which occur secondary to melanoma, lung and breast carcinoma are multiple and tend to be < 3 cm in diameter. Bilateral involvement is seen in 50% of cases. Metastases from the gastrointestinal tract, especially the colon, tend to be large and may mimic renal-cell carcinoma.

Metastases seldom distort the renal outline and central necrosis and calcification are uncommon. For these reasons, the appearance of metastases may be subtle on unenhanced scans but after injection of intravenous contrast medium they do enhance slightly, appearing as areas of low attenuation compared with normal enhancing parenchyma (Choyke et al 1987). Contrast-enhanced CT is the most sensitive technique available for demonstrating metastases (Choyke et al 1987, Pollack et al 1987).

Transitional-cell carcinomas

Although transitional-cell carcinoma generally appears as a filling defect within the collecting system, occasionally it is bulky, infiltrative and mimics renal-cell carcinoma (Ambos et al 1977). However, unlike renal-cell carcinoma, transitional-cell carcinoma spreads by infiltration, preserving the renal outline.

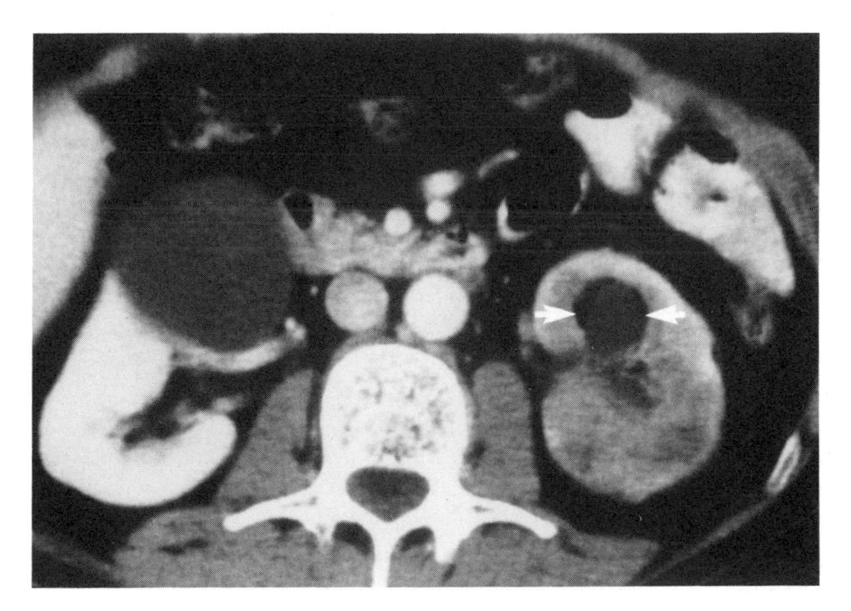

Fig. 13.3 Transitional-cell tumour infiltrating the left kidney and preserving the renal outline shown here after contrast enhancement injection. There is an associated dilated calyx (arrowed) and a large right renal cyst.

Since these tumours arise from the pelvicalyceal system, they usually appear as solid masses in the region of the renal sinus on CT (Fig. 13.3). After contrast medium injection, normal parenchyma is often seen enveloping the central poorly enhancing tumour. An associated dilated calyx is common. All these features suggest a transitional-cell carcinoma rather than a renal-cell carcinoma. CT reliably demonstrates extrarenal extension, venous involvement and local nodal invasion. Involvement of the pararenal space occurs most commonly at the renal hilum (Gatewood et al 1984).

Wilms' tumour

The peak age incidence for Wilms' tumour is between 30 months and 3 years (Kirks et al 1987). The vast majority of Wilms' tumours are sporadic but at least 1% are familial and 5% are bilateral.

The characteristic appearance on CT is of a low attenuation soft-tissue intrarenal mass which is well defined and frequently has a pseudocapsule. It may contain calcification and cystic areas caused by haemorrhage and necrosis (Fig. 13.4). Fibrous stroma and a varying amount of fat may also be present within the mass.

Evaluation of the extent of tumour is important for planning surgery, determining prognosis and assessing response. CT is substantially more

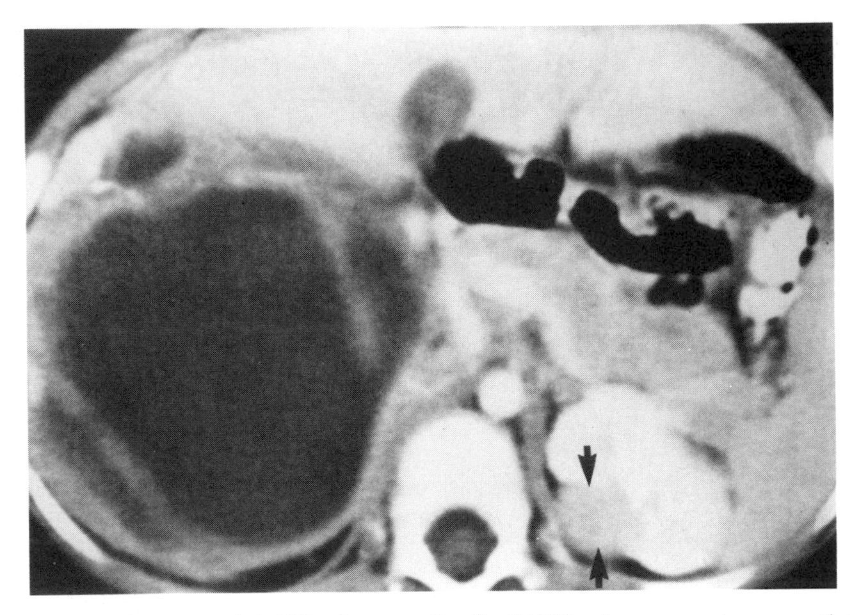

Fig. 13.4 Large cystic right Wilms' tumour. Small solid Wilms' tumour can be seen on the posterior aspect of the left kidney (arrowed).

accurate than ultrasound for assessing perinephric extension and nodal involvement (Siegel et al 1982, Reiman et al 1986). A limiting factor with CT is the difficulty encountered in the detection of involved nodes in children with minimal retroperitoneal fat. Good results have been achieved with both CT and ultrasound for detecting inferior vena caval invasion.

Most authorities recommend ultrasound as the initial screening investigation to evaluate an abdominal mass in children and CT for staging if ultrasound suggests a Wilms' tumour. CT is also superior for evaluating the contralateral kidney (Reiman et al 1986) (Fig. 13.4).

Lung metastases are present at the time of diagnosis in 8–15% of children and CT should be undertaken even if the conventional chest radiograph is normal (Kirks et al 1987).

BENIGN RENAL TUMOURS

Angiomyolipoma

Angiomyolipoma most commonly occurs as an isolated unilateral lesion in young women, although there is a high incidence of this tumour (80%) in patients with tuberous sclerosis. The sensitive detection of fat by CT makes accurate diagnosis possible and thus obviates the need for surgery in the majority of patients (Fig. 13.5).

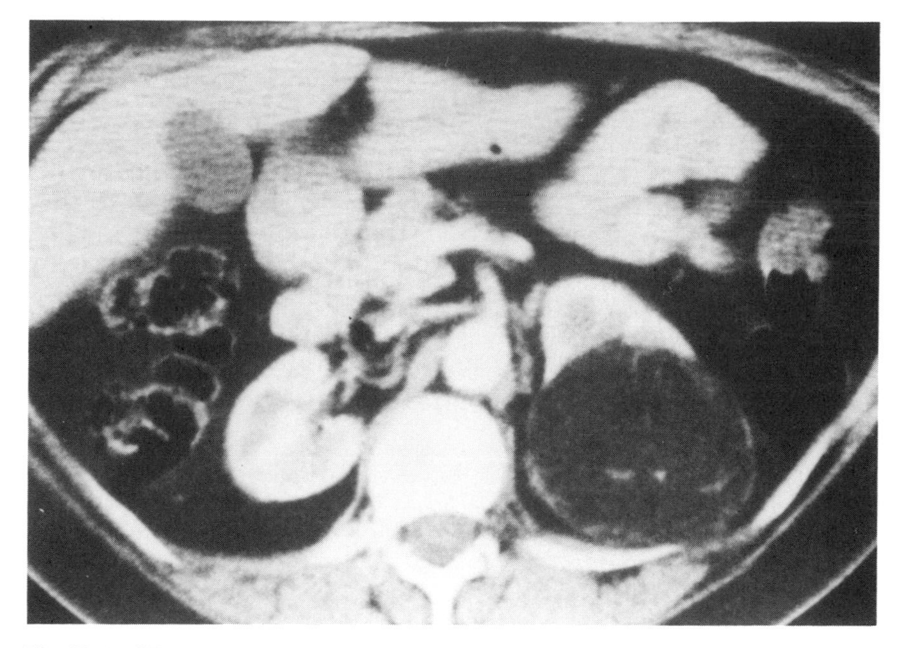

Fig. 13.5 CT scan showing a well-circumscribed angiomyolipoma of the left kidney, sharply demarcated from the renal parenchyma, non-enhancing with strands of soft tissue intermingled within the mass.

Typically, the lesion is a well circumscribed, fat-containing mass totally or partially confined to the renal parenchyma and sharply demarcated from it (Fig. 13.5). An extrarenal pattern of growth occurs in about 25% of cases; the tumour blends with the perirenal fat and the lateral extent of the lesion cannot be established (Saksouk et al 1984). The fatty component usually predominates and shows a density similar to normal subcutaneous or retroperitoneal fat. The smooth muscle and vascular components are seen as strands of soft-tissue density intermingled within the mass. Rarely, the lesion has insufficient fat to be characterized on CT and will appear as a solid mass. In this situation malignancy cannot be excluded.

For small lesions < 2 cm in diameter the use of 2–5 mm CT overlapping slices on unenhanced scans usually allows the fat content to be appreciated. This is important because identification of fat within a renal mass excludes the possibility of a renal-cell carcinoma (Saksouk et al 1984).

Occasionally, the CT diagnosis of angiomyolipoma is not clearcut. Haemorrhage within the lesion may mask the fat component and the diagnosis on CT is then impossible. Rarely, renal angiomyolipoma may involve regional lymph nodes and mimic metastatic malignancy (Harrison & Dyer 1987). Confusion can also be caused when the stromal content of Wilms' tumour contains enough fat to be recognized on CT (Fishman & Garfinkel 1984).

Other benign neoplasms

In general, benign tumours are small lesions which do not distort either the internal architecture or the contour of the kidney. They include adenomas, fibromas, myomas and angiomas. Although adenomas are considered to be benign there is some doubt about their true nature and histologically they may be indistinguishable from a renal-cell carcinoma (Harrison & Dyer 1987). Oncocytoma is an adenoma arising from the proximal tubular cells.

A benign tumour appears on CT as a focal mass with a distinct margin, smooth contour and an homogeneous internal structure. Most are isodense with normal renal parenchyma on unenhanced scans but an oncocytoma may contain a central stellate scar (Quinn et al 1984). Enhancement following contrast medium injection is homogeneous and less dense than the surrounding parenchyma.

Inflammatory mass lesions

Acute focal bacterial nephritis

Bacterial infection of the renal parenchyma may result in a sequence of changes from a solid parenchymal mass (acute focal bacterial nephritis) to suppuration and abscess formation (Harrison & Dyer 1987). CT can accurately demonstrate these changes. 80% of renal and perirenal abscesses develop by direct extension from the renal pelvis and

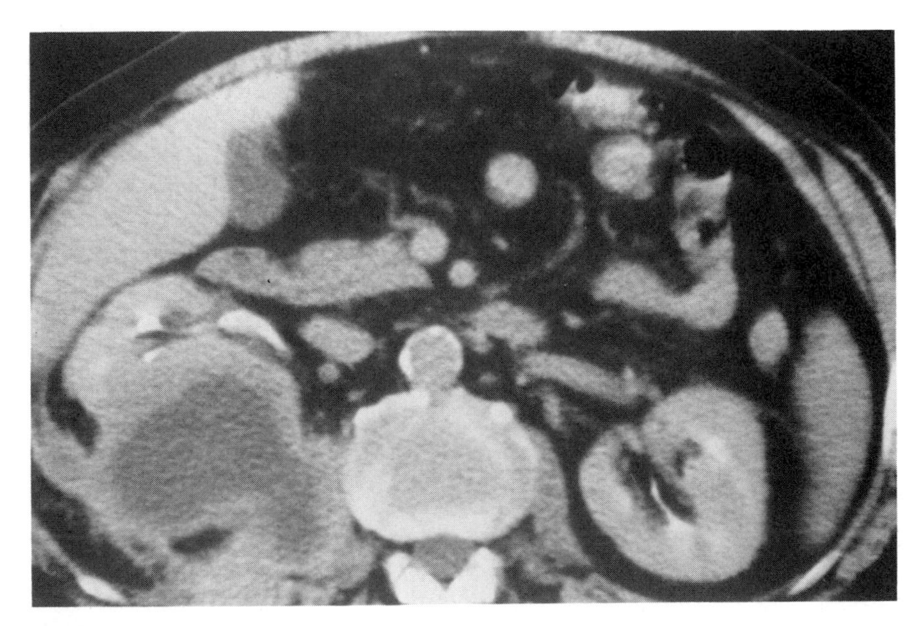

Fig. 13.6 Right renal abscess with thick, irregular enhancing walls and central low-density contents, extending into the psoas and quadratus lumborum muscles.

most are associated with calculus obstruction of the renal pelvis (Davidson 1985b).

The clinical presentation may be surprisingly non-specific with only minimal fever and leucocytosis and up to 20% of abscesses have negative urinalysis and culture (Morehouse et al 1986). In such patients, distinction from malignancy may be difficult.

The mass in focal bacterial nephritis is usually poorly defined, lobar in distribution and often wedge-shaped. It is of relatively low density and enhances inhomogeneously, often with a striated appearance after contrast medium injection. At this stage the lesion cannot be drained. Necrosis and suppuration will lead to a renal abscess if treatment is ineffective.

Renal abscess

Renal abscesses are usually well defined with irregular thick walls which enhance after contrast medium injection in about 50% of cases (Harrison & Dyer 1987) (Fig. 13.6). The contents of an abscess do not enhance and gas bubbles within the mass are unusual (Morehouse et al 1986). An abscess is often accompanied by fascial thickening with perirenal and pararenal extension of the inflammatory process. Frequently the appearance of an abscess is very similar to a renal-cell cancer with central necrosis. Needle aspiration is almost always indicated for diagnostic purposes. CT may also be used to guide catheter drainage.

Xanthogranulomatous pyelonephritis

Xanthogranulomatous pyelonephritis develops as a complication of chronic infection in a collecting system which has been partially obstructed for a long time, usually by a stone. Most commonly, the whole kidney is involved and appears enlarged with dilated calyces containing material of attenuation values slightly less than, or similar to, that of water. The renal pelvis is contracted and in > 75% a stone is seen. Less commonly, the disease is localized, affecting a single calyx or group of calyces. On CT, thinning of the parenchyma is seen around the dilated calyces and this often enhances intensely with contrast medium, probably reflecting the inflammatory nature of the tissue in the calyceal wall and renal parenchyma.

CONCLUSION

CT has been welcomed by clinicians and radiologists alike because it is a highly accurate method of detecting and evaluating solid renal masses. Although in some patients inflammatory solid renal masses can be distinguished from malignant tumours, particularly if the clinical findings are taken into account, confirmation by needle aspiration is required.

Another limitation of CT is the inability to distinguish a small renal-cell carcinoma from a benign lesion and in these patients surgery is mandatory. CT is the best method currently available for staging renal-cell carcinoma and for assessing postoperative recurrence.

REFERENCES

Ambos M A, Bosniak M A, Madayag M A, Lefleur R S 1977 Infiltrating neoplasms of the kidney. American Journal of Roentgenology 129: 859–864

Amendola M A, Ree R L, Pollack H M et al 1988 Small renal carcinomas: resolving a diagnostic dilemma. Radiology 166: 637–641

Bracken R B 1987 Renal carcinoma: clinical aspects and therapy. Seminars in Roentgenology 22: 241–247

Choyke P L, White M E, Zeman R K, Jaffe M H, Clark L R 1987 Renal metastases: clinico-pathological and radiologic correlation. Radiology 162: 359–363

Curry N S, Schabel S I, Betsill W C 1986 Small renal neoplasms: diagnostic imaging, pathologic features and clinical course. Radiology 158: 113–117

Davidson A J 1985a Diagnostic set: large unifocal, unilateral. In: Davidson A J (ed) Radiology of the Kidney. W B Saunders, Philadelphia, p 350

Davidson A J 1985b Diagnostic set: large unifocal unilateral. In: Davidson A J (ed) Radiology of the Kidney. W B Saunders, Philadelphia, p 365

Fishman E K, Garfinkel D J 1984 Computed tomography of Wilms' tumour. In: Siegelman S S, Gatewood O M B, Goldman S M (eds) Computed Tomography of the Kidneys and Adrenals. Contemporary Issues in Computed Tomography. Churchill Livingstone, New York, pp 145–158

Gatewood O W B, Goldman S M, Marshall F F, Siegelman S S 1984 Computed tomography of transitional-cell carcinoma of the kidney. In: Siegelman S S, Gatewood O M B, Goldman S M (eds) Computed Tomography of the Kidneys and Adrenals. Contemporary Issues in Computed Tomography. Churchill Livingstone, New York, pp 81–112

Harrison R B, Dyer R 1987 Benign space occupying conditions of the kidney. Seminars in Roentgenology 22: 275–283

Kirks D R, Kaufman R A, Babcock D S 1987 Renal neoplasms in infants and children. Seminars in Roentgenology 22: 292–302

Levine E 1987 Renal-cell carcinoma: radiological diagnosis and staging. Seminars in Roentgenology 22: 248–259

Marshall F F 1984 Adult renal carcinomas—clinical and surgical considerations. In: Siegelman S S, Gatewood O M B, Goldman S M (eds) Computed Tomography of the Kidneys and Adrenals. Contemporary Issues in Computed Tomography. Churchill Livingstone, New York, pp 31–50

Morehouse H T, Weiner S N, Hoffman-Tretin J C 1986 Inflammatory disease of the kidney. Seminars in Ultrasound, CT and MR 7: 246–259

Parienty R A, Pradel J, Parienty I 1985 Cystic renal cancers: CT characteristics. Radiology 157: 741–744

Pollack H M, Banner M P, Amendola M A 1987 Other malignant neoplasms of the renal parenchyma. Seminars in Roentgenology 22: 260–274

Quinn M J, Hartman D S, Friedman A C et al 1984 Renal oncocytoma: new observations. Radiology 153: 49–53

Reiman T A H, Siegel M J, Shackleford G D 1986 Wilms' tumour in children: abdominal CT and ultrasound evaluation. Radiology 160: 501–505

Reznek R H, Webb J A W, Mootoosamy I, Richards M A 1988 Computed tomography in renal and perirenal lymphoma. British Journal of Radiology 61: 775

Robson C J, Churchill B M, Anderson W 1969 The results of radical nephrectomy for renal-cell carcinoma. Journal of Urology 101: 297–301

Saksouk F A, Fishman E K, Siegelman S S 1984 Computed tomography of angiomyolipoma. In: Siegelman S S, Gatewood O M B, Goldman S M (eds) Computed Tomography of the Kidneys and Adrenals. Contemporary Issues in Computed Tomography. Churchill Livingstone, New York, pp 69–80

Siegel M J, Balfe D M, McClennan B L, Levitt R G 1982 Clinical utility of CT in paediatric

retroperitoneal disease: five years' experience. American Journal of Roentgenology 138: 1011–1017
Webb J A W, Murray A, Bary P R, Hendry W F 1987 The accuracy and limitations of ultrasound in the assessment of venous extension in renal carcinoma. British Journal of Urology 60: 14–17
Weyman P J, McClennan B L, Stanley R J, Levitt R G, Sagel S S 1980 Comparison of computed tomography and angiography in evaluation of renal-call carcinoma. Radiology 137: 417–424
Zeman R K, Cronan J J, Rosenfield A T et al 1985 Imaging approach to the suspected renal mass. Radiologic Clinics of North America 23: 503–529
Zeman R K, Cronan J J, Rosenfield A T, Lynch J H, Jaffe M A, Clark L R 1988 Renal-cell carcinoma: dynamic thin section CT assessment of vascular invasion and tumour vascularity. Radiology 167: 393–396

14. Adrenal imaging

T. H. M. Falke and A. P. van Seters

INTRODUCTION

CT has been the most significant advance in successful visualization of adrenal gland morphology and it is now generally agreed that CT should be used as the initial screening procedure to visualize adrenal gland disorders. The major limitations of CT include difficulty in identifying tumours < 5 mm in diameter and the inability to distinguish small benign masses from malignancy.

ANATOMY

Each adrenal gland lies in the perinephric space, is firmly attached to Gerota's fascia by fibrous bands and is usually separated from the kidney by an intervening capsule.

The adult adrenal gland has a tripartite structure consisting of head, body and tail, and portions of the gland extend laterally to form the alae. The head of the adrenal gland is the most caudal part.

The shape of the normal adult adrenal shows considerable variation on cross-section depending on slice orientation and level of imaging (Wilms et al 1979) (Fig. 14.1).

Right adrenal gland

The right adrenal gland is situated above the upper pole of the right kidney and posterior to the inferior vena cava. Cranially and laterally the gland is in close relation with the posterior segment of the right lobe of the liver. The right adrenal is triangular and has a smooth anterior surface. The anteroposterior axis of the gland courses parallel to the crus of the diaphragm in an oblique plane, angulated 45° with respect to the sagittal plane. The tail of the right adrenal gland is visualized on the most cephalad slices. Adrenal pseudomasses may be simulated on an imaging modality by the close anatomical relationship of normal or diseased surrounding structures, such as the inferior vena cava, upper pole of the right kidney or the gallbladder (Florijn et al 1980, Papanicolaou & Pfister 1985).

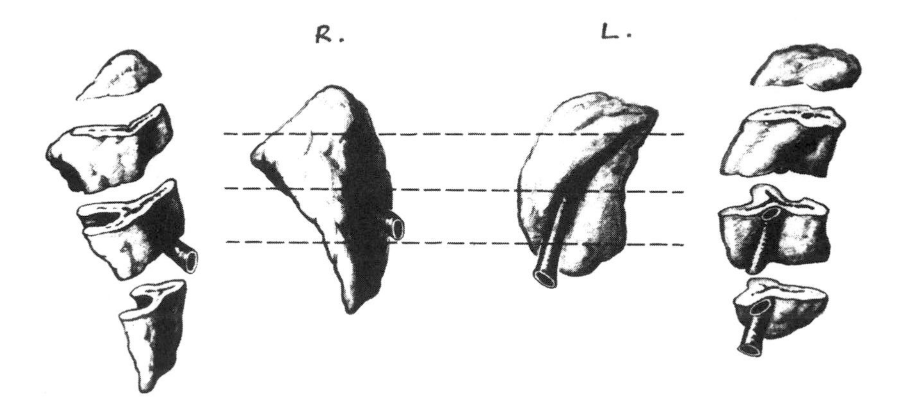

Fig. 14.1 Diagrammatic illustration showing the shape of the normal adult adrenal gland on cross-section.

Left adrenal gland

The left adrenal gland is situated posterior to the splenic vessels and is most often visualized at the level of the pancreatic tail. The head of the left gland is situated anteromedially to the left kidney just above the renal vein and is visualized at a slightly lower level than the head of the right adrenal gland. The left gland is elongated and crescent shaped, with a groove on the anterior surface from which the main suprarenal vein emerges. The course of the left adrenal gland is usually not parallel to the diaphragm. The fundus of the stomach lies anteriorly and cranially to the tail of the left adrenal gland. The close relationship of the adrenal gland to surrounding structures may lead to errors of interpretation. Thus, pancreatic masses, an aneurysm of the splenic artery, an accessory spleen or the upper pole of the left kidney may all be misinterpreted as adrenal masses (Berliner et al 1982).

ADRENAL FUNCTION

The principal steroid hormones are synthesized from a common precursor, (cholesterol) and the hormones so derived are secreted from the three concentric zones of the adrenal cortex; whereas the adrenal medulla produces and secretes the principal catecholamine epinephrine which is derived from the amino acid tyrosine.

The zona glomerulosa (zG) is the outermost zone of the adrenal cortex and cells from this region secrete aldosterone (Neville & O'Hare 1979).

The innermost zones of the adrenal cortex, the zona fasciculata (zF) and the zona reticularis (zR) are responsible for the biosynthesis and secretion of cortisol and the adrenal androgens, dehydroepiandrosterone and androstenedione respectively (Neville & O'Hare 1979).

ENDOCRINE CONDITIONS

Pathology of the adrenal cortex

Cushing's syndrome

The diagnosis of Cushing's syndrome is confirmed by elevated serum cortisol levels and sustained cortisol values following low-dose dexamethasone suppression. The syndrome may be produced by adrenal cortical hyperplasia in response to increased adrenocorticotrophic hormone (ACTH) plasma levels (81%), adrenal adenoma (8–12%) or adrenal carcinoma (8–12%) (Gross et al 1988). ACTH-dependent Cushing's syndrome is usually pituitary driven and in a minority of cases is caused by ectopic ACTH secretion. Ectopic products of ACTH may result from various tumours including oat-cell carcinoma of the lung, pancreatic islet-cell tumour, carcinoid, medullary carcinoma of the thyroid and thymoma (White et al 1982, Howlett et al 1986). Biochemical studies, including determination of plasma ACTH levels and response to high-dose dexamethasone, can be used to separate pituitary-driven Cushing's syndrome and ectopic ACTH-producing tumours from cortisol-producing adrenal neoplasias. The greatest difficulty encountered in establishing a diagnosis through biochemical analysis is the differentiation of pituitary Cushing's disease from ectopic ACTH-producing occult tumours.

The main role of diagnostic imaging of the adrenal gland in Cushing's syndrome is the localization or exclusion of a unilateral adrenal mass (functioning adenoma or carcinoma). Most cortisol-producing adrenal masses are >2 cm in diameter and are therefore well within the range of the spatial resolution of CT (Moss 1983). The absence of a mass on CT almost automatically indicates ACTH-dependent Cushing's disease. However, the presence of a mass on CT may indicate a number of other possibilities. These include an incidental silent adrenal mass, ACTH-producing phaeochromocytoma and a metastasis from an ACTH-producing occult lung carcinoma. In about 20–23% of pituitary-driven Cushing's syndrome bilateral nodular hyperplasia is present. Such cases present a possible pitfall because they may simulate a focal adenoma on CT (Falke et al 1984). Unilateral or bilateral masses encountered in familial Cushing's syndrome due to micronodular adrenocortical dysplasia are too small to be visualized with CT.

In ACTH-dependent Cushing's syndrome adrenal imaging can be helpful to exclude an adrenal tumour and to demonstrate adrenal hyperplasia. Gross enlargement of the glands is suggestive of ectopic ACTH production whereas macronodular hyperplasia points towards pituitary-driven Cushing's syndrome (Doppman et al 1988). In addition, CT may demonstrate a pituitary adenoma or an occult tumour in the thorax or abdomen.

On CT an adenoma usually appears as a well-defined homogeneous mass with a diameter of 2 to 3 cm (Fig. 14.2).

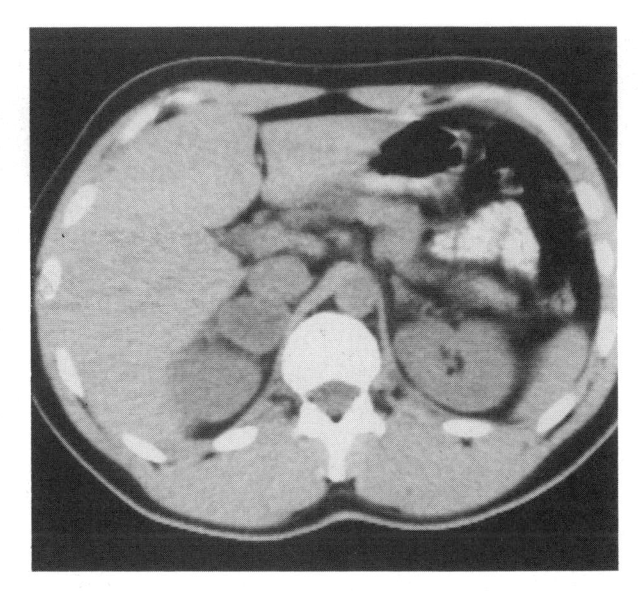

Fig. 14.2 CT scan shows right adrenal adenoma in a patient with Cushing's syndrome.

Hyperplasia results in bilateral adrenal gland enlargement. The shape of the normal gland is maintained and the attenuation values are similar to that of normal soft tissue.

Macroscopic nodular hyperplasia is also bilateral but the glands are irregular in shape and if large enough can be readily identified on CT (Fig. 14.3).

Primary hyperaldosteronism

Primary hyperaldosteronism (Conn's syndrome) is a clinical syndrome that is characterized by excessive production of aldosterone, low plasma renin levels and hypertension. Aetiologies include single aldosterone-producing adenoma (approximately 70%) or bilateral adrenocortical hyperplasia (15–30%) (Vetter et al 1985). In rare cases, primary aldosteronism is caused by macronodular hyperplasia, multiple aldosterone-producing adenomas, extra-adrenal adenoma and unilateral hyperplasia. Adrenal carcinoma producing primary hyperaldosteronism has been reported but is also extremely rare. Postural plasma aldosterone and 18-OH-corticosterone tests provide an indication as to whether the patient has idiopathic hyperplasia or adrenal adenoma.

The main role of CT in the evaluation of patients with primary hyperaldosteronism is the detection of an adenoma (or adenocarcinoma) since these patients with primary hyperaldosteronism caused by tumours can be cured by surgery (Vetter et al 1985).

The average size of aldosteronomas is 1.5 cm and these can be readily

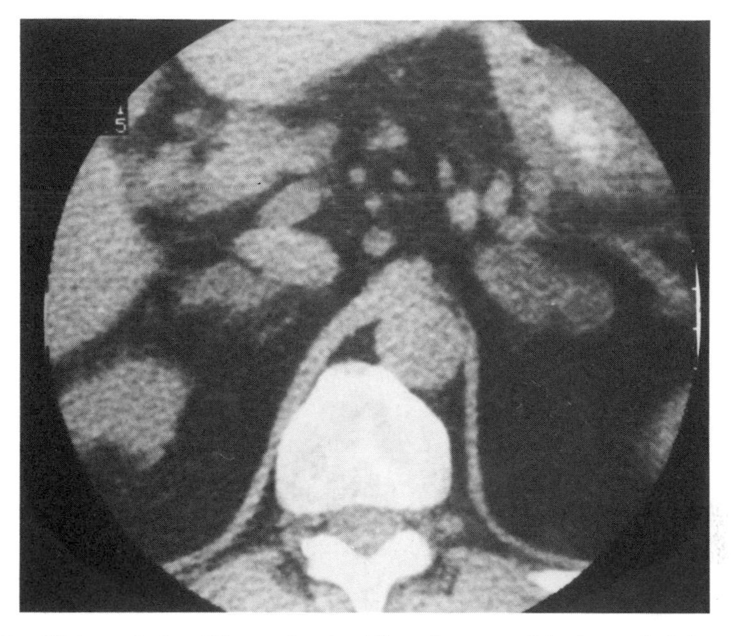

Fig. 14.3 High-resolution CT scan showing bilateral macronodular hyperplasia in Cushing's disease.

shown with CT with an accuracy greater than 83% (Moss 1983) (Fig. 14.4). Most lesions that are missed on CT have a diameter no greater than 1.2 cm and account for about 15–20% of the aldosteronomas (Balkin et al 1985). The inability of CT to detect some of these very small aldosteronomas may necessitate venous sampling (Dunnick et al 1982). Although a small solitary mass of very low density is highly suggestive of an aldosteronoma this finding is inconstant and a small soft-tissue density aldosteronoma cannot be differentiated from a silent adenoma or macronodular hyperplasia (Falke et al 1984).

Primary aldosteronism due to macronodular hyperplasia may occur in a small percentage of cases. Some of the nodules may become large enough to simulate a focal adenoma on CT (Falke et al 1984).

Virilism

In children the clinical picture of virilizing states include (intra-uterine) virilization in females and pseudo pubertas praecox in males. These syndromes are caused by congenital adrenocortical hyperplasia, adrenal adenoma, adrenocortical carcinoma as well as extra-adrenal pathology (e.g. idiopathic polycystic ovary syndrome).

Imaging of both the adrenal and gonadal areas may be required for preoperative diagnosis and localization.

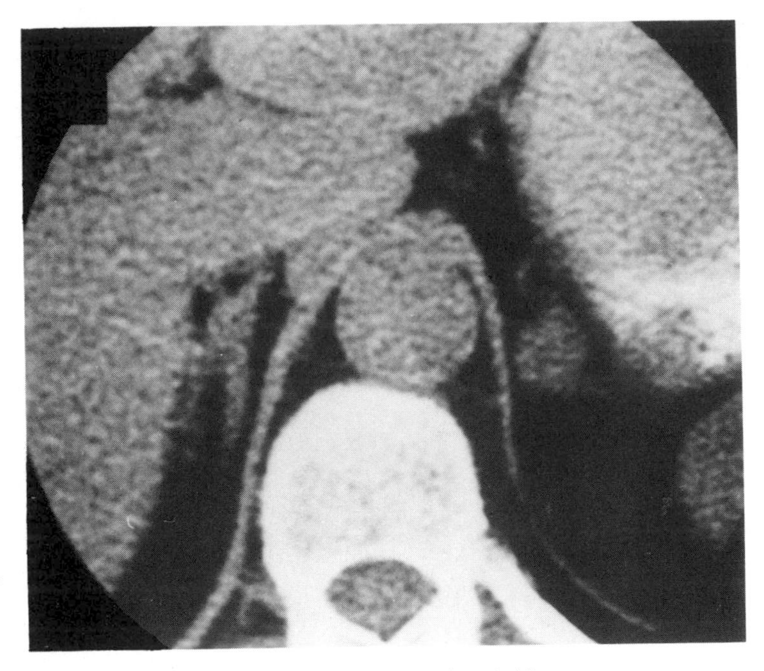

Fig. 14.4 High-resolution CT scan showing a left adrenal aldosteronoma.

Carcinoma

The presenting signs and symptoms of malignant adrenocortical tumours depend on the nature of steroid overproduction, the size of the tumour and the presence of metastases, as well as the sex and age of the patient (Dunnick et al 1982). Among the 'functioning' carcinomas the following syndromes can be recognized: Cushing's syndrome (36%), Cushing's syndrome with virilization (20%), virilization (24%), feminization (6%), mineralocorticoid excess (rarely without overproduction of other steroids) in less than 1%. The remaining tumours are clinically silent and are often referred to as 'non-functioning carcinomas' (13%) (van Slooten et al 1985).

The majority of the carcinomas are large enough to be visualized by conventional radiographic methods such as plain abdominal films or intravenous urography (van Slooten et al 1985). The role of CT is the determination of the adrenal origin of the tumour and the evaluation of tumour extent in relation to surrounding structures (Fig. 14.5). In addition, distant metastases in the liver, lung and bone may be identified.

On CT an adrenal carcinoma appears as a large mass containing areas of low density resulting from haemorrhage and necrosis. Calcification is sometimes seen. A small percentage of tumours invade the inferior vena cava, usually through invasion of the adrenal vein. This can be diagnosed on CT with intravenous contrast medium using dynamic scanning. The

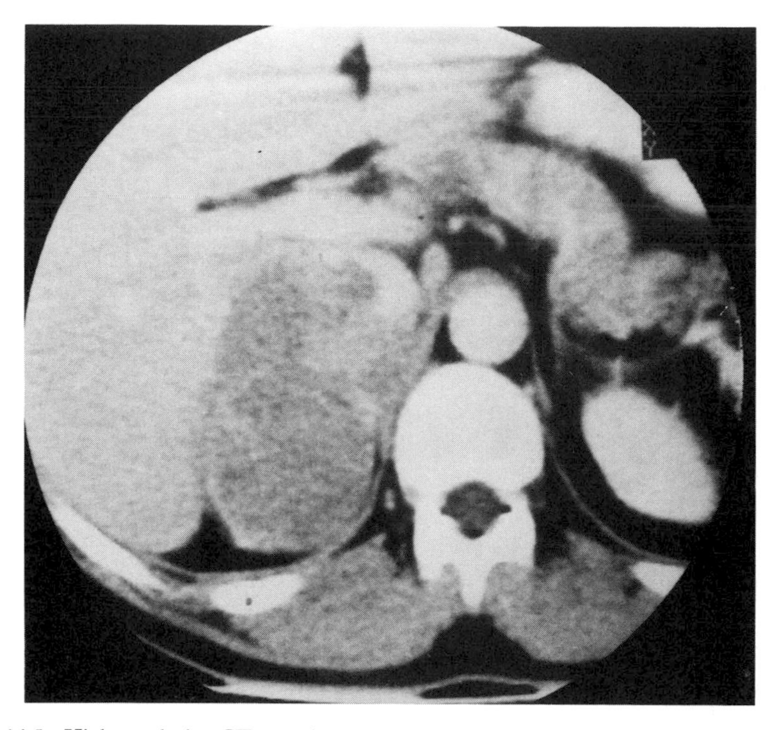

Fig. 14.5 High-resolution CT scan showing a right adrenocortical carcinoma invading the inferior vena cava.

presence of inferior vena caval involvement still warrants surgical resection since complete removal of the thrombus is often feasible (Didier et al 1987).

Cortical disease with hypoadrenalism

Chronic destructive disease Chronic primary hypoadrenalism is a rare condition and in western countries is usually caused by so-called idiopathic atrophy (autoimmune adrenalitis). Up to the 1950s destruction of the adrenal cortex by tuberculosis was the most common cause (Vita et al 1985). Other causes for chronic primary hypoadrenalism are metastatic cancer, Hodgkin's disease, sarcoidosis, amyloidosis, haemorrhage, haemochromatosis and fungal infection (Halvorsen et al 1982, Vita et al 1985, Doppman et al 1988). In contrast to idiopathic atrophy and longstanding tuberculosis, these latter causes are associated with adrenal enlargement.

The main role of CT in patients with chronic primary hypoadrenalism is to detect potentially treatable disease. The presence of adrenal calcification excludes idiopathic adrenal atrophy. Small glands generally indicate either idiopathic atrophy or longstanding tuberculosis and enlarged glands usually indicate early tuberculosis although malignancy should also be considered.

Pathology of the adrenal medulla

Phaeochromocytoma

Phaeochromocytoma occurs in about 0.1% of hypertensive patients. Although the diagnosis of phaeochromocytoma is normally suspected by clinical symptoms (sweating, tachycardia and headache), the features are non-specific and variable. Patients with a phaeochromocytoma usually display various elevated patterns of urine and plasma catecholamines and their metabolites. Symptoms of catecholamine excess may be absent and an occasional patient may have normal or equivocal catecholamine levels. Even when strict criteria are applied for the diagnosis of phaeochromocytoma a substantial number of patients not suffering from the condition will inevitably be imaged (Shapiro et al 1985). The situation is further complicated because silent adenomas are seen with an increased frequency in patients with hypertension.

In adults 90% of the phaeochromocytomas are located in one adrenal gland and 10% occur bilaterally. Most ectopic phaeochromocytomas are located in the abdomen (90%) almost invariably in the pre-aortic ganglia in the vicinity of the renal hilum. Unusual locations include the chest and urinary bladder (Bravo & Gifford 1984). The incidence of malignant phaeochromocytomas is 10% and frequent sites of metastases are bone, lymph nodes, lung and liver. Malignant venous involvement into the inferior vena cava may occur by direct invasion through the venous wall or by extension along the adrenal veins.

The importance of the detection of phaeochromocytomas lies in the fact that hypertension, caused by phaeochromocytoma, is surgically curable in the majority of patients but if unrecognized carries very high morbidity and mortality.

As the majority of phaeochromocytomas are about 5–6 cm in diameter and located in the adrenal gland or adrenal area most of them are detected on CT (Welch et al 1983, Blickman & Falke 1985). They appear as soft-

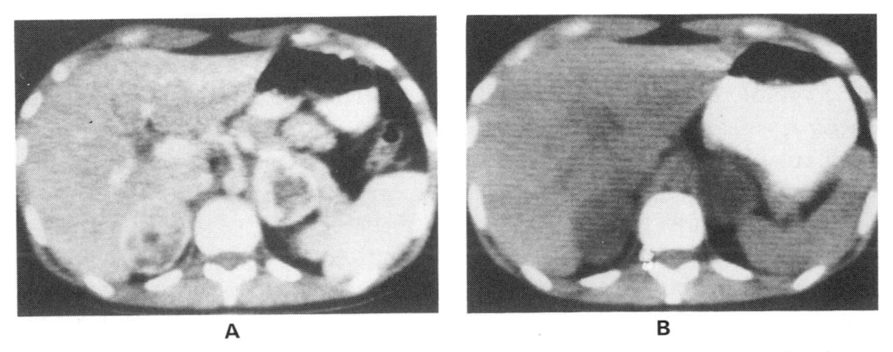

Fig. 14.6 Bilateral adrenal phaeochromocytoma. **A** Before contrast enhancement. **B** After contrast enhancement.

tissue masses which frequently contain an area of central low density. After injection of intravenous contrast medium peripheral enhancement of the thick rim is seen (Fig. 14.6). The accuracy of CT for detecting phaeochromocytomas is approximately 96% (Moss 1983).

In patients with associated neurocristopathies (MEN II syndrome, neurofibromatosis and von Hippel-Lindau syndrome) the incidence of adrenal and extra-adrenal phaeochromocytomas is high. In MEN II syndrome the adrenals are usually involved by bilateral medullary nodular hypertrophy (Cho et al 1980) which may be visible on CT as diffuse adrenal enlargement.

Neuroblastoma and ganglioneuroma

Neuroblastoma is a common tumour in children under 5 years old (85%). Prognosis depends on the age of the child but is usually poor after the neonatal period. Differentiation to a more benign ganglioneuroma may occur and all intermediate levels of differentiation between the neuroblastoma and ganglioneuroma are referred to as ganglioneuroblastoma. The tumours arise from primordial neural crest cells and are found in a variety of locations, the adrenal medulla or adjacent retroperitoneum accounting for the origin of 50–80% of them.

CT is indispensable for diagnosing these tumours (Siegel et al 1982). The technique demonstrates the extent of the primary tumour and thus, provides valuable information for predicting resectability.

SILENT ADRENAL DISORDERS

Silent adenomas

The incidence of silent adenomas at autopsy ranges from 3% for macronodules to 66% for microscopic nodules (Neville 1978). Large nodules with a diameter of 1–3 cm are reported as incidental findings in 0.6–1% of routine upper abdominal CT studies (Mitnick et al 1983) (Fig. 14.7). There is an increased incidence of silent adenomas in patients with lung cancer but CT is unable to distinguish a silent adenoma from an adrenal metastasis and biopy is required if a definitive diagnosis is crucial to patient management (Oliver et al 1984).

Adrenal cyst

Cysts may be of any size and in most instances are unilateral. Adrenal cysts are usually incidental findings on CT or ultrasound. Large cysts are occasionally complicated by haemorrhage which may result in the onset of acute symptoms (Fig. 14.8). An aldosteronoma with unusually low

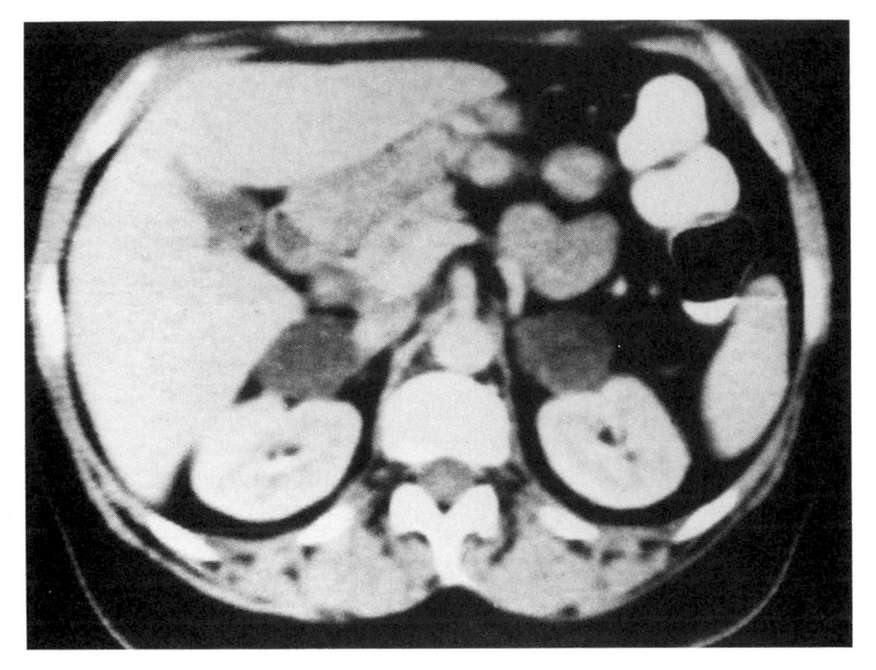

Fig. 14.7 Contrast-enhanced CT scan demonstrates bilateral silent adenomas incidentally discovered in a patient with a suspected malignancy in the digestive tract. There is no enhancement of the lesions.

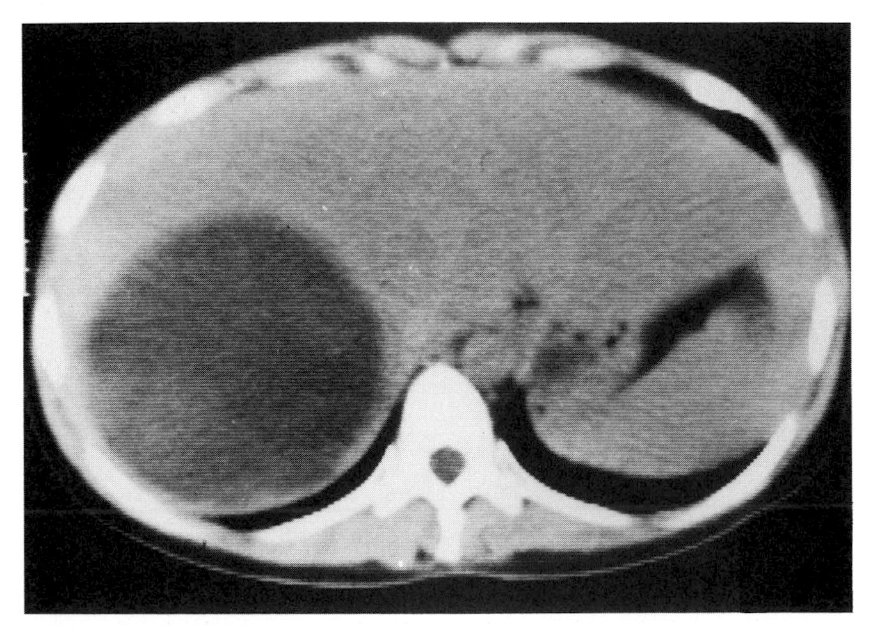

Fig. 14.8 Right adrenal cyst in a patient with acute onset of symptoms.

attenuation values, caused by a high lipid content, may simulate a cystic lesion (Schaner et al 1978).

Angiomyolipoma

Adrenal angiomyolipomas are benign tumours which are comprised of fat and bone marrow elements. An angiomyolipoma containing macroscopic quantities of non-fatty material (such as blood, calcium or myeloid tissue) may have a non-specific appearance on CT if fat is not detectable (Vick et al 1984). Before CT and ultrasound small angiomyolipomas were rarely discovered but large tumours may bleed giving rise to clinical symptoms (Liebman & Srikantaswamy 1981). Angiomyolipomas may be associated with endocrine abnormalities (e.g. Addison's disease, Cushing's disease and Conn's syndrome).

Lymphoma

Involvement of the adrenals by lymphomatous tissue is common with an incidence of 24.9% in reported autopsy series. The glands are enlarged and may retain their normal shape or become round/oval masses similar to other adrenal tumours (Jafri et al 1983).

Metastases

The adrenals are a common site for metastasis. Among the various primary tumours from which they originate the most common are cancer of the lung, kidney, breast, digestive tract, melanoma and ovary. Adrenal metastases are usually clinically silent and seldom cause hypoadrenalism due to parenchymal destruction (Meyer et al 1983).

CONCLUSION

CT has made a dramatic impact on imaging the adrenal glands. The technique reliably detects adrenal masses down to the size of about 1 cm and the demonstration of normal adrenal glands excludes a mass. CT is complementary to biochemical analysis in patients with hormone-secreting syndromes, frequently identifying the nature and cause of the underlying pathology.

REFERENCES

Balkin P W, Hollifield J W, Winn S D, Shaff M I 1985 Primary aldosteronism: computerized tomography preoperative evaluation. South Medical Journal 78: 1071–1074

Berliner L, Bosniak M A, Megibow A 1982 Adrenal pseudotumours on computed tomography. Journal of Computer Assisted Tomography 6: 281–285

Blickman J G, Falke T H M 1985 Computed tomography of pheochromocytoma. Annals of Radiology 28: 447–452
Bravo E L, Gifford R W 1984 Pheochromocytoma: diagnosis, localization and management. New England Journal of Medicine 311: 1298–1303
Cho K J, Freier D T, McCormick T et al 1980 Adrenal medullary disease in multiple endocrine neoplasia type II. American Journal of Roentgenology 134: 23–29
Didier D, Racle A, Etievent J P, Weill F 1987 Tumor thrombus of the inferior vena cava secondary to malignant abdominal neoplasms: US and CT evaluation. Radiology 162: 83–89
Doppman J L, Miller D L, Dwyer A L et al 1988 Macronodular adrenal hyperplasia in Cushing disease. Radiology 166: 347–352
Dunnick N R, Doppman J L, Gill J R, Strott C A, Keiser H R, Brennan M F 1982 Localization of functional adrenal tumors by computed tomography and venous sampling. Radiology 142: 429–433
Falke T H M, te Strake L, van Seters A P 1984 CT of the adrenal glands: adenoma or hyperplasia? Radiology 153: 358
Florijn E, Falke T H M, Scholten E T 1980 Computed tomography of the adrenals. Diagnostic Imaging 49: 273–282
Gross M D, Shapiro B, Sandler M P, Falke T H M, Shaff M I 1988 Localization of adrenocortical and sympathomedullary disorders. In: Sandler M P (ed) Nuclear medicine, magnetic resonance imaging, computed tomography, ultrasonography. Williams & Wilkins, Baltimore (in press)
Halvorsen R A Jr, Heaston D K, Johnston W W, Ashton P R, Burton G M 1982 CT guided thin needle aspiration of adrenal blastomycosis. Journal of Computer Assisted Tomography 6: 389–391
Howlett T A, Drury P L, Perry L, Doniach I, Rees L H, Besser G M 1986 Diagnosis and management of ACTH-dependent Cushing's syndrome: comparison of the features in ectopic and pituitary production. Clinical Endocrinology 24: 699–713
Jafri S Z H, Francis I R, Glazer G M, Bree R L, Amendola M A 1983 CT detection of adrenal lymphoma. Journal of Computer Assisted Tomography 7: 254–256
Liebman R, Srikantaswamy S 1981 Adrenal myelolipomas demonstrated by computed tomography. Journal of Computer Assisted Tomography 5: 262–263
Meyer J E, Halperin E C, Levene S R, Stomper P C 1983 Adrenal insufficiency secondary to metastatic lung carcinoma: CT aided diagnosis. Journal of Computer Assisted Tomography 7: 1107–1108
Mitnick J S, Bosniak M A, Megibow A J, Naidich D P 1983 Non-functioning adrenal adenomas discovered incidentally on computed tomography. Radiology 148: 495–499
Moss A A 1983 Computed tomography of the adrenal glands. In: Moss A A, Gamsu G, Genant H K (eds) Computed Tomography of the Body. W B Saunders, Philadelphia, pp 837–876
Neville A M 1978 The nodular adrenal. Investigative Cell Pathology 1: 99–111
Neville A M, O'Hare M J 1979 Aspects of structure, function and pathology. In: James V H T (ed) The Adrenal Glands. Raven Press, New York, pp 1–15
Oliver T W Jr, Bernardino M E, Miller J I, Mansour K, Greene D, Davis W A 1984 Isolated adrenal masses in non-small-cell bronchogenic carcinoma. Radiology 153: 217–218
Papanicolaou N, Pfister R C 1985 Adrenal pseudotumor: gallbladder simulating a right adrenal mass. CT: The Journal of Computerized Tomography 9: 171–172
Schaner E G, Dunnick N R, Doppman J L, Strott C A, Gill J R Jr, Javadpour N 1978 Adrenal cortical tumors with low attenuation coefficients: a pitfall in computed tomography diagnosis. Journal of Computer Assisted Tomography 2: 11–15
Shapiro B, Copp J E, Sisson J C, Eyre P L, Wallis J, Beierwaltes W H 1985 Iodine-131 Metaiodobenzylguanidine for the locating of suspected pheochromocytoma: experience in 400 cases. Journal of Nuclear Medicine 26: 576–585
Siegel M J, Balfe D M, McClennan B L, Levitt R G 1982 Clinical utility of CT in pediatric retroperitoneal disease: 5 years experience. American Journal of Roentgenology 138: 1011–1017
van Slooten H, Schaberg A, Smeenk D, Moolenaar A J 1985 Morphologic characteristics of benign and malignant adrenocortical tumors. Cancer 55: 766–774
Vetter H, Fischer M, Galanski M et al 1985 Primary aldosteronism: diagnosis and noninvasive lateralization procedures. Cardiology 72: 57–63

Vick C W, Zeman R K, Mannes E, Cronan J J, Walsh J W 1984 Adrenal myelolipoma: CT and ultrasound findings. Urologic Radiology 6: 7–13

Vita J A, Silverberg S J, Goland R S, Austin J H M, Knowlton A I 1985 Clinical clues to the cause of Addison's disease. American Journal of Medicine 78: 461–466

Welch T J, Sheedy P F II, van Heerden J A, Sheps S G, Hattery R R, Stephens D H 1983 Pheochromocytoma: value of computed tomography. Radiology 148: 501–503

White F E, White M C, Drury P L, Fry I K, Besser G M 1982 Value of computed tomography of the abdomen and chest in investigation of Cushing's syndrome. British Medical Journal 284: 771–774

Wilms G E, Baert A L, Marcal G, Goddeeris P G 1979 Computed tomography of normal adrenal glands: correlative study with autopsy specimens. Journal of Computer Assisted Tomography 3: 467–469

15. Blunt abdominal trauma

James W. Walsh

INTRODUCTION

Including both accidental and intentional injuries, physical trauma is the principal cause of death among Americans during the first four decades of life. 10% of trauma deaths occurring annually in the United States are secondary to abdominal injury. Since many patients are victims of multiple injuries, the clinical signs and symptoms of the abdominal component of the injury may be masked by more obvious or compelling injuries elsewhere.

CT is a rapid, comprehensive and accurate non-invasive imaging technique for evaluating the abdominal viscera, retroperitoneum, abdominal wall and pelvis (Federle 1983, Kaufman et al 1984, Federle & Brant-Zawadzki 1986, McCort 1987). CT has largely replaced scintigraphy and ultrasound for diagnosing the presence and extent of blunt abdominal injuries and the technique often has an immediate impact on individual patient care. Arteriography retains a role in imaging of renal vascular injury (Haynes et al 1984, Lang et al 1985), lumbar and iliac artery injury associated with lumbar and pelvic fractures (Sclafini et al 1987) and transcatheter embolization of arterial bleeding sites.

PATIENT SELECTION AND INDICATIONS

Unstable patients with penetrating abdominal wounds or blunt trauma accompanied by hypovolaemic shock or peritonitis are taken directly to surgery. CT is reserved for high-risk, but haemodynamically stable, patients with blunt abdominal trauma. Clinical guidelines to select patients for abdominal CT include:

1. Severe blunt trauma with multiple injuries.
2. Unexplained hypotension.
3. Positive abdominal physical examination.
4. Unreliable physical examination due to an altered sensorium or spinal injury.
5. Unreliable peritoneal lavage due to adhesions from previous surgery.
6. Positive lower chest-abdominal radiographs.

Laboratory guidelines for CT are:

1. Falling haemoglobin (usually 1–2 units).
2. Gross haematuria from a suspected renal cause.
3. Serum hyperamylasaemia.
4. Positive quantitative peritoneal lavage.

Although an elevated serum amylase may indicate a pancreatic injury it can also be associated with small bowel injury or salivary gland injury resulting from severe facial trauma. A positive quantitative peritoneal lavage is $> 100\,000$ RBC/mm^3 or > 500 WBC/mm^3. An elevated intraperitoneal white blood cell count usually indicates a traumatic bowel perforation despite a negative CT scan.

CT is also indicated as an emergency study to evaluate suspected injuries requiring immediate surgical intervention such as pancreatic transection, renal pedicle injury or intraperitoneal bladder rupture. Furthermore, emergency CT may be necessary to assess significant blood loss and hypotension associated with a ruptured spleen, liver or a Malgaigne pelvic fracture.

TECHNIQUE

Careful patient preparation and meticulous technique are vital to successful CT trauma imaging since some traumatic injuries such as linear parenchymal lacerations, pancreatic contusions or bowel and mesenteric injuries may be associated with rather subtle findings.

Oral contrast material can be administered by mouth or nasogastric tube in the emergency room while the patient is stabilizing and undergoing other evaluations. Most centres use 500–900 ml of dilute 2% barium suspension 30–45 minutes before CT examination. Placing obtunded patients in the right lateral decubitus position frequently helps to empty the stomach, fill the duodenum and opacify the small bowel. Water-soluble oral contrast medium is used when a bowel perforation is suspected.

Extraneous objects in the scan field such as ECG leads, intravenous lines and catheter clamps should be removed to prevent streak artefacts which degrade image quality and simulate fracture lines. It is also important to pull the nasogastric tube into the oesophagus, thereby preventing linear artefacts in the upper abdomen due to large air–barium interfaces in the stomach.

Intravenous contrast medium is necessary to maximize the difference between normal contrast-enhancing parenchyma and adjacent low-density lacerations or devascularized parenchyma and intermediate-density haematomas. Intravenous contrast medium is commonly administered as a 100–150 ml bolus of 60% iodine solution or as a 50 ml bolus followed by a rapid drip infusion of 300 ml 30% iodine solution. Many trauma centres now use a mechanical injector to infuse 150 ml of 60% contrast medium at

2–3 ml/sec through a large-bore needle combined with a dynamic study with rapid table incrementation.

The standard abdominal trauma study consists of 8–10 mm thick slices at contiguous 8–10 mm intervals from the domes of the diaphragm inferiorly through the kidneys. This comprehensive survey includes the liver, spleen, pancreas, duodenum and kidneys. In addition, the lower lung fields can be viewed for pneumothorax or haemothorax. In selected cases of suspected pancreatic injury, additional 5 mm slices may be necessary to better define the injury or to exclude fluid pseudotumours due to volume averaging of bowel. If significant lower retroperitoneal or pelvic haemorrhage is suspected, a survey CT can be continued inferiorly to the symphysis pubis at 1–2 cm intervals.

The trauma study can be tailored to include a spine study with a small scan field for lumbar spine fractures or thin sections through the pelvis for three-dimensional multiplanar reconstruction of acetabular fractures.

Finally, it is important to be aware of both a prior peritoneal lavage which affects CT evaluation of a haemoperitoneum and chest and pelvic injuries, which can cause air and fluid accumulations in the abdomen.

SPLEEN

The spleen is the most frequently injured organ in blunt abdominal trauma and is associated with injuries to other organs in 10–18% of cases. The CT manifestations of splenic injury are protean (Federle et al 1987). They include:

1. Haemoperitoneum.
2. Perisplenic blood clot.
3. Low-density linear fracture lines.
4. Blurred, irregular or disrupted splenic margin.
5. Intrasplenic haematoma.
6. Splenic fragmentation.
7. Heterogeneous parenchyma; and/or
8. Subcapsular haematoma.

Perisplenic clot is the most sensitive and specific sign of splenic trauma, even in the absence of visible splenic laceration (Federle et al 1987). Blood clot around the injured spleen differs in appearance from blood in the peritoneal cavity because it is denser (> 60 HU) and more heterogeneous (Fig. 15.1). Subcapsular splenic haematomas are relatively uncommon as an isolated finding but do occur in about 24% of blunt splenic injuries and are usually associated with haemoperitoneum and perisplenic clot. The characteristic CT findings are a crescentic or lentiform low-density fluid collection which flattens or indents the splenic contour and is slightly lower in density than normal contrast-enhanced parenchyma.

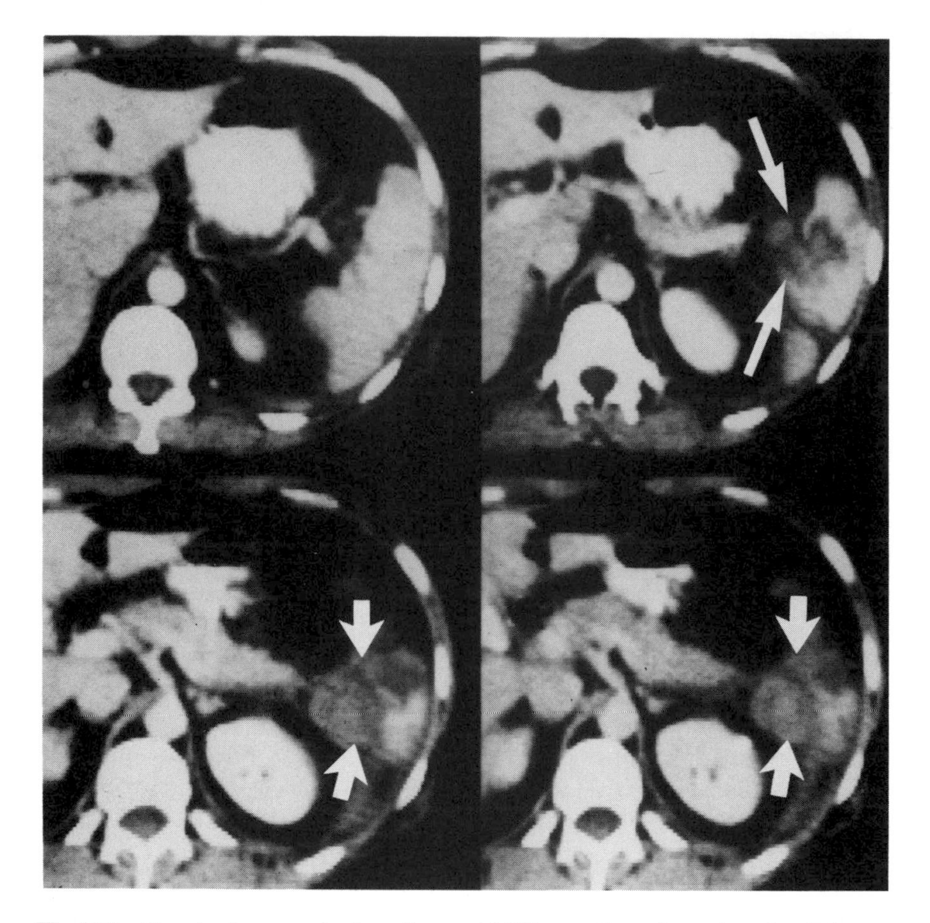

Fig. 15.1 Contained ruptured spleen. Sequential CT scans show disruption of medial splenic border and intrasplenic haematoma (narrow arrows) and inhomogeneous perisplenic blood clot (broad arrows) at inferior spleen tip. Patient treated conservatively after fluid resuscitation for hypotension on admission.

Several pitfalls in CT diagnosis of splenic trauma have been reported (Federle 1983). Normal congenital clefts in the superior, medial and lateral aspects of the spleen may simulate a fracture line. A long extension of the lateral segment of the left lobe of the liver may abut the spleen and be imaged as a thin cleft between these organs. Unlike true splenic lacerations, these anatomical variants are not associated with extracapsular blood collections. Hypotension during the acute trauma period may be associated with decreased splenic blood flow due to sympathetic stimulation and shunting of blood to other organs (Berland & Van Dyke 1985). CT scans through the spleen, during this period may show diffuse hypodensity (20 HU < liver) due to decreased splenic perfusion.

LIVER

Blunt hepatic trauma is the second most common type of intraperitoneal injury and the most common abdominal injury leading to death (10–20% mortality rate). Major burst-type hepatic injuries such as lobar fragmentation, transection and devitalization or 'explosive' liver rupture lead to life-threatening haemorrhage with gross haemoperitoneum and are treated with immediate laparotomy.

The most common liver injury evaluated with CT is an hepatic laceration (Federle 1983, Kaufman et al 1984, Stalker et al 1986). Another less frequent type of injury imaged with CT is a segmental or lobar injury which manifests itself as a large hypodense segment. This type of injury most frequently involves the posterior segment of the right lobe. Isolated subcapsular liver haematomas uncommonly result from blunt trauma. The above types of injury are usually managed conservatively. This is based on the size and extent of liver injury, the amount of associated haemoperitoneum and the clinical course. Surgery may be necessary during the acute injury period for continued haemorrhage, débridement of necrotic tissue and evacuation of large blood clots. Serial follow-up CT scans have become an integral part of conservative treatment and are useful for monitoring both resorption of haemoperitoneum and healing of intrahepatic haematomas, lacerations and fractures (Brick et al 1987, Foley et al 1987) (Fig. 15.2).

Two distinct types of hepatic lacerations may be visualized on CT. First, liver injuries due to compression or deceleration cause thin, linear, branching stellate fractures which parallel the portal or hepatic venous system or surround the intrahepatic inferior vena cava. This type of injury may simulate the CT appearance of dilated bile ducts or may be misinterpreted as normal low-density perivascular fat which marginates major vascular bifurcations. Clues to the CT diagnosis of stellate liver fractures are associated subtle collections of perihepatic haematoma or blood in the

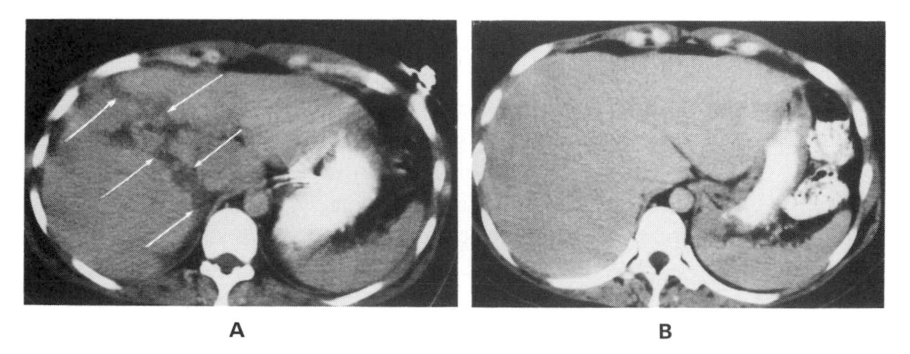

Fig. 15.2 Liver fracture. **A** Oblique liver laceration and fracture (arrows) across right and left lobes treated conservatively. **B** Follow-up CT 8 weeks later shows complete healing.

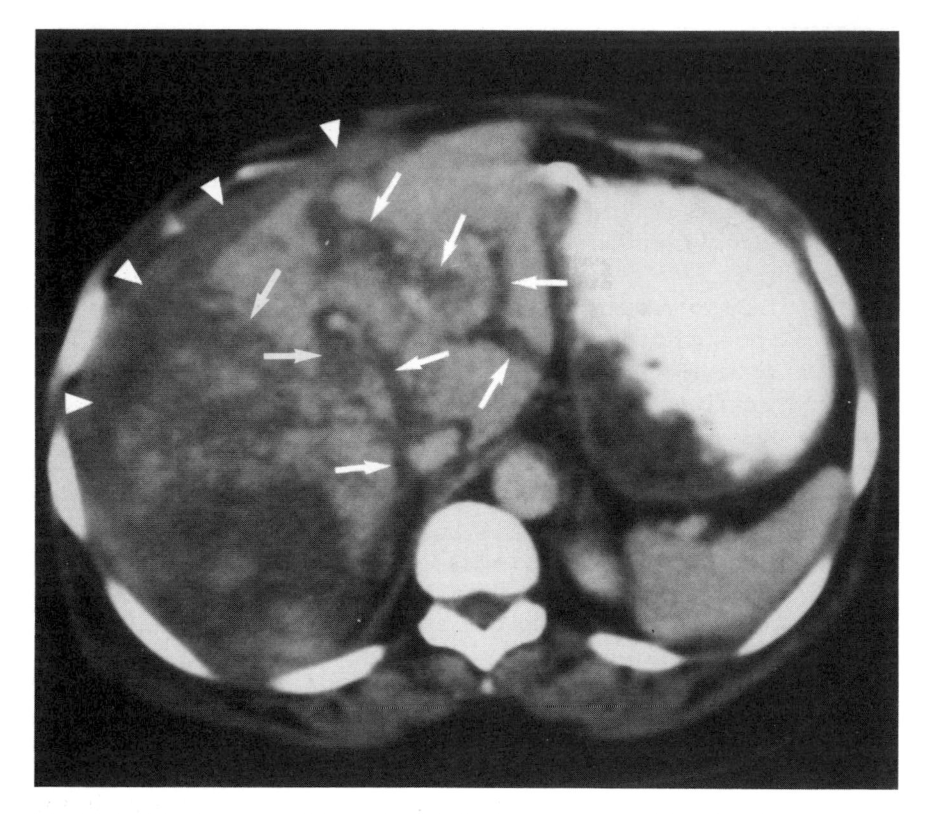

Fig. 15.3 Liver fractures. CT scan through the liver shows a myriad of linear lacerations (arrows) which extend to peripheral liver surfaces and parallel major blood vessels. Most of the right lobe is hypoperfused and there is a small perihepatic haematoma (arrowheads).

posterior subhepatic space. Lacerations which extend between two visceral surfaces indicate a discrete liver fracture (Fig. 15.2).

Secondly, direct blows to the liver tend to tear hepatic parenchyma and cause wide, jagged liver lacerations (Fig. 15.3). CT findings in this type of injury usually consist of irregular non-anatomical fissures or linear collections of low-density haemorrhage within hepatic parenchyma, frequently with small foci of high attenuation representing freshly clotted blood. Since hepatic lacerations may transgress intrahepatic bile ducts, round or oval low-density collections within the hepatic parenchyma may be due to bile pseudocysts or bilomas. Both infected post-traumatic liver haematomas and infected bilomas are amenable to successful percutaneous drainage.

Hepatic parenchymal gas may occur as a manifestation of severe blunt liver trauma without the presence of infection (Panicek et al 1986). Gas bubbles are usually orientated in a straight line along the shear plane of injury.

PANCREAS AND DUODENUM

The pancreas and duodenum are the two most commonly injured structures in the anterior pararenal space because they are located in a vulnerable paramedian position between the lumbar spine and the incoming anterior force. Although pancreatic injuries are uncommon and represent only 3–12% of all abdominal injuries, they are difficult to diagnose, frequently associated with injuries to adjacent organs and carry a mortality rate of 20%. Steering wheel injuries or direct blows to the epigastrium are the major causes of pancreatic trauma. The various types of pancreatic injury include contusion and haemorrhage, pancreatitis and pseudocyst formation, fracture with laceration of the main pancreatic duct and, rarely, complete transection of the gland (Federle 1983). The degree of serum amylase elevation is not commensurate with the degree of injury and significant injury may exist with no elevation at all.

Pancreas

CT diagnosis of pancreatic trauma is dependent upon a good technique with thin slices and recognition of relatively subtle CT findings. A diagnosis of pancreatic contusion or haematoma is made by recognizing a density change in the pancreatic parenchyma as well as focal enlargement. Pancreatic contusions may be hypodense due to oedema or hyperdense due to focal haemorrhage. Traumatic pancreatitis appears as diffuse or focal pancreatic swelling with inflammatory changes or fluid collections in the peripancreatic fat and retroperitoneal spaces. Thickening of the left anterior pararenal fascia may be an associated CT finding. Post-traumatic pseudocysts may form within a few days of traumatic laceration of a pancreatic duct. Pancreatic lacerations or fractures are recognized on CT as hypodense lines or clefts in the gland. Occasionally the plane of laceration may be obscured by internal haemorrhage or oedema. Endoscopic retrograde pancreatography may be necessary to confirm transection of the pancreatic duct.

Federle (1983) has emphasized several important pitfalls in pancreatic trauma diagnosis. Streak artefacts may impair visualization of the critical neck–body region which is the most common site of laceration. A false positive diagnosis of pancreatic laceration may also result from the presence of a vertical low-density plane through the neck of the pancreas. This relatively common normal finding is due to the combination of fat around the mesenteric vessels, physiological thinning of the pancreatic neck and unopacified proximal small bowel.

Unopacified fluid-filled small bowel loops adjacent to the pancreas may also be mistaken for the focal swelling of pancreatitis. Other causes of CT diagnostic errors include intraperitoneal fluid in the lesser sac from another organ injury (e.g. ruptured gallbladder) simulating pancreatitis and a haematoma from adjacent splenic or left renal trauma simulating pancreatic bleeding (Cook et al 1986).

Duodenum

Rupture of the duodenum, although rare, is most frequently seen after automobile accidents with blunt trauma to the upper abdomen. Retroperitoneal perforation is frequently not apparent clinically and delayed diagnosis of duodenal laceration results in a 35–65% mortality. The CT findings of duodenal injury are very subtle and images must be scrutinized carefully on sequential scans.

Oral contrast medium filling the whole of the duodenum is essential. CT diagnosis of duodenal rupture depends on the demonstration of small amounts of extraluminal air and fluid around the second and third portions

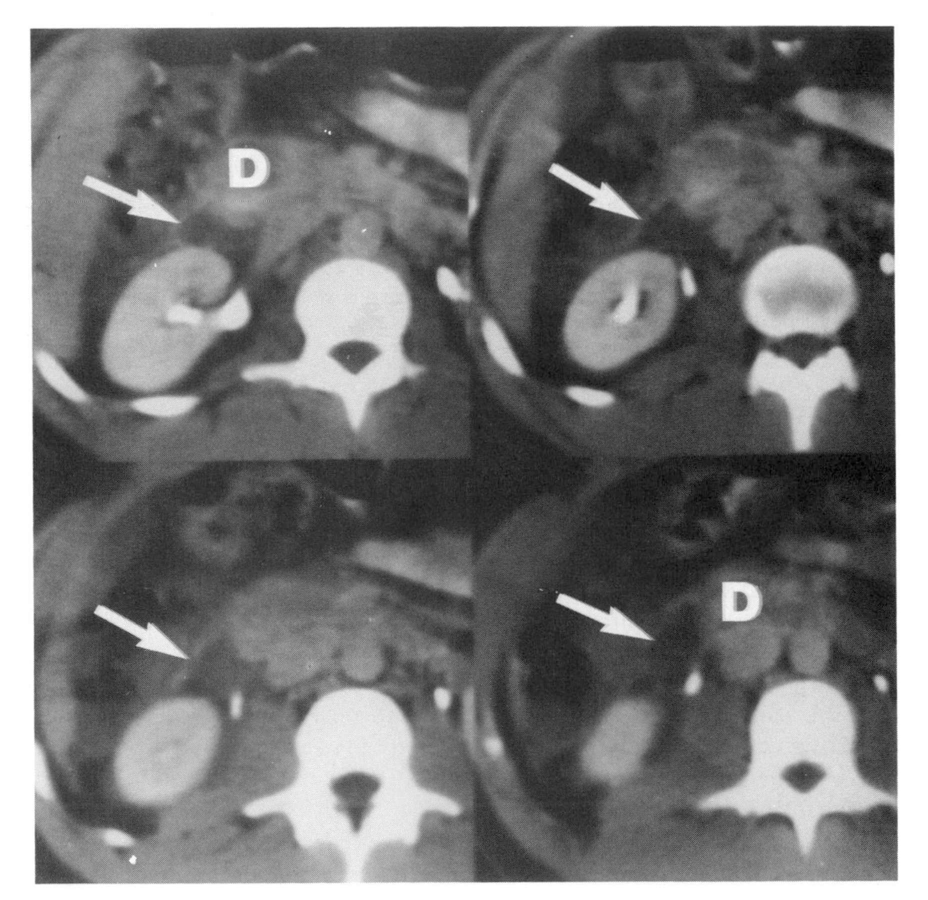

Fig. 15.4 Duodenal rupture. Sequential CT scans through the second and third portions of the duodenum (D) show a small subtle fluid collection (arrows) anterior to the right kidney.

of the duodenum in the right anterior pararenal space (Fig. 15.4). However, caution must be exercised in interpreting periduodenal fluid and gas since traumatic injuries to other body compartments (e.g. pneumothorax or bladder rupture) may be associated with air or fluid collections which have migrated into the retroperitoneum (Cook et al 1986).

MESENTERY AND BOWEL

Blunt trauma to small and large bowel and their mesenteries is uncommon and the sensitivity and specificity of CT diagnosis in these injuries is not known.

Lacerations of small bowel mesenteric vessels may occur with small interloop collections of high density blood surrounded by mesenteric fat (Federle 1983). Rare crush injuries to the small bowel mesentery may be recognized on CT as thickening of the root of the small bowel mesentery just below the third portion of duodenum and anterior to the aorta and inferior vena cava.

Traumatic non-duodenal perforation of the small bowel most commonly involves the proximal jejunum and distal ileum, which are relatively fixed in position, thus predisposing these areas to traumatic injuries.

The CT findings of small or large bowel blunt trauma are mass effect or thickening of the bowel wall, distortion or obliteration of gut lumen and an intramural high-density mass representing the intramural haematoma. All of these CT findings are subtle and their recognition is dependent upon adequate amounts of intra-abdominal fat and excellent bowel opacification with oral contrast material. Even with adequate preparation CT may be false negative for both small and large bowel perforation or transection (Cook et al 1986).

KIDNEY

Blunt renal injuries are quite common and are associated with other clinically significant injuries in 10–20% of cases. The major mechanisms of injury are deceleration, direct blows to the flank and fractures of the lower ribs and/or lumbar transverse processes. Minor renal injuries (contusion, incomplete laceration, intrarenal–extrarenal haematoma) comprise 75–85% of cases. Major renal injuries (complete laceration, fracture) occur in 10% of cases. Catastrophic renal injuries (shattered kidney, vascular pedicle injury) occur in 5% of cases and require urgent surgery. There is a growing national trend towards conservative management for most renal injuries, even in some cases of complete laceration or renal fracture (Fig. 15.5).

Excretory urography is still the screening procedure of choice and adequately depicts the extent of renal injury in 70–85% of cases, despite its non-specific findings. CT is most useful for evaluating patients with

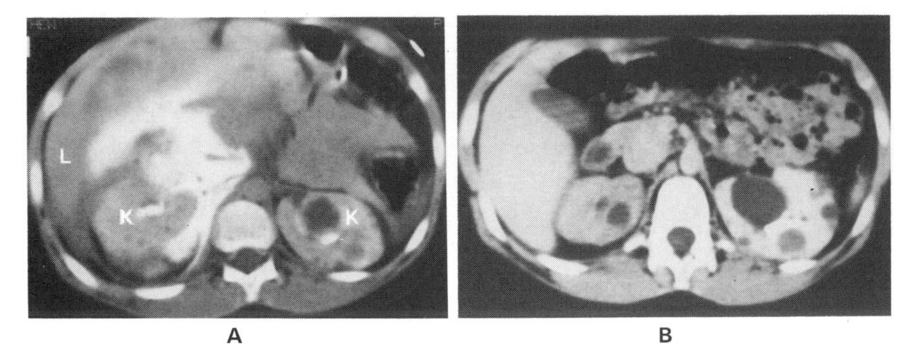

Fig. 15.5 Complete renal laceration. **A** CT scan through kidneys (K) with multiple cysts and inferior liver (L) shows gross extravasation of contrast medium throughout right retroperitoneal spaces. **B** CT scan 4 months later shows complete healing without surgical intervention.

continued gross haematuria, a falling haemoglobin and/or a positive urogram for a major renal injury. Renal angiography retains a supplementary role in renal trauma for definitive diagnosis of subintimal tear, pseudoaneurysm, arteriovenous fistula or renal artery severance.

CT findings in renal trauma encompass a wide variety of appearances (Federle 1983). Intrarenal haematomas due to contusion or incomplete laceration are common and appear as rounded areas of decreased attenuation with poorly marginated borders, with or without associated subcapsular and/or perirenal haematomas. Perirenal haematomas are easily recognized as variable density collections of blood confined by Gerota's fascia. Incomplete renal lacerations are recognized on CT as multiple, linear, hypodense clefts in the renal parenchyma without contrast extravasation.

A complete renal laceration is a focal parenchymal injury which has extended into the collecting system and CT will demonstrate extravasation of opacified urine associated with intrarenal and/or extrarenal haematoma (Fig. 15.5). CT usually depicts a renal fracture as a complete separation of upper and lower pole fragments, extravasation of contrast material and a large perirenal haematoma. The separated fragment may not enhance following injection of contrast material indicating devascularization. A shattered kidney implies multiple renal fragments separated by multiple clefts.

The least common blunt renal injury is a segmental or global renal infarct. A segmental renal infarct is caused by segmental occlusion of polar arterial branches. CT demonstrates a peripheral, hypodense wedge-shaped area with sharply demarcated borders. These CT features, as well as absence of associated subcapsular or perinephric haematoma, help to distinguish a segmental infarct from the more common intrarenal haematoma. These patients should be followed with serial CT to assess reperfusion of the infarcted area or persistent ischaemia associated with the development of hypertension which necessitates subsequent heminephrectomy.

Traumatic occlusion of the main renal artery is seen predominantly in young males and has a strong association with automobile–pedestrian accidents and high vertical falls. This vascular pedicle injury is due to either vascular avulsion or arterial thrombosis and results in a global infarct. The CT findings of global infarction are diagnostic and consist of a thin rim of perfused cortical tissue surrounding an area of non-perfused central renal parenchyma. This constellation of CT findings has been called the CT 'cortical rim sign' (Haynes et al 1984).

RETROPERITONEUM/FLANK/ABDOMINAL WALL

In patients who have been subjected to blunt trauma and have unexplained hypotension or haemorrhage in a clinically occult site, CT is a useful method of investigation. The technique may delineate extensive haemorrhage in the retroperitoneal spaces, in the rectus muscle sheath, in muscles of the abdominal wall, false pelvis or gluteal compartments and also in subcutaneous fat of the abdomen and pelvis (Fig. 15.6). Although this clinical situation is uncommon, these CT findings have an immediate

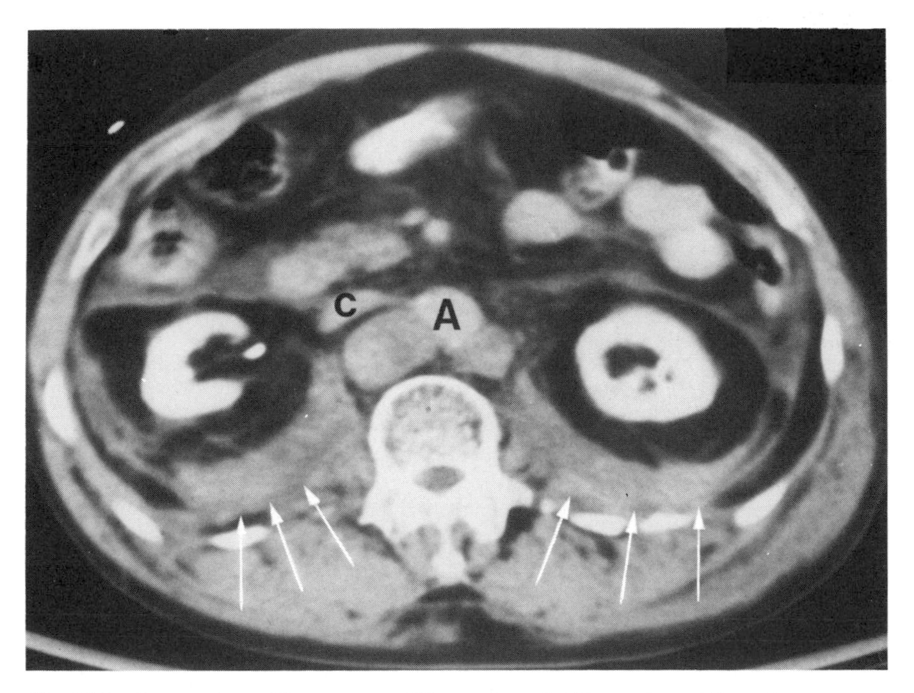

Fig. 15.6 Retroperitoneal haematoma. CT scan through kidneys shows bilateral posterior pararenal haematomas (arrows) and round haematomas posterior to the inferior vena cava (C) and aorta (A).

impact on patient management. CT diagnosis of contained haemorrhage in these anatomical compartments obviates exploratory laparotomy which may otherwise be performed to exclude intraperitoneal injury as the source of occult blood loss.

OCCULT CANCER

Several patients have been encountered who have incurred serious injury associated with blunt trauma to occult malignant tumours, such as Wilms' tumour, hepatoma, renal-cell carcinoma or soft-tissue sarcomas (Cook et al 1986). Neoplasms should be suspected when a contrast-enhanced mass with round margins distinct from adjacent haemorrhage is detected on CT scans. Mild trauma resulting in apparently severe organ injury or haemorrhage should also raise the suspicion of an underlying occult neoplasm.

CONCLUSION

The technological advances, in terms of superb image quality and fast scan times, have rendered CT an excellent method of evaluating patients who have suffered blunt abdominal trauma. The increased utilization of CT during recent years has led to a broad experience which has been correlated with the physiological condition of the patient and together these have provided the foundation on which management decisions are based (Brick et al 1987). This cost-effective role of CT has led to a decreased incidence of unnecessary laparotomy, shorter hospital stays for patient observation and earlier and more specific surgical intervention in appropriate cases (Foley et al 1987).

REFERENCES

Berland L L, Van Dyke J A 1985 Decreased splenic enhancement on CT in traumatised hypotensive patients. Radiology 156: 469–471

Brick S H, Taylor G A, Potter B M, Eichelberger M R 1987 Hepatic and splenic injury in children: role of CT in the decision for laparotomy. Radiology 165: 643–646

Cook D E, Walsh J W, Vick C W, Brewer W H 1986 Upper abdominal trauma: pitfalls in CT diagnosis. Radiology 159: 65–69

Federle M P 1983 Computed tomography of blunt abdominal trauma. Radiologic Clinics of North America 21: 461–475

Federle M P, Brant-Zawadzki M 1986 CT in the evaluation of trauma. 2nd edn. Williams & Wilkins, Baltimore

Federle M P, Griffiths B, Minagi H, Jeffrey R B Jr 1987 Splenic trauma: evaluation with CT. Radiology 162: 69–71

Foley W D, Cates, J D, Kellman G M et al 1987 Treatment of blunt hepatic injuries: role of CT. Radiology 164: 635–638

Haynes J W, Walsh J W, Brewer W H, Vick C W, Allen H A 1984 Traumatic renal artery occlusion: CT diagnosis with angiographic correlation. Journal of Computer Assisted Tomography 8: 731–733

Kaufman R A, Towbin R, Babcock D S et al 1984 Upper abdominal trauma in children: imaging evaluation. American Journal of Roentgenology 142: 449–460

Lang E K, Sullivan J, Frentz G 1985 Renal trauma: radiologic studies. Radiology 154: 1–6
McCort J J 1987 Caring for the major trauma victim: the role for radiology. Radiology 163: 1–9
Panicek D M, Paquet D J, Clark K G, Urrutia E J, Brinsko R E 1986 Hepatic parenchymal gas after blunt trauma. Radiology 159: 343–344
Sclafani S J A, Florence L O, Phillips T F et al 1987 Lumbar arterial injury: radiologic diagnosis and management. Radiology 165: 709–714
Stalker H P, Kaufman R A, Towbin R 1986 Patterns of liver injury in childhood: CT analysis. American Journal of Roentgenology 147: 1199–1205

16. Interventional CT

N. Reed Dunnick

INTRODUCTION

Percutaneous procedures guided by radiological imaging modalities have proved to be a safe and efficacious adjunct to patient care. Aspiration biopsies can provide a tissue diagnosis without surgery and percutaneous drainage procedures have become the treatment of choice for a wide variety of abscesses. Additional techniques, such as percutaneous nephrostomy, biliary or even pancreatic drainage, can be performed under CT guidance, but the multiple manipulations required and ease of performance under fluoroscopic guidance makes CT unnecessary for most cases. This chapter discusses general principles of interventional techniques for percutaneous biopsy and abscess drainage. Common complications and contraindications for these procedures are also addressed.

ABDOMINAL ABSCESS: DETECTION AND DRAINAGE

The detection and treatment of abdominal abscesses has undergone a dramatic evolution in recent years and radiology has been at the centre of this change (Gerzof et al 1979, Haaga & Weinstein 1980). Transverse imaging modalities, computed tomography (CT) and ultrasound (US), enable us to detect abnormal fluid collections without having to rely upon secondary signs of mass effect or abnormal gas collections. Percutaneous aspiration provides confirmation of the diagnosis as well as material for culture. Large-bore catheters can be used to evacuate and drain abscess cavities (Bernardino et al 1984, Johnson et al 1985, Mueller et al 1986, Casola et al 1987, Mueller et al 1987). These improved methods of diagnosis and treatment, coupled with better patient support and more refined antibiotics, have resulted in a marked reduction in the mortality of abdominal abscesses (Saini et al 1983, van Sonnenberg 1984).

Definition

An abnormal fluid collection may arise from a variety of aetiologies. Trauma which results in haemorrhage and laceration of abdominal organs

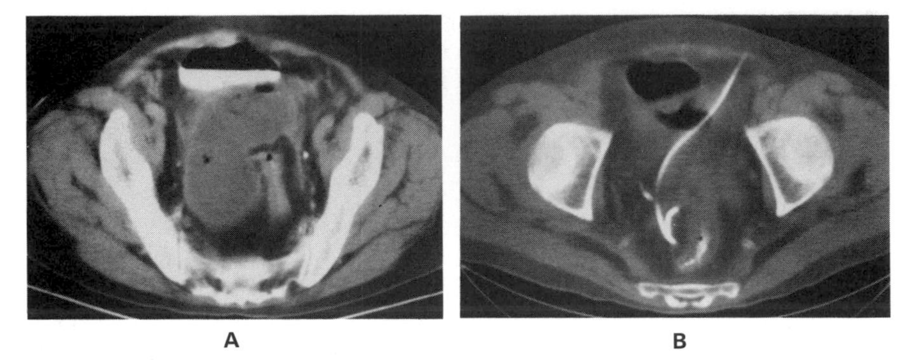

Fig. 16.1 **A** CT scan showing an abnormal fluid collection in the pelvis which is suspicious of an abscess. It has a thick wall, mass effect and contains a small amount of gas. **B** Percutaneous drainage completely evacuated the cavity and resulted in cure.

or ducts may create a fluid collection of urine, bile or lymph. Furthermore, fluid collections may arise as a result of inflammation, such as pancreatitis, or as a manifestation of systemic disease, as in ascites. These abnormal fluid collections conform to normal anatomical spaces and do not have mass effect. They are often recent in onset and may or may not be infected.

An abscess is an abnormal fluid collection which has a well-defined thick wall, does not conform to normal anatomical spaces and has mass effect (Fig. 16.1a). An abscess may begin as an abnormal fluid collection, which becomes infected. It may arise from adjacent infection or may result from infection of a fluid-filled cavity, such as a renal cyst or pancreatic pseudocyst. This distinction is pertinent, as an abscess can usually be cured by percutaneous drainage while an abnormal fluid collection without a defined wall is likely to recur (Fig. 16.1b).

Detection

An abnormal gas collection seen on an abdominal radiograph is often the first radiographic sign indicating the presence of an abscess. However, the majority of abdominal abscesses detected by CT and US do not contain gas (Fig. 16.2). In fact, these modalities are so sensitive for detecting abnormal fluid collections that the most common problem is in differentiating an abscess from an uninfected collection, such as a lymphocoele, pseudocyst or localized ascites (Torres et al 1986). This distinction can be made by aspirating the fluid collection and examining it by inspection, Gram stain and culture (Mueller et al 1984).

The choice of the radiographic modality used to detect an abscess depends upon the individual patient and suspected location. However, in general, CT is the preferred modality (Glass & Cohn 1984, Mandel et al 1985). CT provides useful information about other abdominal organs and most patients do have associated disease. CT demonstrates the most

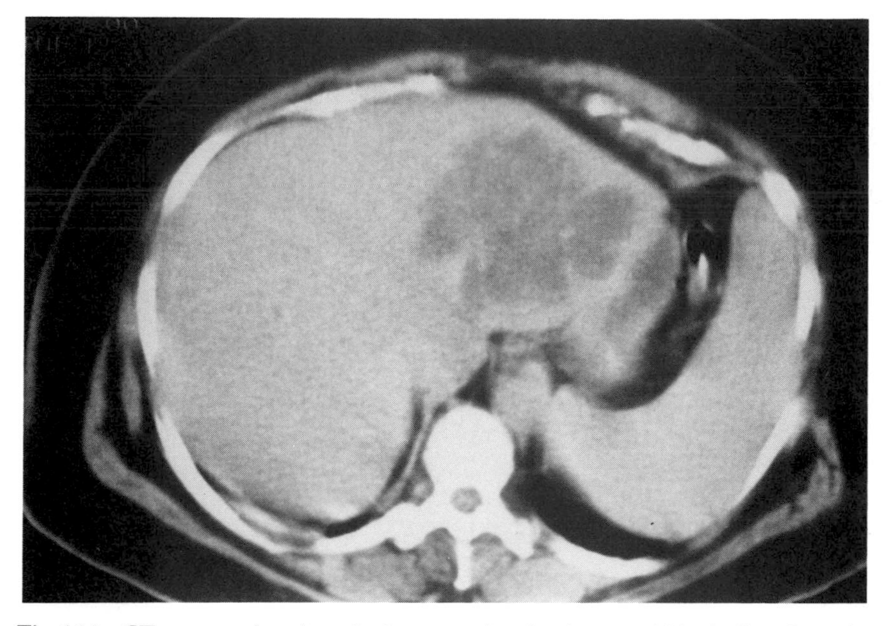

Fig. 16.2 CT scan reveals an hepatic abscess as a low density area within the liver. Several internal septations are seen but the locules usually intercommunicate allowing successful percutaneous drainage.

desirable route for placement of a drainage catheter as well as the location of the catheter side holes. The size of the abscess cavity, as well as the distance from other structures and the skin, can be precisely measured from the CT image. If surgery is needed, CT provides the anatomical information often requested by surgeons prior to operating.

US is also a useful modality for the detection of an abdominal abscess and has several advantages over CT (Nosher et al 1986). US examination of any specific area is usually faster than an abdominal CT examination, especially if a CT technologist must be called to perform the study. If aspiration is performed, US is a more efficient means of guiding the needle than CT. When percutaneous abscess drainage is performed, the size of the cavity can easily be monitored with US, which is also more efficient and less costly than CT.

Percutaneous abscess drainage

If a diagnostic aspiration of a suspected abdominal abscess is undertaken, the same route should be used that will provide therapeutic drainage. This route should: (i) be as direct as possible; (ii) remain extraperitoneal; (iii) avoid other organs; and (iv) allow for dependent drainage (Butch et al 1986). These are guidelines and not absolute rules but adherence to them will improve therapeutic success.

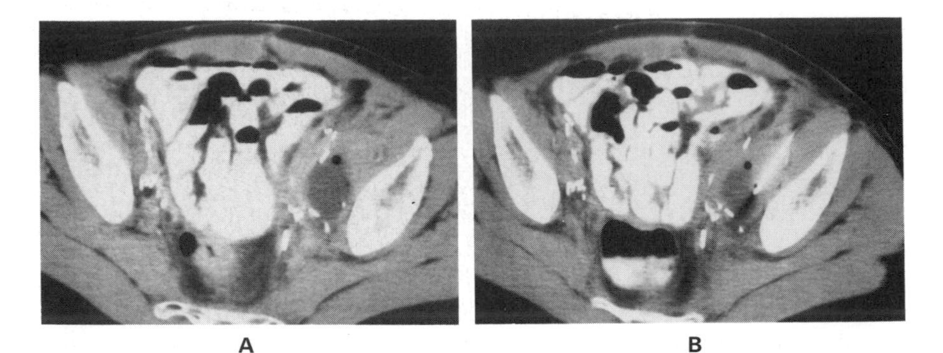

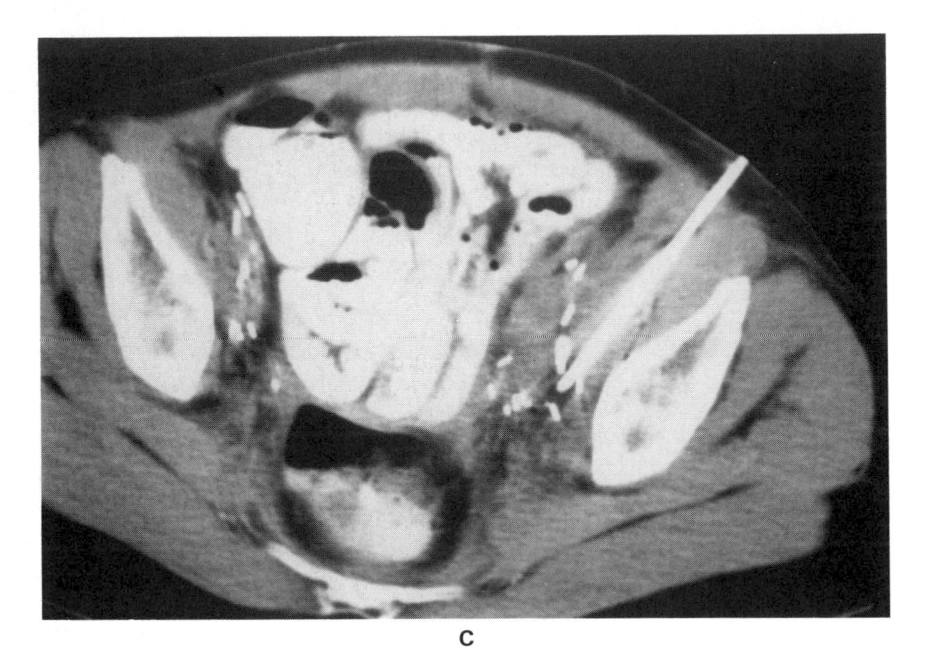

Fig. 16.3 **A** CT scan showing an abnormal fluid collection suggestive of an abscess at the site of previous surgery. **B** Percutaneous aspiration with an 18-gauge needle confirmed purulent material. **C** A 10 French drainage catheter was used to evacuate the cavity.

The initial puncture to drain an abdominal abscess can be performed in several ways. If the aetiology of the fluid collection is uncertain, a diagnostic tap with a small needle may be appropriate. This will cause the least damage to structures traversed. However, if the material within it is viscous, it may not flow through a small gauge needle. It is generally preferable to use an 18-gauge needle to increase the likelihood of withdrawing enough material to be diagnostic.

If the diagnosis of an abscess is almost certain based on the radiographic findings and clinical setting, the initial pass may be made with a trocar catheter. This avoids the multiple manipulations needed when the Seldinger technique is used after a diagnostic aspiration, and is easier and faster to perform. The trocar technique is most often employed when the abscess is: (i) relatively close to the skin; (ii) large; and (iii) away from critical structures.

The most common approach to a suspected abdominal abscess is to make an initial puncture with an 18-gauge needle and withdraw 5–10 ml for inspection, Gram stain and culture (Fig. 16.3). If the fluid is clear it is cultured and Gram stained. In these cases, a small catheter is sometimes left in place to drain the collection until the culture results are known. However, it is preferable to aspirate the cavity completely, if possible, and remove the catheter rather than risk infection of a previously sterile fluid collection.

If the diagnostic aspiration yields purulent material the procedure is extended to the placement of a large-bore catheter. Since the aspiration is usually guided by CT or US, the patient must be transported to a fluoroscopy suite. This can be done most safely by passing a 0.038 inch angiographic guidewire through the needle and coiling it in the abscess cavity. The needle is removed, the guidewire taped in place and the patient can be transported without dislodging the wire or lacerating tissues with the needle tip. Once in the fluoroscopy suite, a series of fascial dilators can be used to enlarge the tract before placing the drainage catheter. This catheter should be large enough to drain the viscous abscess material, yet have side holes confined to a relatively small area so they will not migrate outside the abscess as the cavity shrinks. In most cases, at least a 10 French catheter is required and larger catheters should be used if needed (Gobien et al 1985).

After positioning the drainage catheter in the cavity, the contents should be evacuated as completely as possible (Mueller et al 1984). After initial aspiration, saline lavage is often useful to further eliminate purulent material. Introducing dilute contrast material is valuable, as it defines the extent of the cavity to compare with the CT or US examination, and to use as a baseline for future monitoring. The catheter tip is then placed in the most dependent portion of the cavity and the catheter connected to a bag for external drainage. Since these collections are usually not bloody, irrigation is not necessary to prevent clotting and obstruction of the tube.

Experienced interventionalists may be comfortable in performing the catheter exchanges in the CT or US suite, without the help of fluoroscopy. This can usually be done safely and has the advantage of allowing an immediate repeat scan to determine the size of the abscess cavity after initial drainage.

Patient monitoring

Most patients will experience a dramatic response to evacuation of the abscess cavity. With successful drainage and appropriate antibiotic cover, most patients can be cured in 5–12 days and surgery is not required. The drainage from the abscess will stop, the fever and leucocytosis will subside and the catheter may be removed. In most patients a follow-up CT or US examination is not needed to confirm that the abscess cavity has been completely drained.

Persistence of the abscess suggests a high viscosity which is resistant to drainage, a loculated component which does not readily communicate with the primary collection or infection by multiple organisms, not all of which are susceptible to the antibiotic cover (Lang et al 1986, Lieberman et al 1986). Repeat examination with CT or US with a further culture of the drainage material should readily identify these problems (Papanicolaou et al 1984).

The most difficult abscesses to drain effectively are infected organized haematomas and not all of them can be managed by percutaneous drainage.

PERCUTANEOUS BIOPSY TECHNIQUES

The value of CT in the diagnosis and delineation of disease processes is firmly established. However, the CT appearance is usually non-specific and further tissue characterization is often needed (Sundaram et al 1982, Bernardino 1984). Percutaneous biopsy with cytological or histological evaluation is often definitive. Although this can usually be performed safely and efficiently, care should be taken in choosing the most appropriate needle and route for biopsy.

Biopsy needle

There is a huge selection of needles which may be used to obtain a satisfactory biopsy specimen. They vary in length, diameter and design of needle tip. In general, the larger the diameter of the needle, the larger the specimen obtained. Furthermore, Haaga et al (1983) have shown that when needles of the same size are compared, larger specimens can be obtained with a more acute bevel angle (Andriole et al 1983).

In most clinical settings, cytology will be sufficient. However, occasionally a histological specimen may be needed. Although tissue satisfactory for histology can be obtained with 22-gauge needles using a 'core technique', larger calibre needles are often required (Wittenberg et al 1982).

One of the most critical aspects in selecting the needle is the location of the tissue to be biopsied. On the one hand, if the biopsy target is adjacent to other critical structures, especially arteries, the use of a small-calibre needle will be safer. On the other hand, if the target is small and deep within the body, it may be difficult to position a fine needle in the lesion as these small needles tend to deviate ('bow') from their intended path. Although adequate positioning can almost always be accomplished, it may require many passes which involves a great deal of scanner time.

Since there are so many different needles from which to choose it is probably prudent to select a few with different characteristics and become adept in their use. The author's personal preferences for aspirating needles include the 22-gauge Chiba, the 20-gauge Bernardino–Sones and the 20-gauge Rotex (screw biopsy) needles. The Chiba is a thin needle with an acute bevel angle. It can be passed into or through almost any tissue with a very low complication rate. Despite its small size, a high diagnostic accuracy is obtained when adequately positioned within the tumour. When aspirating deep lesions, there is a tendency for this needle to 'bow' which may be frustrating when trying to position the tip within the mass. However, this characteristic can be used to advantage when the target lies behind a structure you wish to avoid. Since the needle tends to 'bow' away from the bevel, a curved path may be obtained.

The Bernardino–Sones needle is slightly larger and is designed with the cutting edge smaller than the barrel. This allows a core of tissue to be removed which may actually be larger than the cutting edge. The larger size and stiffer shaft of this needle facilitate needle placement. One of these two needles is adequate for the vast majority of soft-tissue mass biopsies. However, the Rotex needle with its unique screw type stylet may occasionally be useful for obtaining small chunks of tissue.

Larger cutting needles are used when a large sample of tissue for histological evaluation is needed. These include, the Lee, Trucut and Ackerman needles. Greater care must be taken in precise placement of these needles as a large core of tissue is removed and may include portions of a duct or blood vessel wall.

Guiding modality

The choice of radiological modality used for guidance is determined by the equipment available and the target lesion. Lung and bone biopsies are usually performed with fluoroscopic guidance. CT can provide valuable anatomical information to help select the safest needle path (Fig. 16.4). Biopsies of liver or pancreatic lesions can often be performed most expeditiously under ultrasound control. Retroperitoneal biopsies including adrenal masses, para-aortic lymph-nodes or soft-tissue masses may require CT for adequate needle placement. We have also found that precise anatomical delineation with CT may allow a biopsy to be undertaken with fluoroscopic guidance using bony landmarks.

The accuracy of percutaneous needle biopsy depends upon the placement of the needle, the quality of the specimen aspirated, the skill of the cytologist and the selection of lesions accepted for biopsy. CT is the most valuable guiding modality for needle positioning. Not only can the location of the needle tip be precisely determined but CT can often identify the ideal location within the mass by avoiding areas of tumour necrosis.

The quality of tissue removed can be affected by the biopsy technique

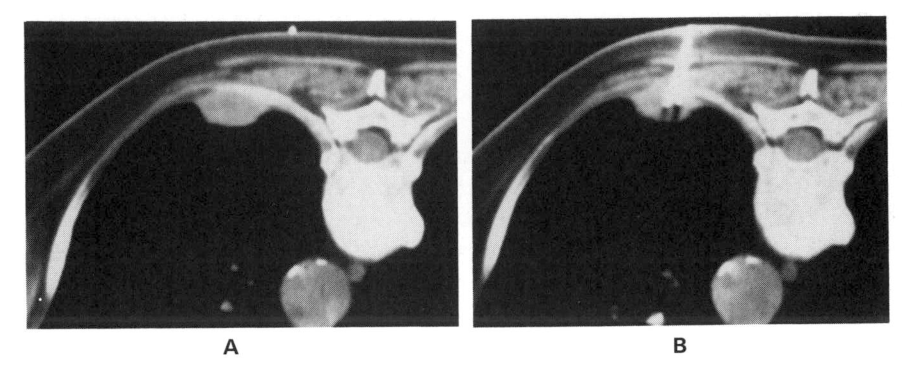

Fig. 16.4 **A** Pleural based lesions are often biopsied under CT guidance as the lesions are easier to see than with fluoroscopy. **B** Clear visualization of the needle and the lesion allows an extrapleural approach.

(Hueftle & Haaga 1986). Most operators prefer to apply suction continuously while moving the needle up and down through the tumour. Rotation of the needle, particularly with the acute angle bevel, may also help to increase the aspirated material. Care should be taken, however, not to aspirate material from adjacent organs as this may be very confusing for the cytologist.

Specific biopsy sites

Percutaneous lung biopsies are routinely performed under fluoroscopic guidance (Lalli et al 1978). However, if a lesion can be seen in only one plane, CT is useful to determine the 'depth' of the lesion (Cohan et al 1984).

Mediastinal biopsies are routinely done with CT guidance but large masses which have borders safely away from major vessels can be biopsied with fluoroscopy. In such cases, CT is required to determine the biopsy site and route prior to fluoroscopic control.

Focal liver lesions are amenable to biopsy with either CT or· US (Fig. 16.5). The location of the liver adjacent to the diaphragm results in large respiratory excursions, so patient co-operation is required. Most operators prefer to avoid the pleura so an angled approach is often selected. Since the liver provides a good ultrasonic window, it is preferable to attempt liver biopsies with ultrasonic guidance.

Pancreatic biopsies remain some of the most difficult. The variable size, shape and enhancement of the pancreas obscures delineation of the mass. Tumours may also evoke a significant inflammatory response and cannot always be distinguished from focal pancreatitis by CT. Furthermore, the complications of pancreatitis and fistula formation by leaking pancreatic enzymes are peculiar to this organ.

The kidney is not biopsied as often as other areas as it is more amenable to surgery. The presence of a normal contralateral kidney allows removal of

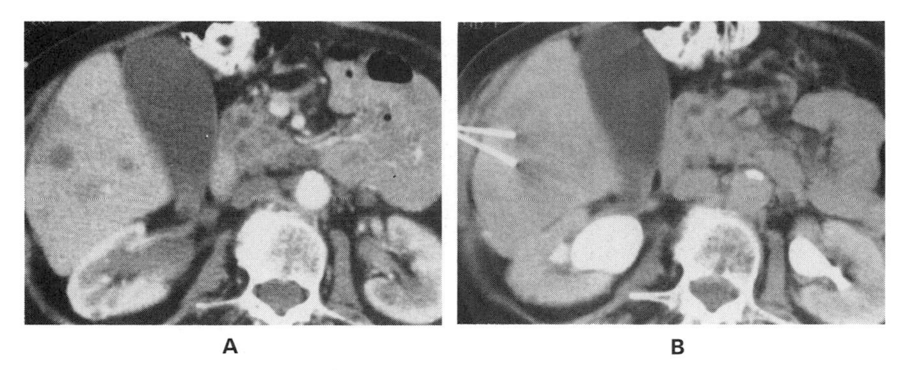

Fig. 16.5 **A** CT scan showing several focal liver lesions. **B** Percutaneous aspiration biopsy confirmed metastatic disease.

the involved kidney. Since a negative biopsy does not exclude malignancy, many urologists prefer to undertake a radical nephrectomy or open biopsy rather than percutaneous aspiration when renal adenocarcinoma is suspected.

Adrenal masses, on the other hand, are among the most frequently biopsied lesions. The adrenal gland is a common site of metastases from a wide variety of primary tumours. However, benign adrenal masses, such as non-functioning adenomas, are also common and thus the presence of an adrenal mass in a patient with an underlying malignancy does not necessarily mean metastatic disease (Berkman et al 1984).

Other retroperitoneal masses including para-aortic and pelvic lymph-node biopsies (Fig. 16.6) are usually performed with CT guidance. A larger tissue sample is required for the diagnosis of malignant lymphoma than that needed for the diagnosis of metastatic carcinoma. It is also much easier for the cytologist to confirm metastatic disease when the primary tumour is known than to make the original malignant diagnosis. Care must be taken to avoid the great vessels, particularly if large cutting needles are used.

Bone biopsies can be considered in two categories. If there is extensive bone destruction, the lesion can be approached as a soft-tissue mass and a small needle such as a 22-gauge Chiba may suffice (Ayala & Zornoza 1983). If the lesion is osteoblastic or more centrally located and protected by normal cortex, a sturdy cutting needle such as an Ackerman is required. After removing the bone core, it is often helpful to obtain an aspirate of the medullary component (Hewes et al 1983). Several different tissue samples are often useful to help the pathologist diagnose primary bone tumours.

Complications

The type and frequency of complications depend upon the organ biopsied, the size and nature of the lesion, the type of needle used and the status of the

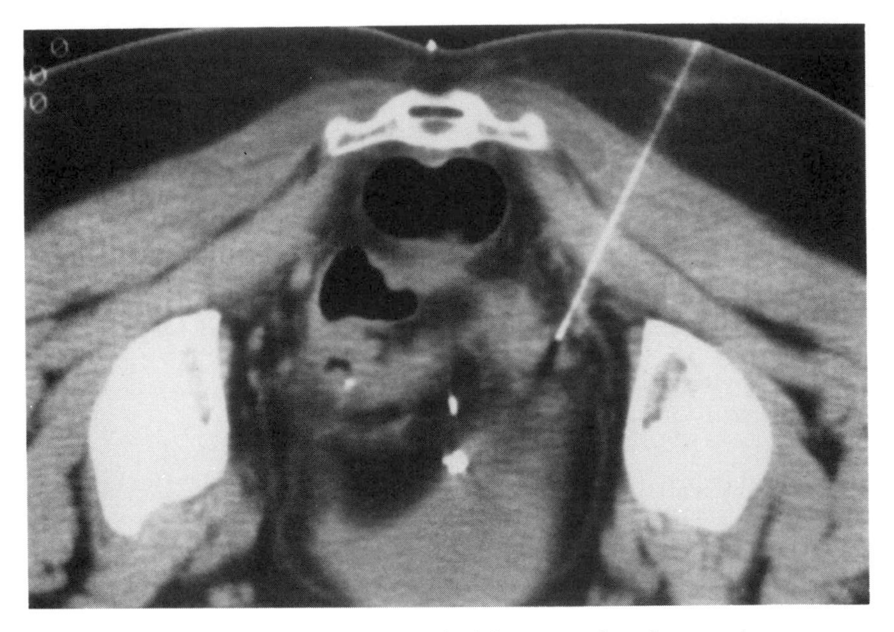

Fig. 16.6 CT-guided percutaneous biopsy of pelvic mass confirmed metastatic tumour.

patient (Yankaskas et al 1986). Mediastinal, lung and lesions in the upper abdomen near the diaphragm often result in pneumothorax. The author has a 25% rate of pneumothorax for percutaneous lung biopsies (Perlmutt et al 1986). Although many of these are small and resolve spontaneously, others require chest tube insertion. The Trocar style chest tube with a Heimlich valve is easy to insert under fluoroscopy and effective in eliminating the pneumothorax.

Bleeding is another common complication. This is rarely a significant problem when fine needles are used, but can be life-threatening in patients who have clotting dysfunction. Bleeding parameters, including prothrombin time, partial thromboplastin time and a platelet count, should be checked if there is any suspicion of abnormal clotting factors.

CONCLUSION

The use of CT for guiding percutaneous interventional procedures has increased its value beyond that of a morphological imaging modality. Frequently, a definitive diagnosis can be reached by CT-guided biopsy after the initial examination has demonstrated the lesion and CT now plays a central diagnostic and therapeutic role in the management of patients with intra-abdominal abscesses.

REFERENCES

Andriole J G, Haaga J R, Adams R B, Nunez C 1983 Biopsy needle characteristics assessed in the laboratory. Radiology 148: 659–662
Ayala A G, Zornoza J 1983 Primary bone tumors: percutaneous needle biopsy. Radiology 149: 675–679
Berkman W A, Bernardino M E, Sewell C W, Price R B, Sones P J Jr 1984 The computed tomography-guided adrenal biopsy. Cancer 53: 2098–2103
Bernardino M E 1984 Percutaneous biopsy. American Journal of Roentgenology 142: 41–45
Bernardino M E, Berkman W A, Plemmons M, Sones P J Jr, Price R B, Casarella W J 1984 Percutaneous drainage of multiseptated hepatic abscess. Journal of Computer Assisted Tomography 8: 38–41
Butch R J, Mueller P R, Ferrucci J T Jr et al 1986 Drainage of pelvic abscesses through the greater sciatic foramen. Radiology 158: 487–491
Casola G, van Sonnenberg E, Neff C C, Saba R M, Withers C, Emarine C W 1987 Abscesses in Crohn Disease: percutaneous drainage. Radiology 163: 19–22
Cohan R H, Newman G E, Braun S D, Dunnick N R 1984 CT assistance for fluoroscopically guided transthoracic needle aspiration biopsy. Journal of Computer Assisted Tomography 8: 1093–1098
Gerzof S G, Robbins H A, Birkett D H, Johnson W C, Pugatch R D, Vincent M E 1979 Percutaneous catheter drainage of abdominal abscesses guided by ultrasound and computed tomography. American Journal of Roentgenology 133: 1–8
Glass C A, Cohn I Jr 1984 Drainage of intra-abdominal abscesses: a comparison of surgical and computerized tomography guided catheter drainage. American Journal of Surgery 147: 315–317
Gobien R P, Stanley J H, Schabel S I et al 1985 The effect of drainage tube size on adequacy of percutaneous abscess drainage. Cardiovascular Interventional Radiology 8: 100–102
Haaga J R, LiPuma J P, Bryan P J, Balsara V J, Cohen A M 1983 Clinical comparison of small- and large-caliber cutting needles for biopsy. Radiology 146: 665–667
Haaga J R, Weinstein A J 1980 CT-guided percutaneous aspiration and drainage of abscesses. American Journal of Roentgenology 135: 1187–1194
Hewes R C, Vigorita V J, Freiberger R H 1983 Percutaneous bone biopsy: the importance of aspirated osseous blood. Radiology 148: 69–72
Hueftle M G, Haaga J R 1986 Effect of suction on biopsy sample size. American Journal of Roentgenology 147: 1014–1016
Johnson R D, Mueller P R, Ferrucci J T Jr et al 1985 Percutaneous drainage of pyogenic liver abscesses. American Journal of Roentgenology 144: 463–467
Lalli A F, McCormack L J, Zelch M, Reich N E, Belovich D 1978 Aspiration biopsies of chest lesions. Radiology 127: 35–40
Lang E K, Springer R M, Glorioso L W III, Cammarata C A 1986 Abdominal abscess drainage under radiologic guidance: causes of failure. Radiology 159: 329–336
Lieberman R P, Hahn F J, Imray T J, Phalen J T 1986 Loculated abscesses: management by percutaneous fracture of septations. Radiology 161: 827–828
Mandel S R, Boyd D, Jaques P F, Mandell V, Staab E V 1985 Drainage by hepatic, intra-abdominal and mediastinal abscesses guided by computerized axial tomography. American Journal of Surgery 145: 120–123
Mueller P R, Saini S, Wittenberg J et al 1987 Sigmoid diverticular abscesses: percutaneous drainage as an adjunct to surgical resection in 24 cases. Radiology 164: 321–325
Mueller P R, Simeone J F, Butch R J et al 1986 Percutaneous drainage of subphrenic abscess: a review of 62 patients. American Journal of Roentgenology 147: 1237–1240
Mueller P R, van Sonnenberg E, Ferrucci J T Jr 1984 Percutaneous drainage of 250 abdominal abscesses and fluid collections. Part II: Current procedural concepts. Radiology 151: 343–347
Nosher J L, Needell G S, Amorosa J K, Krasna I H 1986 Transrectal pelvic abscess drainage with sonographic guidance. American Journal of Roentgenology 146: 1047–1048
Papanicolaou N, Mueller P R, Ferrucci J T Jr et al 1984 Abscess-fistula association: radiologic recognition and percutaneous management. American Journal of Roentgenology 143: 811–815
Perlmutt L M, Braun S D, Newman G E, Oke E J, Dunnick N R 1986 Timing of chest film

follow-up after transthoracic needle aspiration. American Journal of Roentgenology 146: 1049–1050

Saini S, Kellum J M, O'Leary M P et al 1983 Improved localization and survival in patients with intra-abdominal abscesses. American Journal of Surgery 145: 136–142

Sundaram M, Wolverson M K, Heiberg E, Pilla T, Vas W G, Shields J B 1982 Utility of CT-guided abdominal aspiration procedures. American Journal of Roentgenology 139: 1111–1115

Torres W E, Evert M B, Baumgartner B R, Bernardino M E 1986 Percutaneous aspiration and drainage of pancreatic pseudocysts. American Journal of Roentgenology 147: 1007–1009

van Sonnenberg E, Wing V W, Casola G et al 1984 Temporizing effect of percutaneous drainage of complicated abscesses in critically ill patients. American Journal of Roentgenology 142: 821–826

Wittenberg J, Mueller P R, Ferrucci J T Jr et al 1982 Percutaneous core biopsy of abdominal tumors using 22 gauge needles: further observations. American Journal of Roentgenology 139: 75–80

Yankaskas B C, Staab E V, Craven M B, Blatt P M, Sokhandan M, Carney C N 1986 Delayed complications from fine-needle biopsies of solid masses of the abdomen. Investigative Radiology 21: 325–328

17. Staging of gynaecological malignancy

James W. Walsh

INTRODUCTION

Over the past 10 years CT has become the primary imaging modality for staging female pelvic malignancies because of its ability to display pelvic tumour and surrounding organs and to detect occult non-palpable pelvic and abdominal metastases. In comparison to clinical staging techniques, CT gives complementary information and is more accurate for demonstrating advanced disease. CT is most efficacious in evaluating patients with a difficult or equivocal pelvic examination or for staging poorly differentiated cancers with a high propensity for lymph-node or abdominal metastases. When CT is used as the first radiological staging test in these clinical situations, the information obtained may eliminate the need for an excretory urogram and barium enema. CT-guided biopsy is an extension of the diagnostic study and may confirm metastatic disease to the peritoneal cavity and retroperitoneum.

TECHNIQUE

A standard pelvic and abdominal CT technique can be used for staging most pelvic cancers, but variations in procedure for optimizing individual studies and for tailoring the examination to the particular tumour will be stressed. Contrast opacification of distal small bowel and colon is essential when performing a diagnostic pelvic CT study. At the author's institution patients normally receive 450 ml of a 2% oral barium suspension the evening preceding the examination to opacify the colon and an additional 450 ml of oral contrast 45 minutes prior to the scan to fill small bowel loops in the pelvic peritoneal pouches. In individual cases of suspected tumour involvement of the rectum, an optional 200 ml dilute contrast enema with air insufflation can be administered. In patients with suspected paravaginal and paracervical pathology, a vaginal tampon may be inserted to distend the vagina and to outline it with air.

Intravenous contrast medium is used in the majority of pelvic cancer patients to opacify the bladder and ureters, to differentiate contrast-filled blood vessels from adjacent lymph nodes, to enhance the myometrium and visualize the endometrial cavity, and to delineate hypodense tumour boundaries from contiguous normal organ parenchyma. Intravenous contrast medium is usually administered through a large-bore needle as a 50 ml bolus of 60% contrast followed by a rapid drip infusion of 300 ml of 30% contrast. Recent improved contrast opacification techniques combine the use of a mechanical contrast injector with a dynamic scan programme and rapid table incrementation. Usually 50 ml of 60% contrast medium is administered as a bolus injection followed by injection of 100 ml of 60% contrast at the rate of 2 ml/s.

Scan collimation of 8–10 mm is adequate for most pelvic CT studies. However, with the advent of newer high resolution CT scanners it is now possible to take thinner (3–5 mm) slices through the tumour thereby visualizing local tumour extension more precisely. This eliminates the problem of volume averaging of tumour and adjacent normal structures which occurs with thicker slices. Thinner slices are particularly useful for detecting subtle parametrial tumour extension from cervical carcinoma which may be imaged on only one or two scans.

Contiguous 8–10 mm scans are taken from the level of the ischial tuberosities cephalad to the iliac crest. Scanning the lower pelvis first optimizes uterine enhancement and vascular opacification is also maximized which facilitates metastatic node detection. Thin slices through the tumour are added as needed. Scans are then taken at 2 cm intervals from the iliac crest to the diaphragm to survey the retroperitoneum and abdomen for metastatic disease. If the bladder and pelvic ureters are not well opacified on initial pelvic scans, it is a simple 'trick of the trade' to take a few more scans at the end of the study. Sometimes tumour invasion of the bladder from cancer of the cervix is better seen adjacent to a contrast-filled urinary bladder. Also, parametrial tumour extension from cervical carcinoma may be better delineated when it surrounds contrast-filled distal ureters.

Table 17.1 FIGO classification for cervical and endometrial cancer

CERVICAL CANCER	
Stage I	Tumour confined to cervix
Stage IIA	Involvement of upper third of vagina
Stage IIB	Parametrial extension but not to the pelvic side wall
Stage IIIA	Involvement of lower third of vagina
Stage IIIB	Pelvic side wall extension or hydronephrosis
Stage IVA	Bladder or rectal involvement
Stage IVB	Para-aortic or inguinal lymph-node enlargement (> 1.5–2.0 cm) or intraperitoneal metastases
ENDOMETRIAL CANCER	
Stage I	Tumour confined to corpus
Stage II	Tumour involving corpus and cervix
Stage III	Tumour extension to parametria, adnexae, pelvic side wall or pelvic nodes
Stage IVA	Bladder or rectal involvement
Stage IVB	Metastases to para-aortic lymph nodes, peritoneal cavity, omentum or liver

CERVICAL CARCINOMA

Based on 1988 United States cancer statistics, cervical carcinoma is the eighth most common female cancer. The tumour characteristically spreads locally to the vagina or to the parametria and pelvic side wall and metastasizes to pelvic and para-aortic lymph nodes.

CT stage criteria in cervical carcinoma are based on the International Federation of Gynecology and Obstetrics (FIGO) classification (Table 17.1; Fig. 17.1). Although the FIGO classification does not include pelvic lymph-node metastases, CT detection of pelvic lymph-node enlargement is considered a Stage IIIB tumour, i.e. analogous to pelvic side wall spread.

Radical hysterectomy with lymph-node sampling or radiation therapy are treatment options for Stages I–IIA, whereas radiation therapy is the treatment of choice for Stages IIB–IVA. Stage IVB is treated with extended field radiotherapy and/or chemotherapy.

In comparison with surgical staging of cervical carcinoma, the clinical staging error rate is 24–39%. The most common errors are failure to recognize parametrial tumour extension or to detect pelvic and para-aortic lymph-node metastases. Since clinical staging has decreasing accuracy with more advanced tumours, CT is an excellent complementary staging procedure because of its high accuracy in detecting advanced disease

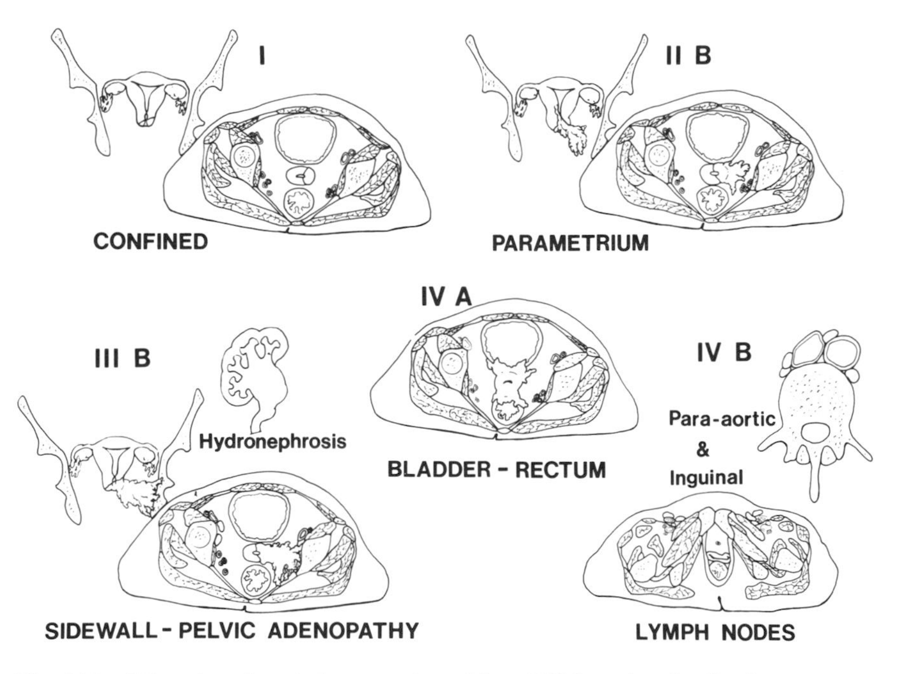

Fig. 17.1 CT staging of cervical cancer adopted from FIGO staging classification.

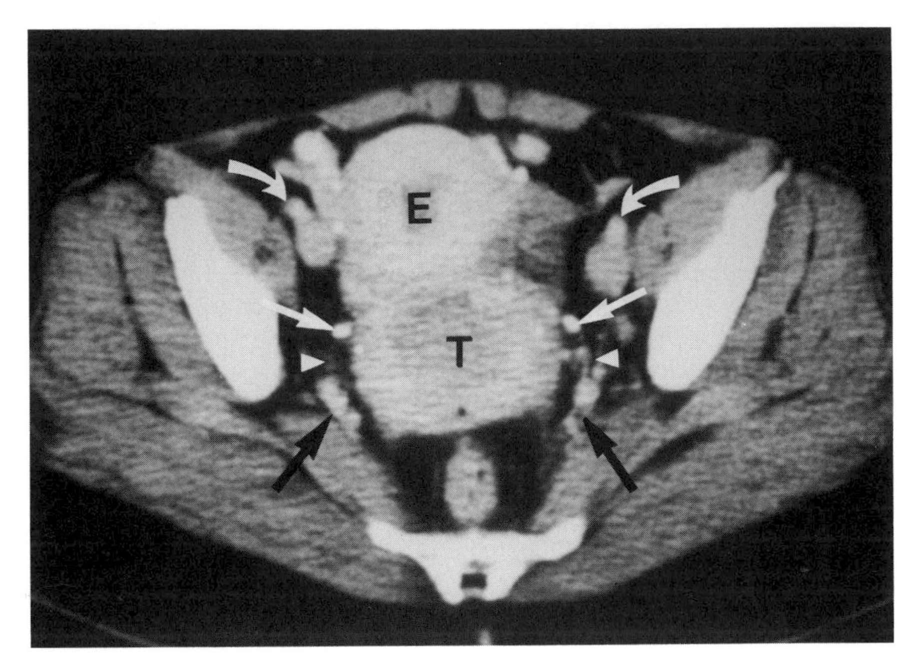

Fig. 17.2 CT Stage IB endocervix cancer. CT scan through uterine fundus and endometrial cavity (E) shows a barrel-shaped hypodense tumour (T) expanding but confined to the endocervix with normal peripheral cervical stroma and normal peri-ureteral fat planes (white arrows). External iliac vessels (curved arrows), small paracervical vessels (arrowheads) and inferior gluteal vessels (black arrows) anterior to piriformis muscles are well opacified with intravenous contrast from this dynamic scan.

(Walsh & Goplerud 1981, Villasanta et al 1983). CT is not routinely indicated for staging early (Stage IB–IIA) tumours, unless they are bulky and/or poorly differentiated, because clinical staging with pelvic examination by experienced gynaecological oncologists has a higher accuracy rate.

The primary goal of CT staging is to differentiate tumour confined to the cervix from tumour which has invaded the parametria. CT criteria for a tumour confined to the cervix (Fig. 17.2) are:

1. Smooth, well-defined peripheral cervix margins.
2. Absence of prominent parametrial soft-tissue strands.
3. No parametrial soft-tissue mass.
4. Preservation of the peri-ureteral fat plane.

Normal round, broad, cardinal and uterosacral ligaments should not be mistaken for lateral tumour extension. The characteristic CT findings of cervical cancer are a solid mass > 3.5 cm in AP diameter enlarging the cervix with hypodense areas in the tumour mass due to necrosis and ulceration. The mass shows diminished intravenous contrast enhancement compared to normal cervical stroma (Fig. 17.2). Myometrial intravenous contrast enhancement is necessary to differentiate normal uterine margins from irregular hypodense borders due to tumour infiltration of parametrial fat. Clinically unsuspected endometrial fluid collections and uterine enlargement due to tumour obstruction of the endocervical canal are also occasionally detected.

Vick et al (1984) defined the CT criteria for parametrial tumour invasion as follows:

1. Irregularity or poor definition of the lateral cervix margins.
2. Prominent parametrial soft-tissue strands.
3. Obliteration of the peri-ureteral fat plane.
4. An eccentric soft-tissue mass.

A parametrial soft-tissue mass and loss of the peri-ureteral fat plane are essential for a definitive CT diagnosis of parametrial tumour extension. CT Stage IIB tumours should also have a demonstrable fat plane greater than 3–4 mm separating the parametrial mass from the pelvic side wall. Caution must be exercised in interpreting loss of the cervical border and minimal soft-tissue infiltration of the para-uterine fat since parametritis, secondary to a previous uterine dilatation and curettage, or cervical conization can mimic the CT findings of parametrial tumour invasion.

Pelvic side-wall tumour extension (Stage IIIB) is characterized by confluent, irregular, linear parametrial soft-tissue strands or by confluent solid tumour which incorporates the obturator internus and piriformis muscles of the pelvic side wall and obliterates their fat planes. CT detection of hydronephrosis with or without pelvic side wall extension indicates a Stage IIIB tumour.

CT criteria for bladder/rectal involvement (Stage IVA) are focal loss of the perivesical/perirectal fat plane accompanied by asymmetric wall thickening, nodular indentations or serrations along the bladder/rectal wall and an intraluminal tumour mass (Fig. 17.3).

CT has a significant overstaging error rate (40–72%) in clinical Stage IB tumours due to a false positive diagnosis of parametrial tumour extension (Grumbine et al 1981, Walsh & Goplerud 1981, Villasanta et al 1983).

Other limitations of CT staging include understaging IIB–IIIB tumours due to microscopic spread and difficulty in diagnosing transmural-mucosal invasion of the bladder and rectum.

ENDOMETRIAL CANCER

Carcinoma of the endometrium is the most common invasive cancer of the female genital tract and the fourth most frequent cancer in women. Since initial symptoms are usually postmenopausal bleeding, patients often seek medical care when the cancer is at an early stage. Thus, the value of CT staging in this malignancy is limited because a high percentage of patients

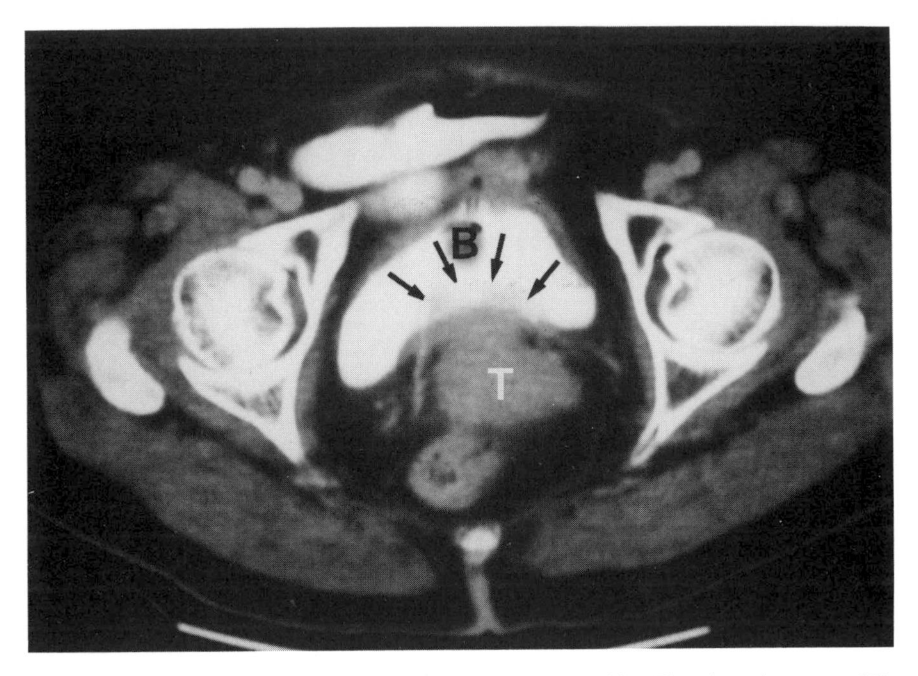

Fig. 17.3 CT Stage IVA cervix cancer. CT scan through bladder (B) and cervix tumour (T) show anterior tumour growth thickening posterior bladder wall with extension into the lumen (arrows).

have early stage disease (70–80%) and do not need imaging studies before hysterectomy.

CT stage criteria are developed from the FIGO classification (Table 17.1; Fig. 17.4). The most common metastatic spread pattern of endometrial adenocarcinoma is regional dissemination via parametrial lymphatics to pelvic and retroperitoneal lymph nodes. There is a much higher incidence of lymphatic or haematogenous metastases in carcinomas with deep myometrial invasion and a poorly differentiated histology. Other less common metastatic routes are penetration of the uterine serosa to seed the peritoneal cavity and local spread to the broad ligament, fallopian tube or ovary. Distant spread via ovarian lymphatics occasionally leads to upper retroperitoneal or supraclavicular lymph-node deposits and haematogenous spread to lung, brain and bone is seen in advanced disease.

Total abdominal hysterectomy and bilateral salpingo-oophorectomy with or without radiation therapy is the treatment of choice in medically operable Stage I–II patients. In Stages III and IV treatment options are combined surgery and irradiation versus irradiation alone.

In two series with CT-surgical staging comparison data, CT had an overall accuracy of 84–88% for staging endometrial cancer (Walsh & Goplerud 1982, Balfe et al 1983). Other data from these studies showed that CT had an 83–92% accuracy in showing tumour confined to the uterus and

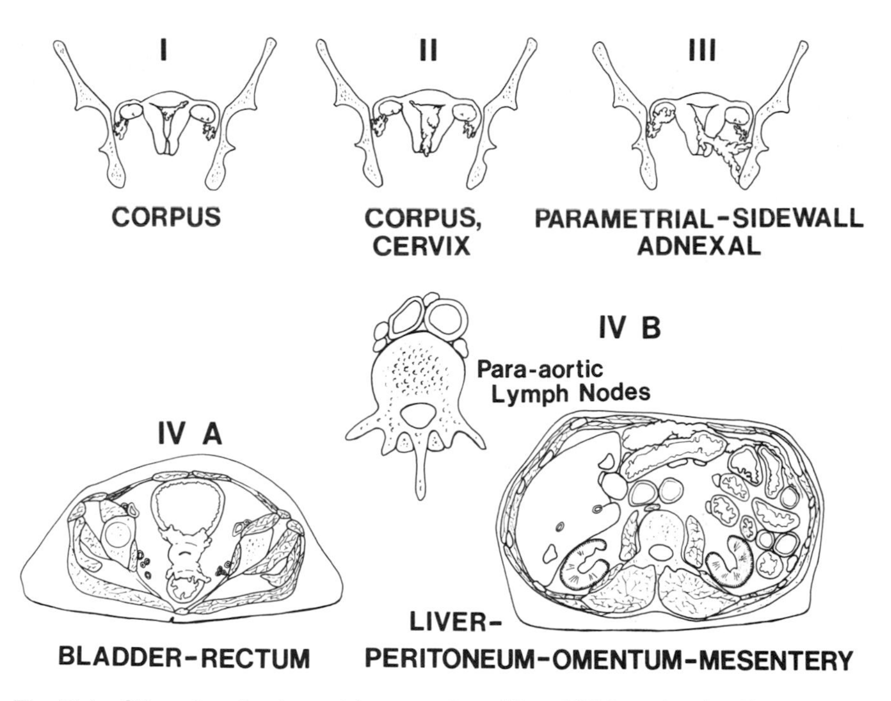

Fig. 17.4 CT staging of endometrial cancer adapted from FIGO staging classification.

an 83–86% accuracy in demonstrating extra-uterine tumour spread. CT staging is most efficacious for accurately determining stage in patients with an equivocal pelvic examination or a medical contra-indication to surgical staging. It is also helpful for screening for lymphatic metastases in patients with poorly differentiated carcinomas or sarcomas and for non-invasive confirmation of advanced disease (Stage III–IVB).

CT staging of endometrial cancer requires intravenous contrast administration to enhance normal myometrium and to delineate intra-uterine tumour. Enhanced CT demonstrates endometrial tumour as a hypodense mass in the uterine cavity or myometrium, as a fluid-filled uterus due to tumour obstruction of the endocervical canal or vagina, or rarely as a contrast-enhancing lesion in the myometrium. Tumour may be confined to the endometrial cavity and appears as a hypodense polypoid mass surrounded by less dense endometrial fluid (Fig. 17.5). Also, endometrial cancer may focally invade the myometrium and be highlighted by adjacent normal enhanced myometrium. Thus, CT may prove useful for determining the depth of myometrial tumour invasion (Dore et al 1987).

Endometrial tumour involvement of the cervix (Stage II) is characterized on CT as cervical enlargement > 3.5 cm in AP diameter as well as inhomogeneous hypodense areas within the fibromuscular stroma of the cervix. CT

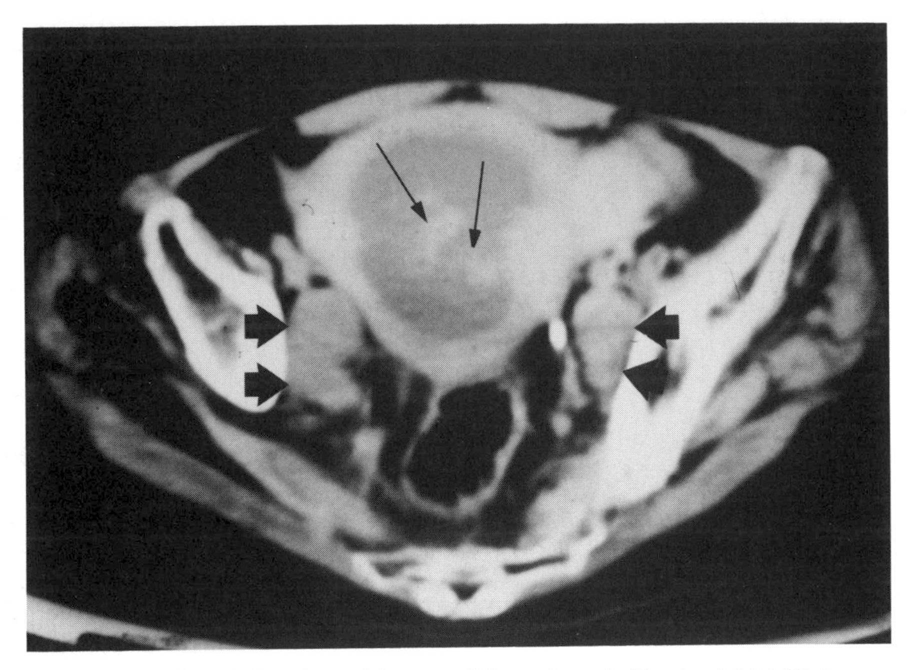

Fig. 17.5 CT Stage IVB endometrial cancer. CT scan through dilated and fluid-filled endometrial cavity containing polypoid tumour (thin arrows) shows bilateral enlarged pelvic lymph nodes (thick arrows). Abdominal scans showed para-aortic lymph-node metastases confirmed by needle aspiration cytology.

reliably identifies tumour confined to the uterus. The CT findings of local extra-uterine endometrial tumour extension (Stage III) are analogous to parametrial and side wall extension seen in cervical cancer (Fig. 17.6). Helpful CT signs to identify a mass as uterine and not ovarian in origin include myometrial wall enhancement, a characteristic pear-shape and midline location and attachments to the round, broad, cardinal or uterosacral ligaments.

UTERINE FLUID COLLECTIONS

Uterine fluid collections are usually due to occlusion of the endocervical canal or vagina from senile contraction, primary or recurrent carcinoma of the cervix or endometrium, radiation therapy or postsurgical scarring. Subsequent accumulation of sterile fluid (hydrometra), pus (pyometra) or blood (haematometra) proximal to the obstruction causes segmental dilation of the uterus and/or proximal vagina. CT demonstrates a fluid-filled ('obstructed') uterus as an enlarged uterus with a distended, fluid-density endometrial cavity surrounded by contrast-enhanced myometrium (Scott et al 1981). In adults, a pyometra or haematometra is usually due to carcinoma of the cervix or endometrium. Occasionally, a grossly distended

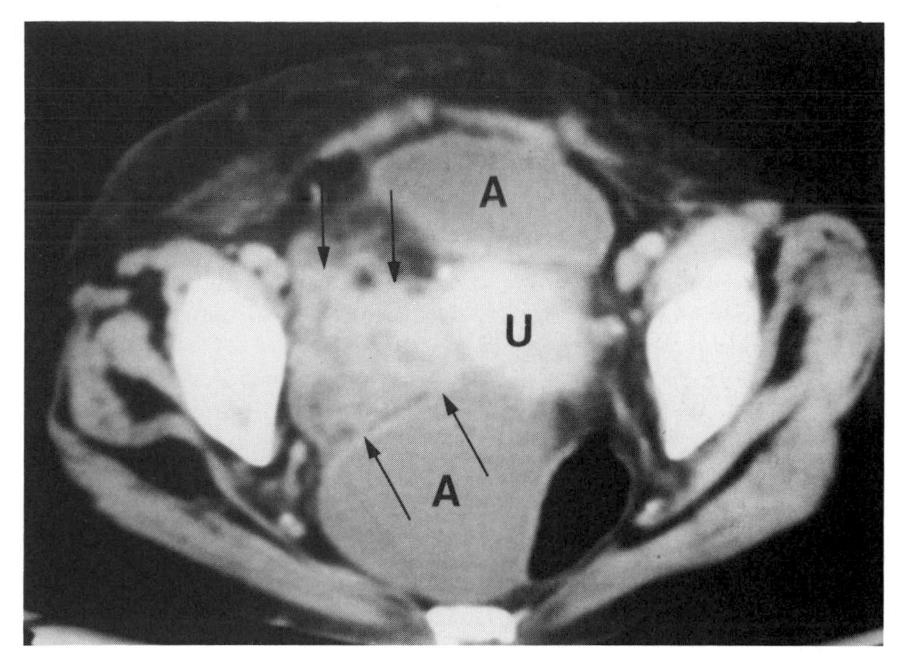

Fig. 17.6 CT Stage IVB endometrial cancer. CT scan through uterus (U) and loculated ascites (A) shows direct tumour extension to right pelvic side wall (arrows). Abdominal scans showed omental metastases.

endometrial cavity with polypoid mural tumour can simulate a cystic ovarian cancer, especially if ascites is present.

OVARIAN CANCER

Ovarian carcinoma is the sixth leading cancer in women and the sixth leading cause of cancer death. Most patients present with a pelvic mass and/or ascites as a manifestation of advanced cancer. Although this tumour may spread locally to the uterus and fallopian tube, metastases most frequently involve the peritoneum, omentum, mesentery and bowel surfaces. Ovarian cancer disseminates primarily by intraperitoneal seeding and surface implantation, less commonly by lymphatic spread and rarely by the haematogenous route.

At most medical centres, CT does not play a major role in the preoperative evaluation of ovarian cancer. When this diagnosis is clinically suspected most patients undergo exploratory laparotomy without extensive preoperative investigation. CT is not as accurate as surgical staging for assessing disease extent because of failure to identify miliary peritoneal seeding and small omental tumour nodules (Amendola et al 1981, Whitley et al 1981). Surgery is both diagnostic and therapeutic by providing a histological diagnosis, an accurate stage, tumour excision and a prognosis based on residual disease. Bilateral salpingo-oophorectomy, hysterectomy, omentectomy, bulk reduction of metastases, peritoneal washings and thorough inspection and/or biopsy of the peritoneum, mesentery, bowel serosa, liver and diaphragm are usually performed.

When preoperative evaluation of a suspected ovarian carcinoma is undertaken, CT has several advantages over clinical assessment. CT is superior to physical examination for detecting ascites and unsuspected metastases to pelvic and para-aortic lymph nodes and to the liver (Johnson et al 1983). In comparison with ultrasound, CT is more accurate for predicting tumour stage and for showing tumour involvement of bowel, pelvic ureter and retroperitoneal lymph nodes (Amendola et al 1981).

In clinical practice, the role of CT in ovarian carcinoma is usually one of characterizing an abdomino-pelvic mass in a symptomatic woman. Familiarity with the CT findings of ovarian cancer are necessary for differential diagnosis of gynaecological pelvic masses. The varied CT appearances of ovarian malignancy (Fig. 17.7a) are as follows:

1. Predominantly cystic mass with thick, irregular wall and/or solid soft-tissue components.
2. Multilocular cyst with internal septations.
3. Predominantly solid mass.
4. Inhomogeneous cystic–solid mass.

Amorphous coarse calcifications can be present either in the cyst wall or within soft-tissue components and are easily detected by CT. Intravenous contrast enhancement may be apparent in the solid components of an ovarian tumour but such enhancement is usually less than that of normal myometrium. Ovarian cancers may be located anywhere in the pelvis or lower abdomen and are most frequently found in the adnexa (ovarian fossa) lateral to the uterus, in the cul-de-sac or over the sacral promontory. They may be bilateral in 20–60% of various histological types. Since metastases

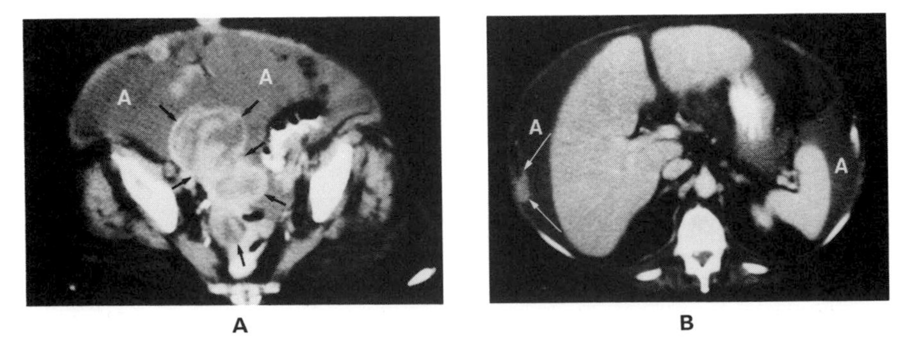

Fig. 17.7 Stage III poorly differentiated endometroid ovarian cancer. **A** CT scan above uterine fundus showed mixed cystic and solid ovarian cancer (arrows) in pelvic inlet surrounded by ascites (A). **B** CT scan through liver and spleen shows peritoneal tumour implant (arrows) outlined by ascites (A).

to the ovary have a CT appearance identical to primary ovarian cancer, images of the stomach and colon should be scrutinized as a possible primary tumour site.

CT may be indeterminate regarding the ovarian versus uterine origin of a pelvic cancer. The major cause for this diagnostic problem is that an ovarian cancer may abut or actually invade the uterus and obscure the intervening para-uterine fat planes. Recognition of the triangular-shaped endometrial cavity and myometrial contrast enhancement are the most important CT findings to differentiate the uterus from a contiguous ovarian cancer.

In addition to assessing the pelvic extent of the primary tumour, CT staging of ovarian cancer requires evaluation of the abdomen for tumour spread to the mesentery, omentum, peritoneum, liver and retroperitoneal lymph nodes.

Mesenteric metastases are recognized on CT as round, 'cake-like' or ill-defined soft-tissue masses surrounded by contrast-filled small bowel loops and mesenteric fat. A less common CT pattern is thickened leaves of the mesentery due to tumour infiltration along mesenteric folds and vessels. Omental metastases are recognized on CT as soft-tissue masses embedded in omental fat anterior to the small bowel and transverse colon in the abdomen or false pelvis. Large confluent omental 'tumour-cakes' may obliterate fat planes between the mass and the anterior abdominal wall due to tumour adhesions and may protrude into the umbilicus.

Peritoneal tumour implants are recognized as 1.5–3.5 cm nodular soft-tissue masses along the lateral peritoneal surfaces of the abdomen. Sub-diaphragmatic peritoneal nodules are best detected between the abdominal wall and the liver in the presence of ascites (Fig. 17.7b). When ascites is present, current high-resolution CT scanners can resolve peritoneal implants as small as 5 mm, but this is the exception rather than the rule. Ovarian cancer commonly implants on the serosal surfaces of the caecum, transverse mesocolon, sigmoid colon or small bowel loops. The major limitation of CT for staging ovarian cancer is its inability to reliably detect visceral or peritoneal tumour implants smaller than 1–2 cm.

Ovarian lymphatic metastases, although uncommon, characteristically skip the pelvic and lower retroperitoneal nodes to involve the upper retroperitoneal and renal hilar nodes directly via gonadal lymphatic spread. Metastases in these nodal sites are readily detected with CT.

CONCLUSION

CT complements clinical staging in patients with gynaecological cancers. Its greatest impact has been in defining the extent of disease in patients with carcinoma of the cervix but it also has an important place in the diagnosis and assessment of ovarian cancer. Although CT is generally not required for staging endometrial tumours the technique may be helpful in selected patients.

In the past few years magnetic resonance (MR) imaging has also become an excellent primary pelvic staging technique with at least an equivalent overall staging accuracy in evaluating cervical and endometrial cancers. However, at present its high cost and lack of general availability preclude its use as a routine staging procedure.

REFERENCES

Amendola M A, Walsh J W, Amendola B E, Tisnado J, Hall D J, Goplerud D R 1981 Computed tomography in the evaluation of carcinoma of the ovary. Journal of Computer Assisted Tomography 5: 179–186

Balfe D M, Van Dyke J, Lee J K T, Weyman P J, McClennan B L 1983 Computed tomography in malignant endometrial neoplasms. Journal of Computer Assisted Tomography 7: 677–681

Dore R, Moro G, D'Andrea F, La Fianza A, Franchi M, Bolis P F 1987 CT evaluation of myometrium invasion in endometrial carcinoma. Journal of Computer Assisted Tomography 11: 282–289

Grumbine F C, Rosenshein N B, Zerhouni E A, Siegelman S S 1981 Abdominopelvic computed tomography in the preoperative evaluation of early cervical cancer. Gynecologic Oncology 12: 286–290

Johnson R J, Blackledge G, Eddleston B, Crowther D 1983 Abdomino-pelvic computed tomography in the management of ovarian carcinoma. Radiology 146: 447–452

Scott W W Jr, Rosenshein N B, Siegelman S S, Sanders R C 1981 The obstructed uterus. Radiology 141: 767–770

Vick C W, Walsh J W, Wheelock J B, Brewer W H 1984 CT of the normal and abnormal parametria in cervical cancer. American Journal of Roentgenology 143: 597–603

Villasanta U, Whitley N O, Haney P J, Brenner D 1983 Computed tomography in invasive carcinoma of the cervix: an appraisal. Obstetrics & Gynecology 62: 218–224

Walsh J W, Goplerud D R 1981 Prospective comparison between clinical and CT staging in primary cervical carcinoma. American Journal of Roentgenology 137: 997–1003

Walsh J W, Goplerud D R 1982 Computed tomography of primary, persistent and recurrent endometrial malignancy. American Journal of Roentgenology 139: 1149–1154

Whitley N O, Brenner D, Francis A et al 1981 Use of the computed tomographic whole body scanner to stage and follow patients with advanced ovarian carcinoma. Investigative Radiology 16: 479–486

18. Staging of bladder and prostate cancer

Janet E. S. Husband

INTRODUCTION

Carcinoma of the bladder and prostate are common tumours, their incidence increasing with age. Carcinoma of the prostate accounted for 12% of all cancers in males in the United Kingdom in 1985 and carcinoma of the bladder accounted for 6% of all male and 2% of all female malignancies. In patients with invasive bladder cancer less than 50% survive five years (Shipley et al 1985) and in those with advanced cancer of the prostate, with no evidence of disseminated disease, 5-year survival rates are also poor (McGowan 1977).

Early bladder tumours can be successfully treated by transurethral resection but more advanced tumours require radiotherapy as well as surgery (Bloom et al 1982). Chemotherapy is also being used with increasing success (Young & Garnick 1988). Surgery offers the best chance of cure for patients with early stage prostatic cancer while radiotherapy and drugs are given for advanced local tumour and disseminated disease.

The majority of bladder tumours (95%) are transitional-cell papillary carcinomas. The remainder are squamous-cell tumours, mixed transitional-cell and squamous-cell tumours, adenocarcinomas or undifferentiated lesions. Prostatic neoplasms are practically always adenocarcinomas. Rare exceptions include sarcomas and leiomyosarcomas.

STAGING METHODS

The TNM classification for staging bladder and prostate cancer is used (UICC 1982) (Table 18.1; Figs. 18.1 and 18.2).

Conventional T staging of bladder cancer is carried out using cystoscopy with biopsy, transurethral resection and bimanual examination under general anaesthesia. Ultrasound techniques may also be useful for evaluating the primary tumour but these have not gained such widespread acceptance as CT.

Staging primary prostate neoplasms still relies heavily on the findings of rectal digital examination, although transrectal ultrasound is now being employed in several centres with excellent results (Salo et al 1987). CT is

Table 18.1 TNM classifications for bladder and prostate cancer (abbrev) UICC 1982

Bladder	
Tis	Carcinoma-in-situ
Ta	Papillary, non-invasive
T1	Lamina propria infiltration
T2	Superficial muscle
T3a	Deep muscle
T3b	Extravesical spread
T4a	Invading prostate, uterus or vagina
T4b	Invading pelvic/abdominal wall
N0	No lymph-node involvement
N1	Involvement of single homolateral node
N2	Involvement of contralateral/bilateral multiple regional nodes
N3	Fixed regional nodes
N4	Common iliac/aortic/inguinal nodes
M0	No metastases
M1	Distant metastases
Prostate	
Tis	Carcinoma-in-situ
T0	No tumour palpable
T1	Tumour surrounded by normal gland
T2	Tumour confined to gland. Smooth nodule deforming contour
T3	Tumour extending beyond capsule $\pm$ seminal vesicle involvement
T4	Tumour fixed or involving adjacent structures
N0	No lymph-node involvement
N1	Involvement of single homolateral node
N2	Involvement of contralateral/bilateral/multiple regional lymph nodes
N3	Fixed regional nodes
N4	Common iliac/aortic/inguinal nodes
M0	No metastases
M1	Distant metastases

used less commonly than for staging bladder tumours and is most useful for assessing advanced disease.

Lymph-node involvement in both bladder and prostate cancer may be detected with CT but lymphography also has an important role.

The detection of distant metastases is based on conventional radiography, ultrasound, radionuclide scanning and occasionally CT.

PATTERNS OF TUMOUR SPREAD

Bladder tumours spread directly by infiltrating through the bladder wall into the perivesical fat and adjacent structures. In early-stage tumours lymph-node metastases are rare but once the primary tumour has spread beyond the bladder wall the incidence of lymph-node metastases rises to about 60% (van der Werf-Messing et al 1982). The lymph nodes first involved which are visible on CT are the hypogastric and obturator nodes. Further spread occurs via the external iliac chain to the para-aortic nodes.

Direct spread of carcinoma of the prostate is similar to carcinoma of the bladder. The primary tumour first distorts the prostatic capsule and then

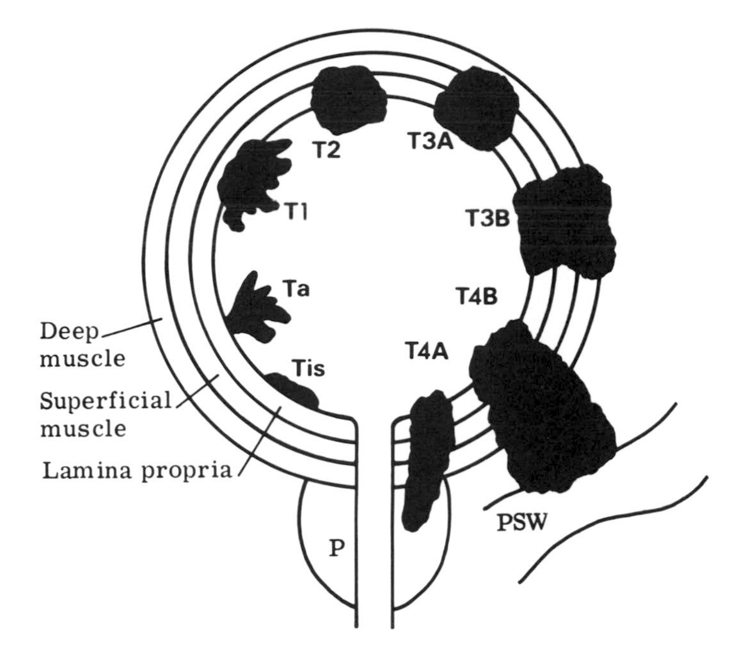

Fig. 18.1 Diagram illustrating T staging for carcinoma of the bladder. Prostate (P), pelvic side wall (PSW). (Reproduced by kind permission of Churchill Livingstone, New York.)

breaks through it into the periprostatic fat and adjacent organs, particularly the seminal vesicles. The pattern of nodal spread is also similar to carcinoma of the bladder with initial involvement occurring in the hypogastric and obturator chain. The incidence of lymph-node metastases is related to periprostatic extension and if the seminal vesicles are involved the incidence of lymph-node deposits is approximately 80% (McLaughlin et al 1976).

The risk of haematogenous spread in both bladder and prostate cancer increases with the size of the primary tumour and the number and size of involved nodes. In carcinoma of the prostate haematogenous spread is common with the predilection for bone. The prostate is surrounded by a rich venous plexus which drains into the internal iliac veins and also communicates with the vertebral venous plexus. This probably accounts for the high incidence of bone metastases (75%) in patients with multiple positive nodes.

TECHNIQUE OF EXAMINATION

Assessment of patients with bladder and prostate cancer should include CT examination of the abdomen for metastatic disease as well as evaluation of the pelvis. In our department a similar technique is used for staging both these tumours.

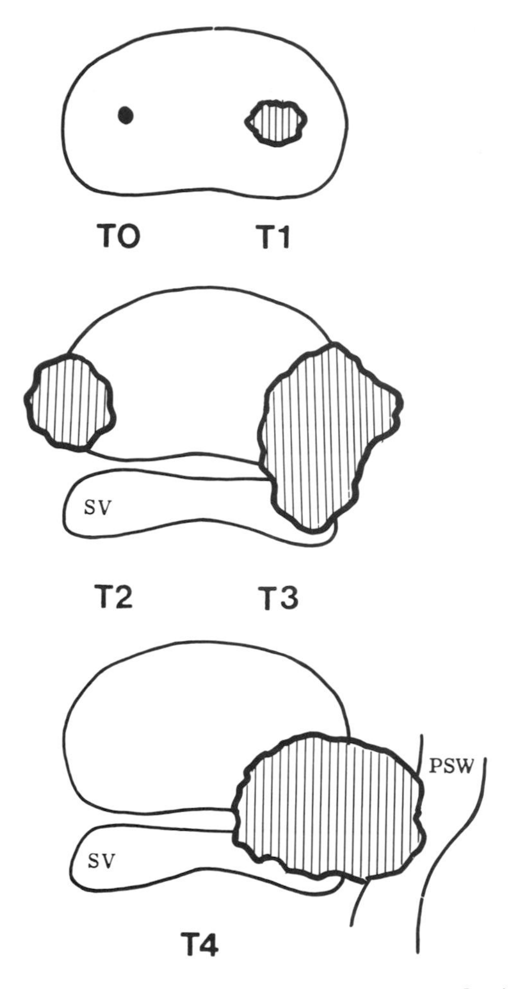

Fig. 18.2 Diagram illustrating T staging for carcinoma of the prostate. Seminal vesicle (SV), pelvic side wall (PSW). (Reproduced by kind permission of Churchill Livingstone, New York.)

The abdomen is scanned first from the domes of the diaphragm to the middle of the fifth lumbar vertebra using 8 mm collimation with a slice interval of 1.4 cm. The pelvis is examined using 8 mm collimation at 10 mm intervals. In addition contiguous 4 mm thick slices are taken through the prostate when examining prostatic cancer patients.

The pelvic scan is undertaken during injection of intravenous contrast medium using dynamic scanning with automatic table movement. A bolus of 50 ml (370 mgI_2/ml) is injected before scanning through the pelvis begins and a further 50 ml is injected during the first two minutes of the pelvic study. The advantages of this technique are:

1. Minimal lymph-node enlargement is easier to identify because the vessels of the pelvic side walls are opacified.
2. Bladder tumours enhance and this facilitates detection of extravesical spread and adjacent organ invasion.
3. In female patients the uterus enhances which helps to identify the organ and its relationship to tumour in patients with large volume extravesical disease.
4. After initial assessment scans can be repeated with contrast medium in the bladder and ureters. This may be useful for identifying a bladder tumour which is difficult to visualize on the initial scan. It may also show ureteric obstruction or involvement by tumour.

THE BLADDER

CT findings

The intraluminal component of a bladder tumour is usually seen as a soft-tissue mass projecting into the bladder lumen (Fig. 18.1) but in some cases the only abnormality identified is an area of localized bladder wall thickening.

CT is impractical for staging tumours less than T3a because early stages of disease cannot be distinguished from each other. The major advantage of CT is the ability to detect extravesical tumour spread thus distinguishing T3a from T3b stage disease (Hodson et al 1979, Jeffrey et al 1981). The earliest sign of extravesical spread on CT is poor definition of the outer aspect of the bladder wall in the region of the tumour with 'whispy' strands of soft tissue extending into the perivesical fat (Fig. 18.3). In more advanced disease an obvious soft-tissue mass is seen extending beyond the bladder wall.

Tumour spread to the pelvic side wall (T4b) appears as a soft-tissue mass extending from the bladder as far as the obturator internus muscle and/or anterior abdominal wall (Fig. 18.4). Invasion of adjacent organs (T4a) may be difficult to identify with CT because there is no clear fat plane between the posterior bladder wall and such structures as the rectum, prostate, uterus and vagina. However, a structure partially or completely surrounded by tumour should be considered as involved. Spread to seminal vesicles is diagnosed if soft tissue obliterates the seminal vesicle fat angle (Fig. 18.5), however, this fat angle may also be lost if the rectum is over-distended or if the patient is scanned in the prone position.

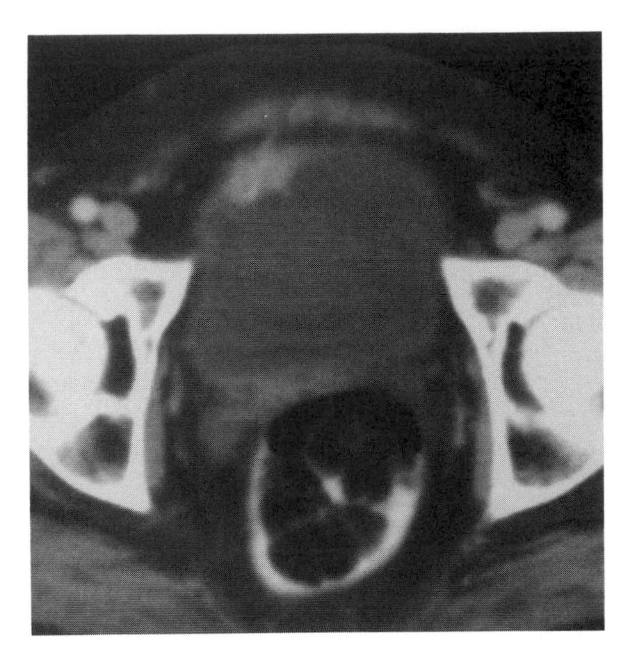

Fig. 18.3 CT scan showing a bladder tumour arising from the anterior bladder wall. Extravesical extension is seen as 'whispy' strands of soft tissue extending into the perivesical fat. Note enhancement of the tumour with intravenous contrast medium.

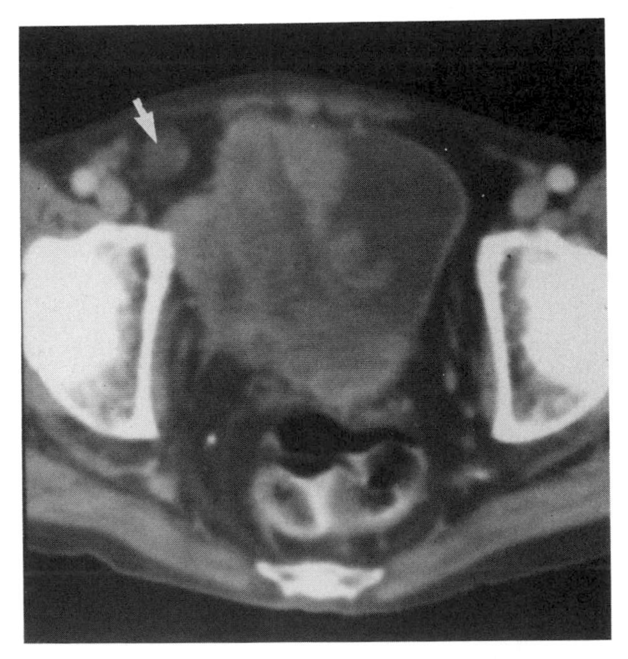

Fig. 18.4 CT scan of a patient with advanced bladder cancer. Tumour extends as far as the pelvic side wall on the right (Stage T4B). Note enlarged lymph node (arrow).

Difficulties of interpretation

1. Detection of early extravesical tumour spread.
2. Detection of adjacent organ involvement.
3. Tumours of the bladder base may be difficult to identify and distinguish from an enlarged prostate. In addition, prostatic invasion by a bladder tumour may be impossible to identify.
4. Tumours of the dome may be difficult to visualize because the surrounding bladder wall has a similar density to tumour.
5. Post-endoscopy. If CT is undertaken within a few days of endoscopy oedema and inflammation may be misinterpreted as tumour. Blood clot may also simulate intraluminal tumour.
6. Post-radiotherapy. Radiotherapy produces bladder wall thickening, reduction in bladder capacity and generalized increase in density of the perivesical fat. These findings make interpretation of post-radiotherapy CT less accurate than in the untreated patient.

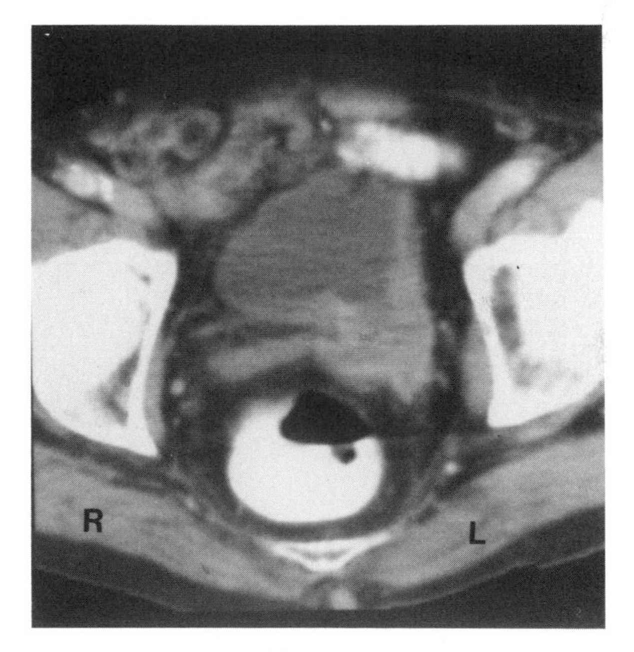

Fig. 18.5 Seminal vesicle invasion on the left in a patient with a tumour arising in the posterior bladder wall. Note loss of the seminal vesicle fat angle on the left compared with the normal fat angle on the right.

Accuracy of CT

The overall accuracy of CT compared with clinical and histopathological staging ranges from 64 to 92% (Koss et al 1981, Morgan et al 1981). Direct comparison of CT between different series is impossible because there are many variable factors. For example in some patients CT is evaluated following radiotherapy and transurethral resection which both lead to errors of overstaging (Kellett et al 1980, Vock et al 1982, Sarno et al 1983). Other causes of over-staging include misinterpretation of normal structures lying adjacent to the bladder wall as tumour, or mistaking the absence of a fat plane between the bladder wall and adjacent organs as evidence of tumour invasion. Under-staging results from failure to identify minimal and microscopic perivesical extension.

The accuracy of CT increases with advanced disease and although errors are inevitable CT is superior to clinical staging in patients with invasive disease.

PROSTATIC CANCER

CT findings

Small tumours (T0, T1) contained within the gland and surrounded by normal prostatic tissue cannot be detected with CT because there is no density difference between the tumour and surrounding prostatic parenchyma. Even those tumours which produce asymmetry of the gland (T2) may be missed unless there is a significant alteration of the prostatic contour. The prostate is usually enlarged in advanced disease (normal range: transverse diameter 3–5 cm, AP diameter 2.5–4.5 cm) but this is not

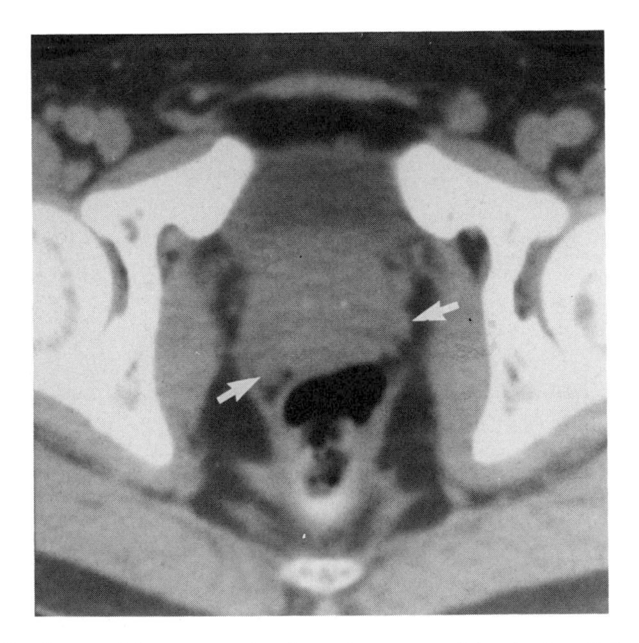

Fig. 18.6 Carcinoma of the prostate showing enlargement of the gland and bilateral extraprostatic spread (arrowed).

always so. Volume estimations of the prostate may be useful for radiotherapy planning and monitoring response to treatment but CT overestimates the volume of the gland because the capsule cannot be distinguished from prostatic parenchyma (Sukov et al 1977). Enlargement of the gland due to tumour cannot be distinguished from enlargement due to benign prostatic hyperplasia. If the two conditions coexist this may also lead to over-estimation of tumour volume.

Local tumour spread usually occurs in the dorsal direction because Denonvillier's fascia is an effective barrier against infiltration by tumour (Schroeder & van der Werf-Messing 1982).

Advanced extraprostatic spread is readily recognized on CT because an irregular soft-tissue mass is seen extending beyond the gland (Fig. 18.6). Minimal extracapsular extension is difficult to identify because there is very little fat between the gland and the levator ani muscles. Furthermore, if the gland is grossly enlarged the capsule may abut against the levator ani and urogenital diaphragm making assessment of early extraprostatic invasion impossible.

Tumour invasion of the bladder lumen produces an irregular intraluminal mass. However, bladder wall thickening may be seen when there is no invasion, presumably due to oedema. Rectal invasion is uncommon but can be diagnosed with CT if there is contiguity between the primary prostate tumour and an intraluminal rectal mass. The recognition of seminal vesicle involvement is important because this cannot be determined on rectal examination. As in bladder cancer, loss of the seminal vesicle fat angle is the crucial sign of invasion.

Accuracy of CT

Staging primary prostatic cancer with CT is more difficult than at any other tumour site in the pelvis which probably accounts for the small number of studies so far reported. The overall accuracy of CT compared with histopathological staging varies from 47 to 73% (Golimbu et al 1981, Emory et al 1983). Although these figures are low compared with those for carcinoma of the bladder the results are significantly better than those for clinical staging alone. Under-staging results from failure to identify extraprostatic spread and is more frequent than errors of over-staging. As with bladder cancer CT is more accurate in advanced than early disease.

LYMPH-NODE INVOLVEMENT

Pelvic lymph nodes 1.5 cm in diameter or greater are generally considered to be abnormal on pelvic CT (Fig. 18.7). However, as CT image quality and techniques have improved, it is now possible to detect lymph nodes which are only about 1 cm in diameter, and a lymph node > 1 cm should therefore be regarded with suspicion.

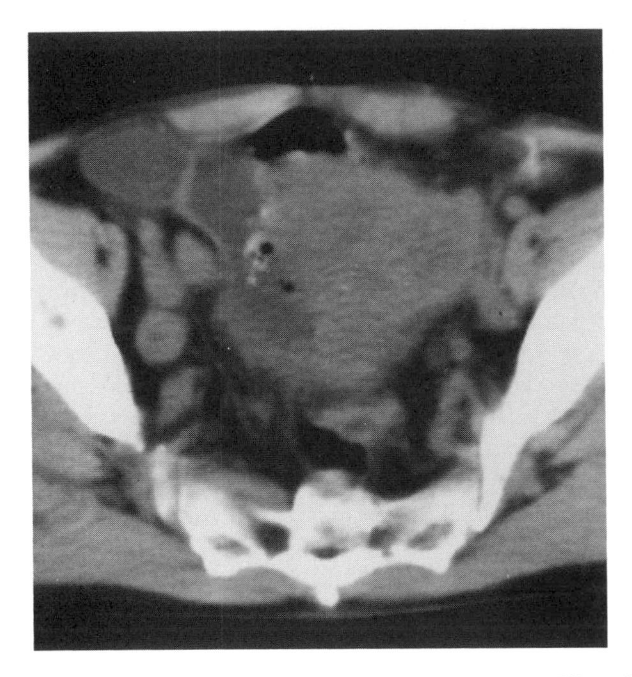

Fig. 18.7 CT scan of a patient with an advanced T4B bladder tumour. Bilateral enlarged lymph nodes are seen in the external iliac, obturator and internal iliac chains. A confident diagnosis of lymph-node metastases can be made.

Minimal degrees of enlargement are easier to identify in the external iliac chains than in the internal iliac group. Asymmetry of the external iliac vascular bundles on comparing one side of the pelvis with the other is a useful sign of minimal lymphadenopathy. If minimally enlarged nodes are identified it should be borne in mind that chronic lymphadenitis, fatty replacement or reactive hyperplasia may produce nodal enlargement and such benign conditions cannot be distinguished from tumour (Fig. 18.8).

Lymphography demonstrates the internal architecture of opacified nodes and in this respect provides more information than CT. Lymphography may therefore enable distinction between metastases and benign lymph-node enlargement and may also demonstrate metastases in normal-sized nodes. Internal iliac and obturator nodes are not usually opacified at lymphography and this is a major disadvantage of the technique in the assessment of bladder and prostatic cancer. With both techniques it should be remembered that a certain percentage of false negative examinations result from microscopic metastases in normal-sized nodes which will not be detected by any imaging modality.

Accuracy

Overall, the accuracy of CT varies from 70 to 93% (Golimbu et al 1981,

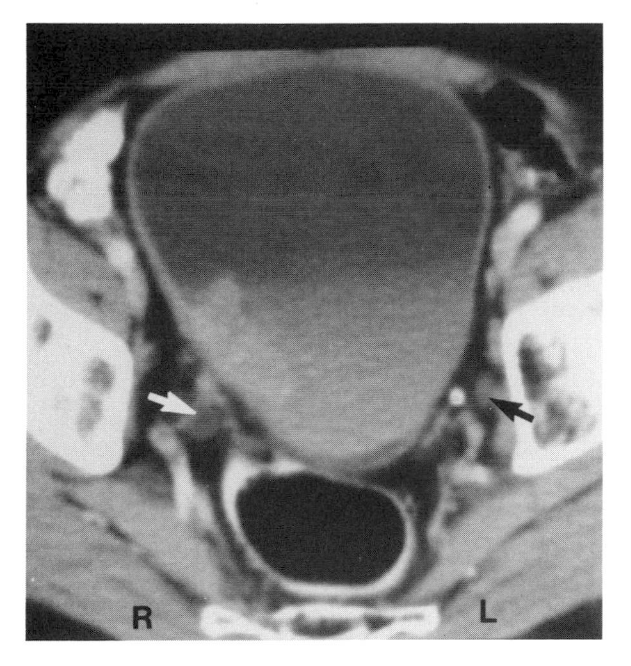

Fig. 18.8 CT scan of a patient with bladder cancer showing the tumour (T). The right ureter is dilated (white arrow). A 1 cm diameter lymph node is seen in the left internal iliac chain but a definite diagnosis of a lymph-node metastasis cannot be made (black arrow).

Levine et al 1981) and these figures compare well with those of lymphography for which accuracies range from 48 to 94% (Wajsman et al 1975, Loening et al 1977). In the light of these results we undertake CT as an initial investigation. In patients with unequivocally positive CT studies CT-guided biopsy can confirm metastatic spread and obviate the need for staging laparotomy. In patients with negative or equivocal CT studies lymphography provides an alternative procedure.

METASTASES

It is beyond the scope of this text to discuss the sites of distant metastases in carcinoma of the bladder and prostate. When staging these patients with CT scans should be reviewed on bone windows and attention also paid to the liver.

CONCLUSION

Advances in scanner technology, together with the wealth of experience in CT which has been gained during recent years have enabled the advantages and limitations of the technique to be clearly defined for staging bladder and prostate cancer.

CT has made an important impact on staging bladder cancer because the presence and extent of extravesical tumour spread can be accurately documented. Furthermore, in those patients undergoing radical radiotherapy CT-integrated planning can be routinely employed (Dobbs & Husband 1985). CT is likely to have an increasing role for monitoring response to chemotherapy as more successful drugs are developed.

CT is of little value for staging patients with tumours < T3A and in this respect the technique has been disappointing. Lymph-node status can be investigated with CT as effectively as with lymphography and consequently there has been a significant reduction in the number of lymphograms performed.

The role of CT for staging prostate cancer is more limited because CT staging is less accurate than for bladder cancer. Its importance lies in the documentation of gross local disease for radiotherapy planning and in the detection of lymph-node metastases.

REFERENCES

Bloom H J G, Hendry W F, Wallace D M, Skeet R G 1982 Treatment of T3 bladder cancer: controlled trial of pre-operative radiotherapy and radical cystectomy versus radical radiotherapy (second report and review). British Journal of Urology 54: 136–151

Dobbs H J, Husband J E 1985 The role of CT in the staging and radiotherapy planning of prostatic tumours. British Journal of Radiology 58: 429–436

Emory T H, Reinke D B, Hill A L, Lange P H 1983 Use of CT to reduce understaging in prostatic cancer: comparison with conventional staging techniques. American Journal of Roentgenology 141: 351–354

Golimbu M, Morales P, Al-Askari S, Shulman Y 1981 CAT scanning in staging of prostatic cancer. Urology 18: 305–308

Hodson N J, Husband J E, Macdonald J S 1979 The role of computed tomography in the staging of bladder cancer. Clinical Radiology 30: 389–395

Jeffrey R B, Palubinskas A J, Federle M P 1981 CT evaluation of invasive lesions of the bladder. Journal of Computer Assisted Tomography 5: 22–26

Kellett M J, Oliver R T D, Husband J E, Kelsey Fry I 1980 Computed tomography as an adjunct to bimanual examination for staging bladder tumours. British Journal of Urology 52: 101–106

Koss J C, Arger P H, Coleman B G, Mulhern C B, Pollack H M, Wein A J 1981 CT staging of bladder carcinoma. American Journal of Roentgenology 137: 359–362

Levine M S, Arger P H, Coleman B G, Mulhern C B, Pollack H M, Wein A J 1981 Detecting lymphatic metastases from prostatic carcinoma: superiority of CT. American Journal of Roentgenology 137: 207–211

Loening S A, Schmidt J D, Brown R C, Hawtrey C E, Fallon B, Culp D A 1977 A comparison between lymphangiography and pelvic lymph node dissection in the staging of prostatic cancer. Journal of Urology 117: 752–756

McGowan D D 1977 Radiation therapy in the management of localised carcinoma of the prostate: a preliminary report. Cancer 39: 98–103

McLaughlin A P, Saltzstein S L, McCullough D L, et al 1976 Prostatic carcinoma: incidence and location of unsuspected lymphatic metastases. Journal of Urology 115: 89–94

Morgan C L, Calkins R F, Cavalcanti E J 1981 Computed tomography in the evaluation, staging and therapy of carcinoma of the bladder and prostate. Radiology 140: 751–761

Salo J O, Kivisaari L, Sakari R et al 1987 Computerized tomography and transrectal ultrasound in the assessment of local extension of prostatic cancer before radical retropubic prostatectomy. Journal of Urology 137: 435–438

Sarno R C, Klauber G, Carter B L 1983 Computer assisted tomography of urachal abnormalities. Journal of Computer Assisted Tomography 7: 674–676

Schroeder F H, van der Werf-Messing 1982 Prostate. In: Halnan K E (ed) Treatment of cancer. Chapman and Hall, London, pp 475–493
Shipley W U, Rose M A, Perrone T, Mannix C M, Heney N M, Prout G R Jr 1985 Full dose irradiation for patients with invasive bladder carcinoma: clinical and histologic factors prognostic of improved survival. Journal of Urology 134: 679–683
Sukov R J, Scardino P T, Sample W F, Winter J, Confer D J 1977 Computed tomography and transabdominal ultrasound in the evaluation of the prostate. Journal of Computer Assisted Tomography 1: 281–289
UICC (International Union Against Cancer) 1982 TNM-Atlas. Illustrated Guide to the TNM/pTNM-Classification of Malignant Tumours. Spiessl B, Hermanek P, Scheibe O, Wagner G (eds). Springer Verlag, Berlin
van der Werf-Messing B, Schroeder R H, Bush H 1982 Bladder. In: Halnan K E (ed) Textbook of cancer. Chapman & Hall, London, pp 457–474
Vock P, Haertel M, Fuchs W A, Karrer P, Bishop M C, Zingg E J 1982 Computed tomography in staging of carcinoma of the urinary bladder. British Journal of Urology 54: 158–163
Wajsman Z, Baumgartner G, Murphy G P et al 1975 Evaluation of lymphangiography for clinical staging of bladder tumors. Journal of Urology 114: 712–714
Young D C, Garnick M 1988 Chemotherapy in bladder cancer: the North American experience. In: Raghavan D (ed) The management of bladder cancer. Edward Arnold (Publishers), pp 245–263

19. Hodgkin's and non-Hodgkin's lymphoma

Graham R. Cherryman

INTRODUCTION

CT scanning is now routinely performed in patients presenting with lymphoma because full radiological assessment of disease extent is useful for selecting the most appropriate therapy and for determining patient prognosis (Kaplan 1980, Meyer et al 1984, Neumann et al 1985, Castellino et al 1986). Furthermore, serial CT studies may be used to monitor response to therapy and evaluate any residual masses (Lewis et al 1982, North et al 1987). Finally, should the patient relapse the information provided by CT is valuable for planning further treatment and for treatment failure analysis (Oliver et al 1983, Heron et al 1988).

Lymphomas are tumours of the immune system and frequently arise in and involve lymph nodes. The cross-sectional imaging capability of CT is ideally suited for the detection of enlarged nodes and, in addition, CT may display extranodal disease.

PATTERN OF TUMOUR GROWTH

Lymph nodes

Four stages of lymph-node involvement may be recognized in patients with lymphoma. Initially tiny, so-called micrometastases, are found in the node which do not produce nodal enlargement. These may be occult or may be detected on lymphangiography but cannot be diagnosed on CT.

Eventually tumour growth within the node is sufficient to produce nodal enlargement and, at this stage involved nodes can be recognized on CT. Standard criteria have now evolved for recognizing nodal enlargement on CT (Castellino et al 1984, Glazer et al 1985) but experienced radiologists may modify these depending on the size of normal nodes seen in their referral population. Furthermore, a knowledge of the patterns of involvement seen in the different lymphomas is helpful for assessing whether a minimally enlarged node is likely to be involved by tumour or not.

In most studies thoracic and axillary nodes are regarded as normal if under 1 cm in diameter, retrocrural nodes are presumed normal if < 0.6 cm in diameter, while in the retroperitoneum and pelvis 1.0 and 1.5 cms are

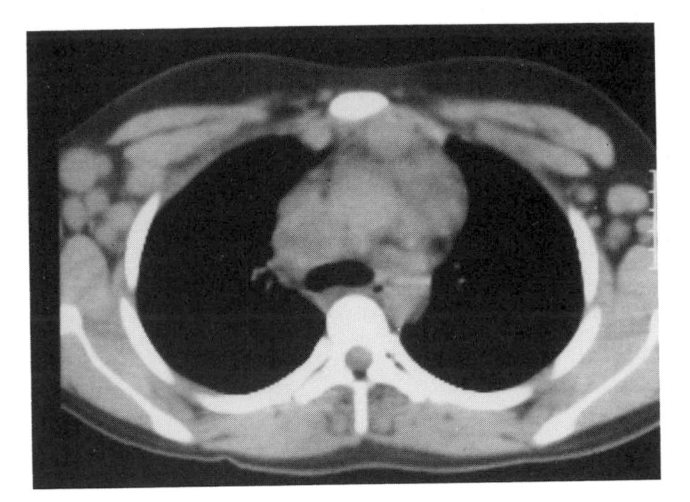

Fig. 19.1 CT scan through the upper mediastinum shows widespread lymphadenopathy. The large mediastinal nodes have a blurred outline indicating extranodal spread of disease. The large axillary nodes have a sharply defined margin indicating that tumour is confined within the nodes.

taken as the upper limit of normal respectively. Nodal assessment on the basis of size remains a difficult choice between high sensitivity (describing a number of non-involved nodes positive) or high specificity (describing a number of smaller, but involved nodes negative). False negative results are not only due to tumour in normal-sized nodes but occur if an enlarged node is not identified or misinterpreted. False positive results occur if nodal enlargement is due to a benign process or if a soft-tissue structure is incorrectly identified as an enlarged node. Interpretative errors can be minimized with careful attention to technique, for example using the prone position to differentiate nodes from unopacified bowel loops and intravenous contrast medium to identify vascular structures and normal variations.

In general, the larger the affected node the easier it is to recognize and the higher the probability that it is involved. However, it should be borne in mind that lymph nodes considered only as suspicious of involvement on CT are unlikely to alter treatment decisions in many patients.

Further tumour growth leads to extension through the capsule of the node and at this time CT shows a blurred outline to the enlarged node (Fig. 19.1). Eventually individual nodes are no longer discernible and the tumour appears as an amorphous soft-tissue mass. Extranodal extension results in involvement of surrounding structures and organs. In most instances it is impossible on CT images to distinguish contiguity from true early invasion. As a general rule lymphoma tends to displace surrounding structures and invasion is a late feature.

Extranodal sites

Spread of lymphoma to extranodal sites is a consequence of vascular invasion. In Hodgkin's disease this is invariably seen after splenic involvement. Non-Hodgkin's lymphomas, especially the higher grade (diffuse) lymphomas, invade local lymphatic and blood vessels. Tumour emboli then disseminate through the circulation and may lodge at different sites within the body (Bragg et al 1986). Extranodal lymphoma can be recognized on CT provided there is either a change in the morphology and/or the density of the involved tissues. The sensitivity of CT scanning varies at different sites within the body and thus CT is of greater value in the brain, soft tissues, lungs, pleura and bones than in the spleen and liver (Amendola 1986).

STAGING CLASSIFICATION

The Ann Arbor staging classification for Hodgkin's disease is most widely used and may also be applied to non-Hodgkin's lymphoma (Table 19.1). Patients with non-Hodgkin's lymphoma fall into two basic groups: (i) follicular (nodular or low grade) lymphomas and (ii) diffuse (intermediate and high grade) lymphomas (Jaffe 1986).

Stage I disease is most typically seen in the patient with unilateral neck node involvement. The prognosis is very good and treatment usually consists of extended field irradiation to the neck and mediastinum. Hodgkin's disease spreads through the body by involvement of contiguous nodal groups and extended field techniques are designed to include any occult disease in adjacent lymph-node groups. Non-Hodgkin's lymphoma does not spread in a predictable manner and treatment choice is more limited because few patients are likely to be cured by local irradiation. For this reason, the Ann Arbor staging system is of less practical value.

In Stage II disease prognosis is related to the number of affected sites and

Table 19.1 Ann Arbor staging classification for Hodgkin's disease

Stage I	Involvement of a single lymph-node group
Stage IE	Involvement of a single extralymphatic organ or site
Stage II	Involvement of two or more lymph-node groups on the same side of the diaphragm
Stage IIE	As in II + localized involvement of an extralymphatic organ or site on the same side of the diaphragm
Stage III	Involvement of lymph-node groups on both sides of the diaphragm
Stage IIIS	As in III + involvement of the spleen
Stage IIIE	As in III + localized involvement of an extralymphatic organ or site
Stage IV	Diffuse or disseminated involvement of one or more extralymphatic organs or sites ± lymph-node involvement

is significantly worse if disease is demonstrated in three or more sites. The choice between radiotherapy, chemotherapy or both is more difficult and it is particularly in these patients that CT scanning may play a key role in treatment choice.

Patients with Stage III and IV disease are treated almost invariably with chemotherapy.

THORAX

Lymph-node involvement

CT scans taken through the anterior mediastinum are critical because it is here that disease is characteristically seen. Indeed, it is exceptional for tumour to be present in the chest without anterior mediastinal involvement. Pulmonary changes in a patient with Hodgkin's disease, in the absence of mediastinal or hilar adenopathy, should be regarded as non-lymphomatous.

CT may reveal mediastinal disease in the patient with a normal chest radiograph. Castellino et al (1986) found CT evidence of mediastinal disease in 14 out of 47 patients with normal chest films. Early involvement of hilar nodes may be difficult to recognize and CT should be performed with intravenous contrast enhancement using dynamic scanning.

A major advantage of CT is the ability to detect lymph-node involvement

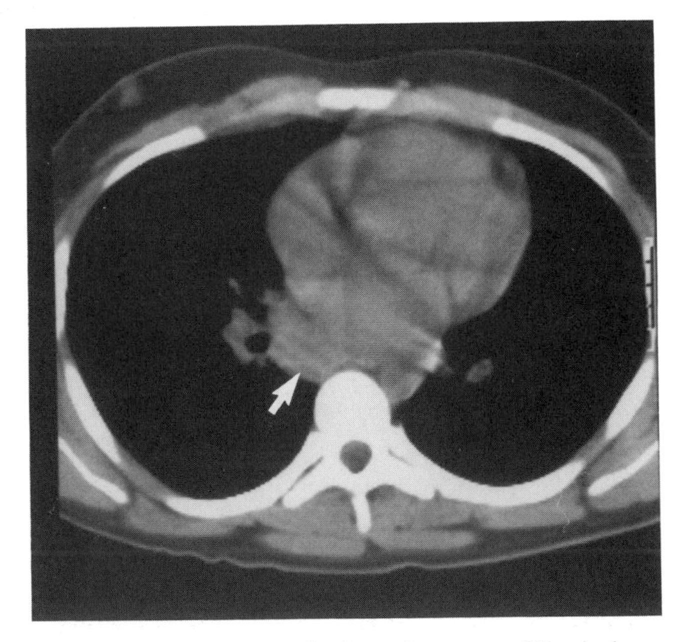

Fig. 19.2 CT scan through the lower mediastinum shows a mass filling in the azygo-oesophageal recess (arrowed).

at sites which are otherwise difficult to evaluate and where the demonstration of disease may lead to a change in management. In this respect evaluation of the subcarinal nodes is important. Lymphadenopathy may be recognized by displacement and even narrowing of the bronchi. A soft-tissue mass may be detected and is most easily recognized when it alters the contour of the azygo-oesophageal recess (Fig. 19.2). The demonstration of retrocrural and diaphragmatic lymphadenopathy is also important because this increases the probability of disease extension into the abdomen. The detection of internal mammary or axillary node enlargement may change treatment by demonstrating disease beyond standard radiotherapeutic fields.

Lung involvement

Pulmonary parenchymal disease is seen in approximately 10% of patients with Hodgkin's disease at the time of diagnosis but is more common at the time of recurrence. Two forms are recognized by the Ann Arbor staging classification: extension from the hilum into one lobe of a single lung (designated by the subscript E) and haematogenous pulmonary spread (Stage IV disease). Our experience suggests that CT is no more sensitive than conventional chest radiography for diagnosing tumour extension from the hilum and almost all patients with demonstrable pulmonary involvement are Stage IV. Typically, disseminated pulmonary involvement is seen on CT as one or more slightly ill-defined nodules (Fig. 19.3), although a

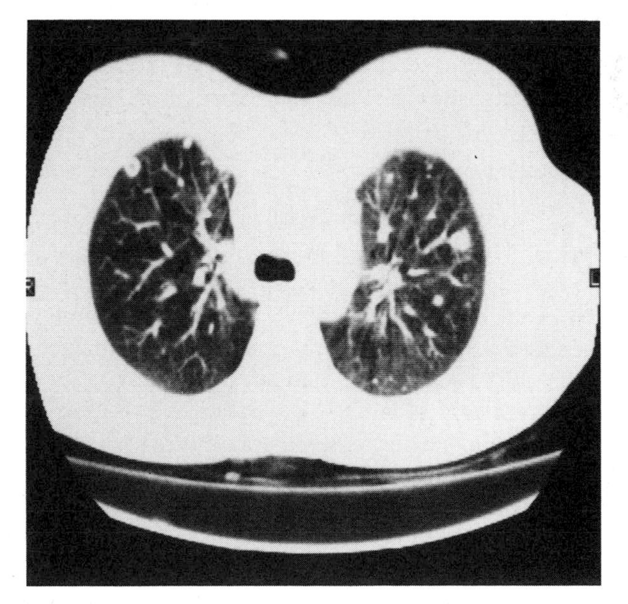

Fig. 19.3 CT scan of a patient with Hodgkin's disease showing multiple ill-defined pulmonary nodules.

wide variety of appearances may be seen including patchy or lobar consolidation, segmental collapse or reticulo-nodular infiltration. It may be very difficult to distinguish pulmonary involvement from inflammatory changes. In many instances these inflammatory changes are associated with benign pleural effusions and only approximately one-third of radiologically demonstrable effusions contain malignant cells on aspiration. Plaques of pleural disease are well seen on CT. They are usually associated with malignant effusions and are a feature of recurrent rather than primary Hodgkin's disease.

The role of CT

Hodgkin's disease

In patients who are to be treated with chemotherapy the immediate contribution of CT is the demonstration of additional sites of disease, which may or may not alter the stage, and the definition of the total tumour bulk.

It is in the patient initially considered for radiotherapy that thoracic CT makes its greatest impact. The demonstration of disease beyond the confines of the standard mantle field is an indication for chemotherapy or combined modality treatment. The Stanford experience showed that thoracic CT resulted in a management change in 15% of patients (Castellino et al 1986).

Treatment response may be judged on serial CT studies. In many instances the CT appearances will return completely to normal and in this regard the greater sensitivity of CT compared with conventional chest films has been welcomed. Residual soft-tissue masses may be seen in some patients and it is difficult to separate those with residual active disease from those with an inert mass (Lewis et al 1982, North et al 1987).

Non-Hodgkin's lymphoma

Non-Hodgkin's lymphoma involves the thorax less frequently than Hodgkin's disease. Those with follicular lymphomas typically have widespread adenopathy at presentation and in most cases the involved nodes are large and obvious on chest radiographs. At present there is no effective treatment which prolongs life and some patients are managed expectantly. CT demonstration of small volume mediastinal disease is therefore of little practical value. Treatment is usually given when symptoms develop and CT may be used to define radiotherapy treatment portals.

Patients with diffuse lymphomas are almost invariably treated with chemotherapy. CT of the thorax may show more extensive disease than is appreciated on chest radiographs but this will not influence management. Detailed CT assessment of the thorax is essential in the small percentage of patients presenting with apparent early stage disease who may qualify for radiotherapy treatment.

ABDOMEN

Lymph-node involvement

Abdominal nodal involvement in patients with non-Hodgkin's lymphoma is frequent. The involved nodes are usually larger than those seen in Hodgkin's disease and the pattern of involved sites also differs (Fig. 19.4). For example, mesenteric node involvement is common (51%) whereas it is rare in Hodgkin's disease (< 4%). Para-aortic lymphadenopathy is seen in half the patients compared to only a 25% incidence in Hodgkin's disease.

Extranodal disease

Typically, Hodgkin's disease in the abdomen spreads through the lymphatic system to involve the spleen and this is more likely if deposits are present in the upper abdominal nodes. Splenic infiltration increases the likelihood of haematogenous dissemination and it is rare for the liver or bone marrow to be involved in the absence of splenic disease. The detection of splenic deposits is therefore important but the results of CT have been disappointing. The typical pattern of splenic and hepatic involvement is multiple small (1–3 mm) metastases which cannot be identified on CT until the deposits are so numerous that generalized organ enlargement occurs (Castellino et al 1984). Although splenic enlargement can be identified it is not a reliable sign of splenic infiltration since approximately one-third of involved spleens are not enlarged. Conversely, one-third of enlarged spleens are not involved by tumour. Occasionally, CT may identify hepatic

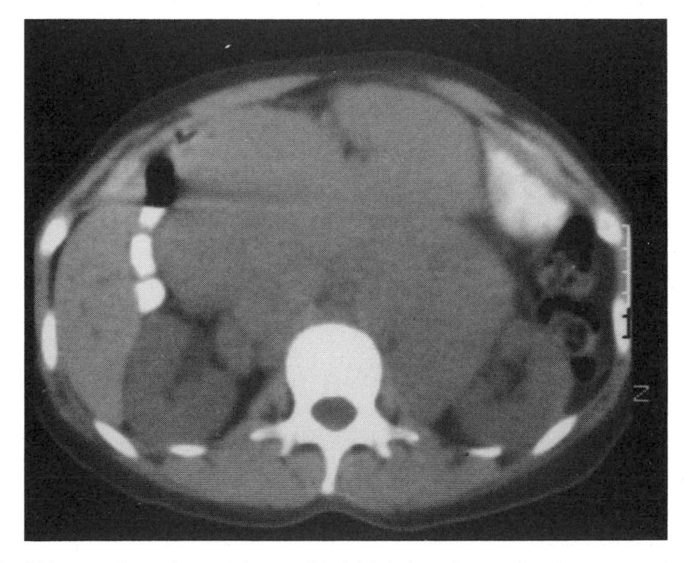

Fig. 19.4 CT scan of a patient with non-Hodgkin's lymphoma showing gross enlargement of retroperitoneal and mesenteric nodes.

and splenic focal lesions but this is uncommon. Other sites of extranodal spread are at presentation but bone metastases and muscle invasion are occasionally identified.

Diffuse lymphomas are frequently extranodal and involvement of the spleen usually produces significant enlargement. Liver metastases are also identified more commonly than in Hodgkin's disease.

Involvement of the gastrointestinal tract may be primary or secondary and bowel wall thickening is the most common finding. This may be associated with regional lymphadenopathy and it is not unusual for enlarged mesenteric nodes and thickened bowel wall to be matted together as a conglomerate tumour mass. The staging of primary extranodal disease is important as complete surgical excision may be curative.

Pancreatic lymphoma is rare and on CT it is usually impossible to differentiate pancreatic infiltration from involvement of peripancreatic nodes. Renal and adrenal lymphoma are manifestations of haematogenous spread and are most commonly seen late in the course of the disease (see Ch. 13 and 14). Occasionally, the ovaries and uterus are infiltrated by tumour in patients with widespread diffuse lymphoma.

Soft-tissue muscle masses are often seen in resistant or recurrent non-Hodgkin's lymphoma, the most frequent site being the ilio-psoas muscle (Fig. 19.5). These masses may invade adjacent bone or extend through the

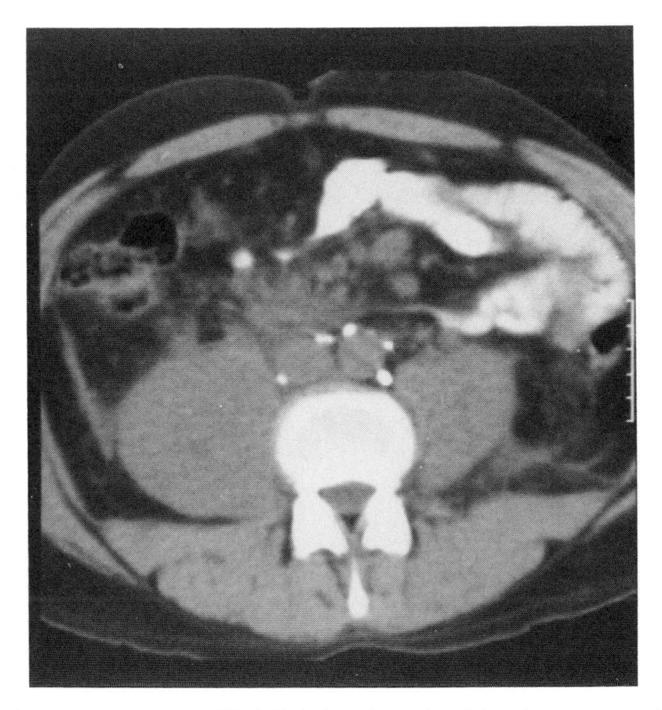

Fig. 19.5 CT scan showing non-Hodgkin's lymphoma involving the psoas muscles.

intervertebral foramina into the spinal canal and care should be taken to review the paravertebral region in all patients. Extradural deposits may also be identified and are of great importance as they may herald both local cord compression and spread of disease within the cerebrospinal fluid.

The role of CT

Hodgkin's disease

Staging laparotomy for Hodgkin's disease is now uncommon in the United Kingdom. This is partly due to changes in treatment policy and partly to the apparent failure of staging laparotomy to confer a survival advantage in patients with negative laparotomies treated with mantle irradiation.

Lymphangiography may detect metastases in normal-sized nodes and for this reason it has a greater sensitivity than CT for staging abdominal Hodgkin's disease (Castellino et al 1984). In patients with Hodgkin's disease, who are to be treated with chemotherapy, the demonstration of abdominal nodal involvement is of most value for assessing prognosis and providing a baseline for post-treatment assessment. CT is the preferred technique and lymphangiography is considered unnecessary. When disease is clinically localized and the proposed treatment is irradiation, the detection of abdominal nodal disease will alter management. In the presence of a normal CT examination it is arguable that lymphangiography will identify a few patients with small volume nodal deposits.

Non-Hodgkin's lymphoma

The ability of CT to demonstrate multiple sites of nodal and extranodal disease has challenged the use of lymphangiography to such an extent that it is now rarely used. As in the thorax, CT is an excellent method for monitoring treatment response and disease progression.

CONCLUSION

CT scanning is an integral part of modern cancer radiology and has a major role in the management of patients with lymphoma. Since the manifestations of lymphoma are protean it is important to identify the clinical question before a CT examination is undertaken. Furthermore, the capabilities and limitations of CT to answer these questions should be thoroughly understood. Close collaboration between the clinician and the radiologist will ensure that the relevant information is obtained from the CT study and that this information is used to best advantage.

REFERENCES

Amendola M A 1986 CT staging of lymphoma. In: Glazer G M (ed) Staging of Neoplasms. Churchill Livingstone, New York pp 147–189

Bragg D G, Colby T V, Ward J H 1986 New concepts in the non-Hodgkin lymphomas: radiologic implications. Radiology 159: 289–304

Castellino R A 1986 Hodgkin Disease: Practical concepts for the diagnostic radiologist. Radiology 159: 305–310

Castellino R A, Hoppe R T, Blank N et al 1984 Computed tomography, lymphography and staging laparotomy: correlations in initial staging of Hodgkin disease. American Journal of Roentgenology 143: 37–41

Castellino R A, Blank N, Hoppe R T, Cho C 1986 Hodgkin disease: contributions of chest CT in the initial staging evaluation. Radiology 160: 603–605

Glazer G M, Gross B H, Quint L E, Francis I R, Bookstein F L, Orringer M B 1985 Normal mediastinal lymph nodes: number and size according to American Thoracic Society Mapping. American Journal of Roentgenology 144: 261–265

Heron C W, Husband J E, Williams M P, Cherryman G R 1988 The value of thoracic computed tomography in the detection of recurrent Hodgkin's disease. British Journal of Radiology 61: 567–572

Jaffe E S 1986 Relationship of classification to biological behaviour of non-Hodgkin's lymphomas. Seminars in Oncology 13: 3–9

Kaplan H S 1980 Hodgkin's Disease. 2nd edn. Harvard University Press, Cambridge

Lewis E, Barnardino M E, Salvador P G, Cabanillas F F, Barnes P A, Thomas J L 1982 Post-therapy CT-detected mass in lymphoma: is it viable tissue? Journal of Computer Assisted Tomography 6: 792–795

Meyer J E, Linggood R M, Lindfors K K, McLoud T C, Stomper P C 1984 Impact of thoracic computed tomography on radiation therapy planning in Hodgkin disease. Journal of Computer Assisted Tomography 8: 892–894

Neumann C H, Parker B R, Castellino R A 1985 Hodgkin's disease and the Non-Hodgkin lymphomas. In: Bragg D G, Rubin P, Youker J E (eds) Oncologic Imaging. Pergamon Press, New York pp 477–501

North L B, Fuller L M, Sullivan-Halley J A, Hagemeister F B 1987 Regression of mediastinal Hodgkin disease after therapy: evaluation of time interval. Radiology 164: 599–602

Oliver T W, Bernardino M E, Sones P J Jr 1983 Monitoring the response of lymphoma patients to therapy: correlation of abdominal CT findings with clinical course and histologic cell type. Radiology 149: 219–224

20. The spine—disc and degenerative disease

Brian Kendall

INTRODUCTION

Modern CT systems provide excellent delineation of the vertebrae, intervertebral discs, thecal sac and epidural fat. Any protrusion of the disc substance outside the line of the vertebral end-plates is demonstrable. It usually extends posteriorly to indent the theca in typical fashion but it may herniate postero-laterally and migrate laterally or, in the lumbar region, cranially to affect an exiting nerve root. In adolescents and young adults it may herniate through the vertebral body near the apophyseal ring and a fragment of the latter and/or the disc may impinge on the theca and/or nerve root (Dietemann et al 1988).

THE ROLE OF CT

Lumbar spine

For patients presenting with lumbago and sciatica, CT is a very satisfactory initial test (Williams et al 1982a). Radiculography, which in disc lesions primarily shows the extrinsic defects on the thecal sac and root sheaths, is roughly equal to CT in overall accuracy (Fries et al 1982). However, interpretation of myelograms is more frequently inconclusive (Raskin & Keating 1982) and more dependent on clinical correlation (Tchang et al 1982). Myelography is invasive and more expensive than CT if the cost of overnight stay is considered. Moreover, 5% of herniated lumbar discs are extremely lateral and neither these nor laterally placed tumours can be shown by myelography (Williams et al 1982a, Osborne et al 1984).

Myelography may be necessary following equivocal or negative CT especially if there are unexplained neurological signs; intrathecal tumours, an important but relatively rare cause of lumbago and/or sciatica, are frequently not revealed by CT without intrathecal contrast medium. However, magnetic resonance (MR) imaging is the preferred modality in this situation and is a major reason why it should ultimately replace CT for routine lumbar spine studies.

Cervical spine

Cervical myelopathy, whether acute or chronic, is most commonly caused by cervical spondylosis or disc protrusion encroaching on a spinal canal of small sagittal diameter. If compression is mainly from the front by disc material and/or osteophytes at one or two levels, especially if there is good clinical correlation, an anterior surgical approach is commonly favoured. More extensive disease, especially when there is associated marked infolding of the dura posteriorly, is more often treated by extensive laminectomy.

When available, MR imaging is the most satisfactory primary study since it can produce a longitudinal image of the spine, cerebrospinal fluid (CSF) and cord in a few minutes without any possibility of inducing deterioration of cord function which occasionally complicates the manipulations of myelography. On a sagittal T1 weighted image the anatomy is displayed like a negative contrast myelogram. The sites of cord compression are revealed and images with the neck in flexion and extension can easily be achieved to show instability and its effect on the cord. Supplementary axial images through the affected levels more accurately depict the compressing agent and the congruous deformity of the spinal cord. Incongruous reduction of cross-sectional area of the cord is indicative of atrophy. Cystic changes and cavitation, including cystic myelomalacia, in which the intramedullary fluid resembles CSF, will tend to return a similar signal. On T2 weighted images local changes in the water content of the discs, which decrease with degeneration and ageing, is evident and the degree of any encroachment of the low signal dura on to the high signal CSF is revealed. Most intramedullary pathologies reflect high signal: myelomalacia as well as demyelination, acute allergic myelitis and intramedullary tumours, which may present with symptoms suggesting cord compression, will be shown and their nature may be suspected in the clinical context.

Where MR imaging is not freely available, myelography from the lumbar route is generally used. The conventional water-soluble myelogram will show impression from the discs on the theca and root sheaths, but the contour of cord deformity and the congruity with the compressing agents and the degree of reduction of cross-sectional area is best shown by computed myelography (CM). Ossification of the posterior longitudinal ligament (Kadoya et al 1978) and degenerative thickening, with or without ossification, of the ligamenta flava, which may act alone as a compressing agent or be associated with spondylosis, are generally better shown by CT than MR imaging (Stollman et al 1987).

Brachalgia, usually with neck pain, is common with spondylosis affecting a non-stenotic cervical spinal canal and with lateral cervical disc protrusions. Many such patients may be adequately elucidated by radiographs followed by CT alone, but myelography is usually performed if surgery is contemplated, and computed myelography will more exactly depict root compression. Currently, MR imaging as routinely performed does not consistently demonstrate the cervical nerve roots but oblique images using sophisticated surface coils are likely to do so in the near future (Leeds & Jacobson 1987).

Thoracic spine

Thoracic cord compression is more commonly caused by extramedullary tumour than by spondylosis or disc protrusion, even though MR imaging studies have shown the incidence of herniated thoracic discs to be several times more frequent than previously demonstrated. Osteomyelitis of the spine is relatively more frequent in this region and, as in the cervical region, intramedullary lesions may simulate compression of the cord.

By far the most satisfactory investigation is MR imaging but, when this is not available, radiographs of the spine are useful for detection of bone destruction by malignant or inflammatory lesions, or erosion by extramedullary tumours. Thoracic discs are commonly calcified in cases with a disc prolapse: they may be subtle to detect on spine radiographs (McAllister & Sage 1976) but are beautifully revealed on CT. Chest radiographs may show lung masses or rib destruction and point to malignant or inflammatory processes.

In patients with a known malignancy, spinal metastases may be confirmed by bone-seeking isotopes and, when symptoms suggest the possibility, osteoid osteoma may be revealed at an early stage before radiographs are positive (Omojola et al 1982).

Once localized, all pathological processes, except intramedullary tumours, are better demonstrated by CT. However, the spinal cord is not shown adequately without intrathecal contrast medium, so that myelography, supplemented as necessary by computed myelography, is usually required prior to surgery.

TECHNIQUE

Lumbar spine

For the lumbar region, most centres adopt the gantry application technique (Hirschy et al 1981) which can be planned accurately following the initial lateral digital image. To show the whole of the intraspinal course of the roots, it is essential that scans cover from the level of the pedicles of the vertebra above and those below each disc, otherwise sequestrated fragments which have migrated away from a disc may not be detected. Some form of magnification/zooming is needed and for this the radiographer should ensure that the patient is central within the gantry. In order to attain parallelism at the L5–S1 disc, the natural lumbar lordosis may be reduced by gentle hip flexion. The best resolution will be produced by thin slices; in the lumbar region a slice thickness of 3–4 mm is an ideal compromise in order to limit the number of slices required to cover the area. Most centres examine the lowest three discs as a routine but also include the upper lumbar discs if clinical signs indicate a high lesion.

Cervical spine

Since most of the movement of flexion and extension takes place at C5–6 and C6–7 levels, cervical spondylosis is most pronounced and soft disc herniations are most frequent at these levels. Postero-anterior and lateral radiographs of the cervical spine are made prior to a cervical study, both to exclude unexpected pathology at other levels and to reveal the extent of spondylosis. The patient is positioned supine, with the knees flexed and the head and neck slightly extended, so as to ensure that a vertical beam will be as close as is practicable to a tangent to the vertebral end-plates. The head and neck are aligned straight, with the midline central, and immobilized using Velcro strapping. The shoulders are depressed by asking the patient to exert gentle traction against a strap looped under the soles of their feet.

Because of the paucity of epidural fat in the lower cervical region, there are advantages in using intravenous contrast medium, either as a bolus alone or followed by drip infusion during the study. Some authorities use contrast enhancement routinely (Sundram 1988) while others, including ourselves, reserve it for particular cases, including all post-operative patients.

The lateral digital image is used to assess the degree of gantry tilt necessary to pass parallel to a suspected disc or to determine the best axis in relation to the general lordosis in which to make serial sections. The cervical vertebral discs may be so narrow, particularly in the presence of spondylosis, which make it impracticable to go through the whole disc even with narrow (1.5 or 2 mm) collimation. Thus, axial slices are usually obtained without gantry tilt, particularly if the cervical lordosis is considerable. CT slices are taken from the fourth cervical to the first thoracic vertebra using 1 or 2 mm contiguous slices; the third and fourth cervical vertebrae are also examined if clinically indicated.

If noise or streak artefacts obscure the level of interest in large patients, it may be necessary to repeat selected slices with increased exposure or using 5 mm collimation.

A similar protocol is used for computed cervical myelography. The appropriate region of clinical interest in the thoracic spine is best examined by overlapping 5 mm sections. The images are viewed and photographed on both soft tissue and bone windows using extended window width (200 HU). The digital radiograph is magnified three times so as to demonstrate clearly the level of the sections without obscuring anatomical landmarks.

The radiation dose to the patient should be maintained low while ensuring diagnostic quality of the examination. This is assured by giving precise instruction to: (i) prohibit swallowing movement and breathing, (ii) protect the pelvis with a lead-rubber apron, (iii) perform a definitive examination using either intrathecal or intravenous contrast as a primary venture when specifically indicated.

Post-processing, particularly image filtration (smoothing), is sometimes useful for showing soft-tissue edges more clearly on noisy images. The thin slice collimation allows the production of high-resolution reformatted images in multiple planes. One pixel thick sagittal reformats may confirm small disc protrusions. With noisy scans, 3–5 pixel thick reformats will improve contrast in the image. Re-reformatted images made in the axis of the disc will further confirm lesions encroaching on the spinal canal and demonstrate the degree of compromise of the spinal canal and the deformity of the spinal cord.

INTERPRETATION

The shape and outline of the spinal canal are ideally shown by high-resolution CT. The anatomy of the spine should be assessed with special reference to the sagittal diameter of the bony canal. In the lumbar region less than 11.5 mm in the mid-plane is significantly narrow (Ullrich et al 1980) but it may reduce to below 3 mm in the lateral thirds before becoming abnormal. In the mid and lower cervical region 15 mm is an adequate sagittal diameter; a developmental sagittal diameter below 12 mm is critically small.

Relatively minor pathological impressions from disc disease, apophyseal joint, osteoarthritis and thickened ligaments may be important in a canal which developmentally has small dimensions. The nature of any stenosis—short pedicles, facet joint osteoarthritis, spondylolisthesis—is evident on CT and the degree of combined bony and soft-tissue stenosis can be reliably estimated.

The disc margins should be related to the shape of the adjacent vertebral end-plates. The normal discs have concave posterior aspects, except L5–S1 which is slightly convex. Projecting disc substance may be contrasted against or efface locally the epidural fat and cause displacement or compression of the dural sac, root sheaths or nerve roots (Fig. 20.1). A disc herniation will usually be evident as a focal protrusion beyond the contours of the end-plates whereas a bulging annulus will extend beyond the end-plate in a circumferential fashion and the degenerate nucleus may contain gas (Williams et al 1982b). Reactive marginal osteophytes, misalignment of vertebrae and buckling of the posterior dura, each of which may contribute to degenerative canal stenosis, are all well shown by CT. Reactive sclerosis within the bodies is usually adjacent to the disc but it may be more extensive and then simulate reaction to inflammation or neoplasm.

An injected disc is usually associated with destruction of the adjacent

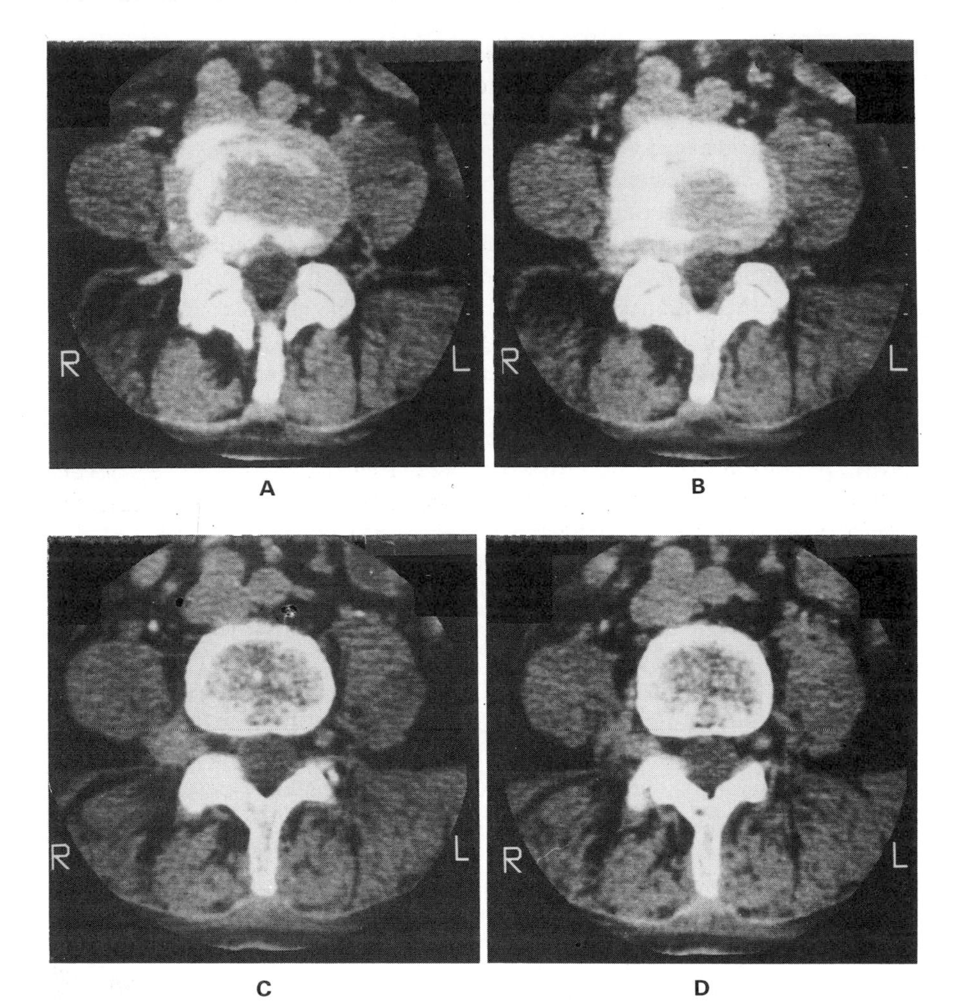

Fig. 20.1 Lateral lumbar disc protrusion (**A, B, C, D**). Contiguous 5 mm sections. The disc protrusion is continuous with similar density to the disc substances (**A & B**). It fills the right intervertebral foramen at the level of the disc, obliterating the fat, and extends superolaterally into the lateral half of the foramen and into the adjacent paravertebral region compressing the exiting nerve root (**C & D**). The disc causes only minimal impression of the right anterolateral aspect of the theca and the significant root compression could not be recognized on myelography.

parts of the vertebral bodies and paravertebral soft-tissue swelling. In tuberculosis, a low-density abscess expanding the psoas or other muscles with an origin from an affected vertebra, may also be shown.

In the mid and lower cervical spine the cervical enlargement of the cord occupies a relatively large proportion of the subarachnoid space and the epidural space tends to be relatively narrow and poorly visualized. For this reason, soft-disc protrusions can be difficult to show on plain CT.

Opacification of the epidural venous plexus may help in their demonstration: the retrocorporeal plexus drains into anterior longitudinal epidural veins which are in a plane medial to the intervertebral foramina and pedicles. Uncinate veins behind the unco-vertebral joints connect the anterior longitudinal veins with the foraminal veins which surround the vertebral arteries and the spinal nerve roots and ganglia. All the veins ultimately drain through the vertebral into the innominate veins to the superior vena cava. Disc bulges and herniations deviate these opacified veins posteriorly and are outlined against them. Cord compression is undoubtedly studied best by computed myelography (Fig. 20.2 a and b). Congruous deformity of the spinal cord with local diminution in cross-sectional area is the definitive sign. This may not reverse or do so incompletely following decompression, suggesting irreversible cord damage. Diminished cord cross-sectional area at uncompressed levels suggests atrophy and contrast accumulation in cord substance indicates myelomalacia (Iwasaki et al 1985).

Protruded thoracic discs are often partly calcified and are easily diagnosed if the calcification is both within the disc space and extending from it into the intraspinal mass. Even when the disc fragment is sequestrated, calcification is frequently still present in the part of the disc remaining within the intervertebral space and within discs at other levels also. The latter may be the only pointer to the diagnosis in the uncommon situation in which a sequestrated fragment is driven well away from a disc space, especially if it comes to lie posterolaterally or penetrates through the dura and may then simulate a meningioma. Computed myelography will

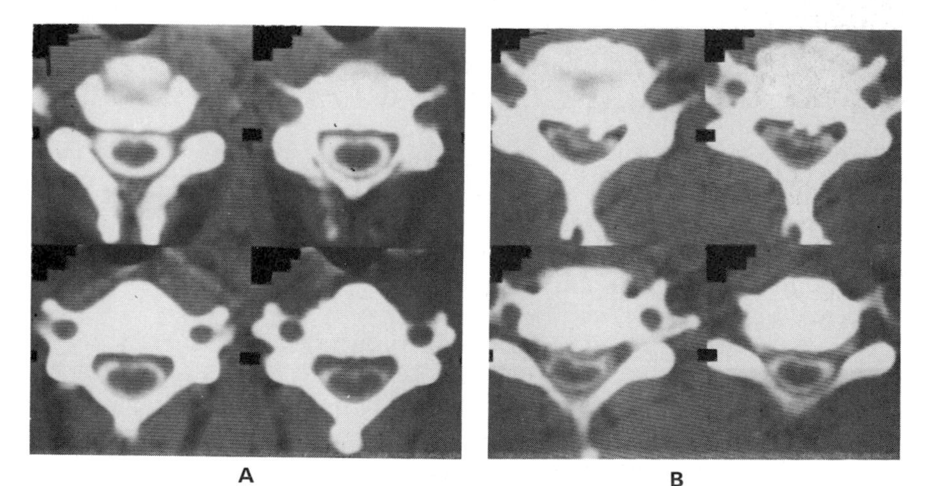

Fig. 20.2 Cervical spondylosis with cord compression. CT myelogram. **A** 1.5 mm contiguous sections at normal level showing size and shape of spinal cord. **B** At level of spondylosis showing posterior osteophytes extending back to narrow the spinal canal and compress the spinal cord. Note marked reduction of the cross-sectional area of the cord and congruous deformity.

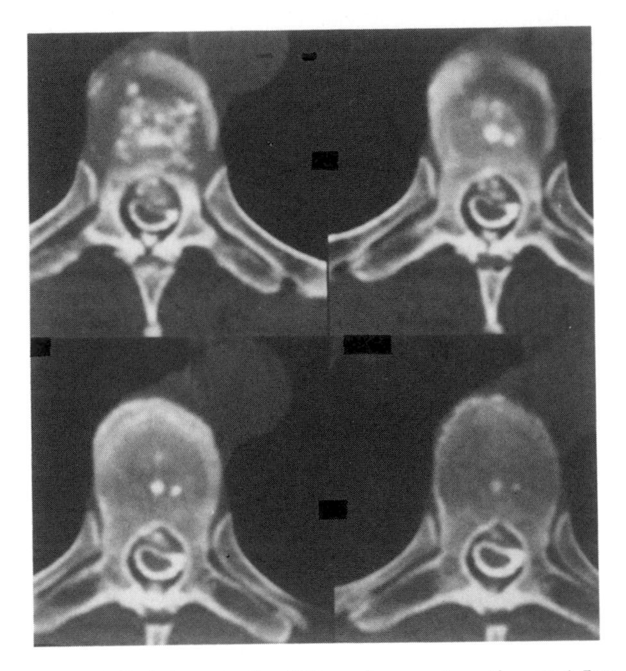

Fig. 20.3 Prolapsed calcified thoracic disc. CT myelogram: 4 contiguous 1.5 mm sections. The disc substance is calcified both within the intervertebral space and within the prolapsed position which fills more than the anterior half of the spinal canal. It displaces the theca and cord posteriorly and the compression causes congruous deformity of the cord.

show the precise relationship of the disc to the cord and the degree of cord compression (Fig. 20.3).

Difficulties of interpretation

There are numerous problems in the interpretation of spinal CT (Teplick et al 1982). Disc degeneration occurs with normal ageing and symptomatic disc lesions are quite common in the lumbar and cervical regions (Wiesel et al 1984). An obvious disc lesion does not necessarily account for the current symptoms and all levels should be carefully studied and abnormalities correlated with clinical signs (Peterson et al 1987).

Overlap of adjacent end-plates due to subluxation of one vertebra on another may result in partial volume averaging causing disc substance apparently to protrude beyond the confines of the disc margins. This can generally be recognized by study of the serial scans.

Differential diagnosis

The differential diagnosis of lesions situated close to the exit foramina, in addition to laterally-sited discs, includes neurofibromata, large dorsal root ganglia and conjoined or developmentally dilated nerve root sheaths. The latter can generally be recognized as expansions of CSF density in the axis of the root sheaths, often with local widening of the lateral part of the spinal canal. If doubt persists MR imaging or myelography will elucidate the problem.

The postoperative spine

The postoperative spine poses particular problems. The surgical defect is apparent and the underlying flaval ligament is absent. The tissue planes around the thecal sac are usually found to be indistinct and the sac itself may be drawn by fibrosis towards the side of the surgical approach. Within such fibrosis a recurrent disc protrusion may present a clearly defined mass continuous with and of the same density as the disc substance. However, it may also be of similar density to the fibrosis and/or be sequestrated. Intravenous enhancement is a useful adjunct in equivocal cases (Dixon & Bannon 1987). The fibrosis should enhance evenly, while disc material does not enhance and contrasts as relatively low density against the fibrous tissue, dura or epidural venous plexus (Schubiger & Valavanis 1982, Braun et al 1985).

CONCLUSION

Disc and degenerative disease involving the vertebrae, intervertebral discs, thecal sac and epidural fat can be elegantly demonstrated with CT provided that meticulous attention is paid to technique. The appropriate use of intravenous and intrathecal contrast medium is essential if optimal results are to be achieved. Even so, CT has significant limitations and the difficulties of interpretation are numerous. There is no doubt that in many situations MR imaging is superior to CT but until MR imaging becomes widely available CT provides an effective alternative.

REFERENCES

Braun I F, Hoffman J C Jr, Davis P C, Landman J A, Tindall G T 1985 Contrast enhancement in CT differentiation between recurrent disk herniation and postoperative scar: prospective study. American Journal of Roentgenology 6: 607–612

Dietemann J L, Runge M, Badoz A et al 1988 Radiology of posterior apophyseal ring fractures: report of 13 cases. Neuroradiology 30: 337–344

Dixon A K, Bannon R P 1987 Computed tomography of the postoperative lumbar spine: the need for an optimal dose of intravenous contrast medium. British Journal of Radiology 60: 215–222

Fries J W, Abodeely D A, Vijunco J B, Yeager V L, Gaffey W R 1982 Computed tomography of herniated and extruded nucleus pulposa. Journal of Computer Assisted Tomography 6: 874–887

Hirschy J C, Leue W M, Berninger W H, Hamilton R H, Abbott G F 1981 CT of the lumbosacral spine: importance of tomographic planes parallel to vertebral end plate. American Journal of Roentgenology 136: 47–52

Iwasaki Y, Abe H, Isu T, Miyasaka K 1985 CT myelography with intramedullary enhancement in cervical spondylosis. Journal of Neurosurgery 63: 363–366
Kadoya G, Nakamura T, Tada A 1978 Neuroradiology of ossification of the posterior longitudinal ligament. Neuroradiology 16: 357–358
Leeds N E, Jacobson H G 1987 Radiology. Journal of the American Medical Association 258: 2287–2289
McAllister V L, Sage M R 1976 The radiology of thoracic disc protrusion. Clinical Radiology 27: 291–299
Omojola M F, Cockshott W P, Beatty E G 1982 Osteoid osteoma: an evaluation of diagnostic modalities. Clinical Radiology 32: 199–240
Osborne D R, Heinz E R, Bullard D, Friedmann A 1984 Role of computed tomography in the radiological evaluation of painful radiculopathy after negative myelogram: foraminal neural entrapment. Neurosurgery 14: 147–153
Peterson O F, Buhl M, Eriksen E F et al 1987 The significance of preoperative radiological examinations in patients treated with Cloward's operation. Acta Neurochirurgica (Wien) 88: 39–45
Raskin S P, Keating J W 1982 Recognition of lumbar disc disease: comparison of myelography and computed tomography. American Journal of Roentgenology 139: 349–355
Schubiger O, Valavanis A 1982 CT differentiation between recurrent disc herniation and postoperative scar formation: the value of contrast enhancement. Neuroradiology 22: 251–254
Stollman A, Pinto R, Benjamin V, Kricheff I 1987 Radiologic imaging of symptomatic ligamentum flavum thickening with and without ossification. American Journal of Neuroradiology 8: 991–994
Sundram S R 1988 Contrast enhanced computed tomography of cervical disc herniation. Radiography 54: 133–142
Tchang S P, Howie J L, Kirkaldy-Willis W H, Paine K W, Moola D 1982 Computed tomography versus myelography in diagnosis of lumbar disc herniation. Journal of Canadian Association of Radiology 33: 15–20
Teplick J G, Teplick S K, Goodman L, Haskin M E 1982 Pitfalls and unusual findings in computed tomography of the lumbar spine. Journal of Computer Assisted Tomography 6: 889–893
Ullrich C G, Binet E F, Sanecki M G, Kieffer S A 1980 Quantitative assessment of the lumbar spinal canal by computed tomography. Radiology 134: 137–143
Wiesel S W, Tsourmas N, Feffer H L, Citrin C M, Patronas N 1984 A study of computer-assisted tomography. 1. The incidence of positive CAT scans in an asymptomatic group of patients. Spine 9: 549–551
Williams A L, Haughton V M, Daniels D L, Thornton R S 1982a CT recognition of lateral lumbar disc herniation. American Journal of Roentgenology 139: 343–347
Williams A L, Haughton V M, Meyer G A, Ho K G 1982b Computed tomographic appearance of the bulging annulus. Radiology 142: 403–408

21. Joint disease

Stephen J. Golding

INTRODUCTION

Cross-sectional display and the ability to demonstrate bone and soft tissue together have made CT a valuable addition to musculoskeletal imaging. It has been shown, using indications proposed by the Society for Computed Body Tomography, that the technique yields unique and valuable information in the majority of cases (Griffiths et al 1981). This review considers the indications for using CT in disease of joints, both those which are applied to joints generally and those which are peculiar to specific joints.

CT may be used to complement conventional radiographs or arthrograms, in which case the conventional examination may be curtailed. Examination techniques vary according to the joint and indication and are described in detail in the references listed.

Ultrasound is complementary to CT, being used to detect effusions, periarticular cysts and lesions of cartilage in selected joints. This technique has the advantage that juxta-articular soft tissues may be examined dynamically (Wilson 1988).

Today, it is short-sighted to discuss the role of CT without considering that of magnetic resonance (MR) imaging. This demonstrates most of the components of joints and discriminates between soft tissues with a contrast resolution that is unequalled by any other technique (Sims & Genant 1986). It is only in the demonstration of intra-osseous detail that MR imaging is inferior to CT. MR imaging is still at an early stage of development but studies of musculoskeletal application have shown impressive progress and when the technique becomes generally available it will clearly make an important impact on orthopaedic medicine.

GENERAL INDICATIONS

Trauma

CT is an accurate method of confirming fractures when these appear equivocal on radiographs and also of assessing fracture dislocations prior to operative fixation. In practice, examination of the hip is the most common, followed by the shoulder, knee and ankle.

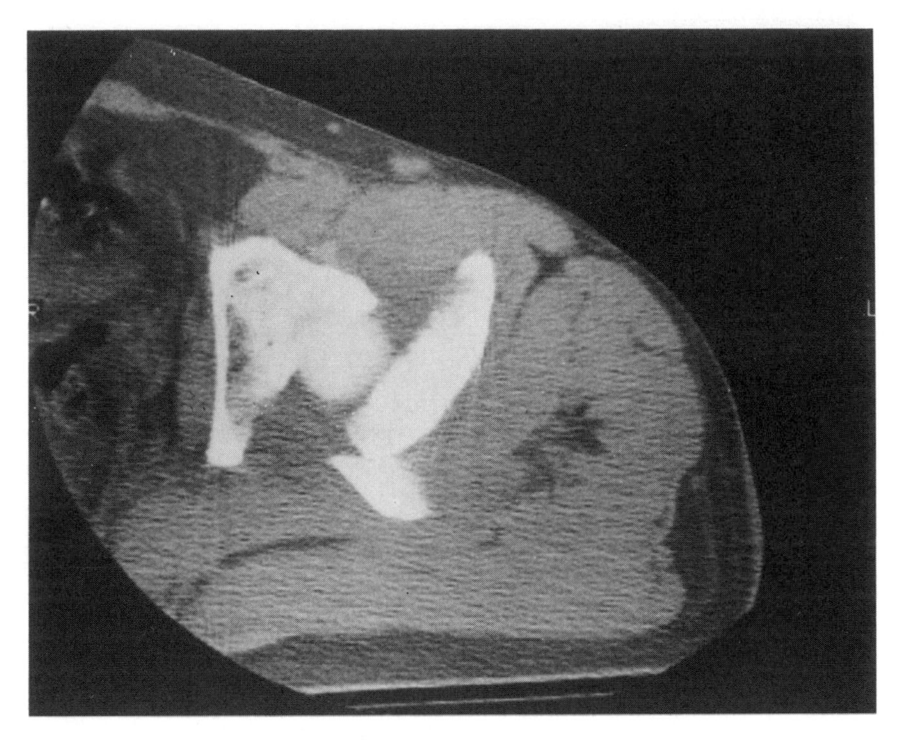

Fig. 21.1 Axial scan showing an oblique fracture of the acetabular roof with subluxation of the femoral head into the defect. The posterior acetabular lip has also fractured and the fragment lies posteriorly.

Fractures which may be detected by CT alone include those of the acetabulum, sacral alae (including sacro-iliac joint diastasis), posterior acetabular lip, tibial plateaux and those involving the subtalar joint (Dalinka et al 1985, Heger et al 1985).

Precise anatomical information is required for the operative fixation of complex fracture dislocations. CT often yields unique information and it has been shown that in the hip the results of examinations may influence surgical management in up to a third of cases (Griffiths et al 1984) (Fig. 21.1). Other instances where CT has been recommended include those around the shoulder, talocalcaneal fractures, particularly those with involvement of the joint, and distal tibial pilon fractures. In all these areas CT provides a reliable basis for surgery (Martinez et al 1985). CT should also be used when apparently simple dislocations fail to reduce, in which case soft tissue or bony fragments may be found within the joint.

Reformatting CT sections to provide three-dimensional views often gives a unique perspective of joint trauma (Fig. 21.2). The demonstration of displaced fractures may be more informative than that on radiographs or axial images, although the latter are better at detecting undisplaced fractures (Burk et al 1985).

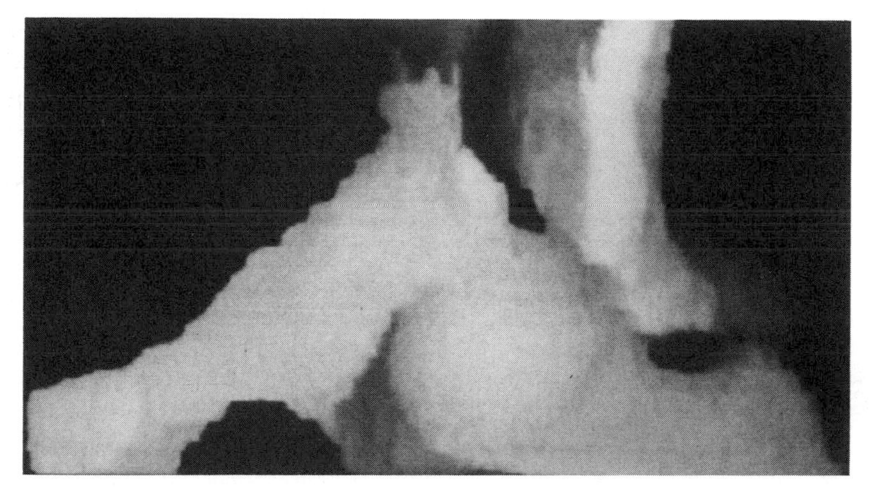

A

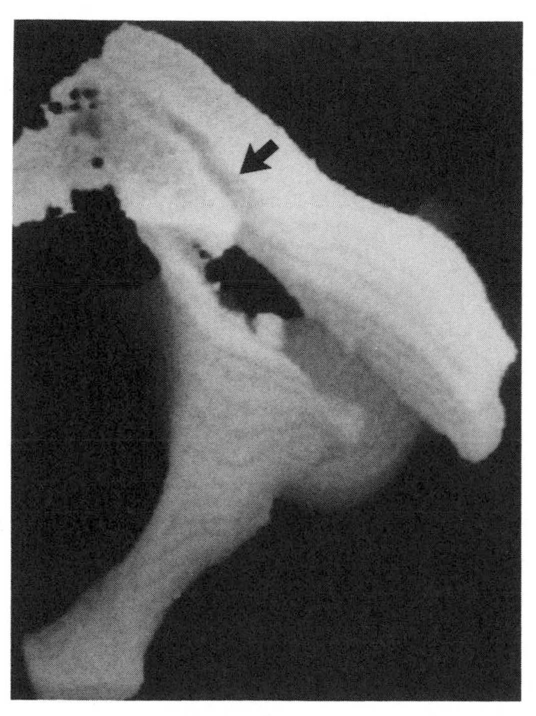

B

Fig. 21.2 Three-dimensional images reformatted from the axial examination shown in Figure 21.1, viewed from in front (**A**) and above (**B**), showing the extent of the fracture and the subluxation of the femoral head into the defect. Note that there is also diastasis of the sacro-iliac joint (arrow).

Injuries of the acetabulum occur most frequently in road traffic accidents and have a significant mortality, being associated with injury to the pelvic viscera. This should be considered in all cases undergoing examination and CT provides the facility to obtain images of the soft tissues at the same time, without additional radiation exposure (Dalinka et al 1985).

Equivocal radiographic appearances

One of the major benefits of CT to the radiologist has been to elucidate suspicious areas on conventional radiographs. Demonstration of pathology by CT is conclusive and disease may also be reliably excluded. Joint lesions which may be detected in this way include early erosive changes in arthritis and osteomyelitis, small neoplasms including metastases and small areas of structural collapse in articular surfaces. The technique is particularly effective for demonstrating lesions around the sacro-iliac joints, a difficult area radiographically (Smith et al 1987).

Juxta-articular neoplasms

CT has an established place in the staging of musculoskeletal neoplasms. Joints may be involved either by direct spread into the joint space or by

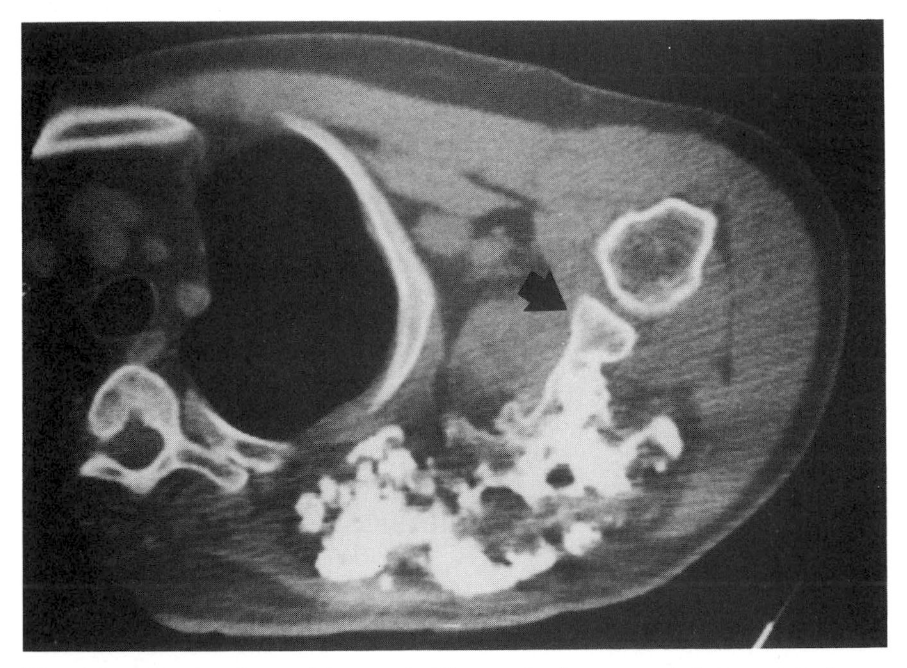

Fig. 21.3 Osteochondroma of the scapula. The examination was carried out to assess the glenoid bone stock (arrow) prior to resection with preservation of the shoulder joint.

infiltration of the capsular tissues. Detection of joint space invasion influences the extent of surgery, in particular the level of excision of malignant tumours. Those which commonly involve the joint directly include osteogenic sarcoma around the knee, Ewing's sarcoma in the ankle, synovial sarcoma and pigmented villonodular synovitis (Martinez et al 1985). Giant-cell tumours are particularly important in the foot and CT is the best technique for demonstrating erosion of subarticular bone (Levine et al 1984).

Although, in general, the appearance of neoplasms does not permit a differential diagnosis to be made, in lesions which occur around joints the technique may give some guidance as to whether the disease is benign or malignant (Yousem & Scott 1987).

CT is not limited to the evaluation of malignant neoplasms and one of the most common applications is the assessment of broad-based osteochondromata as an aid to planning the surgical approach (Fig. 21.3).

Osteonecrosis

It is well established that early avascular necrosis of joints is difficult to detect radiologically. Radiographs become abnormal only when there is established structural collapse. Scintigraphy detects early reactive change in devascularized bone and CT is more sensitive than radiography for detecting subarticular demineralization and structural collapse of articular surfaces. However, it is recognized that early lesions may be missed by CT (Magid et al 1985).

It now seems probable that MR imaging will prove to be the optimal technique for detecting osteonecrosis. More lesions are found with MR imaging than with CT or scintigraphy and a definite change in signal intensity is seen, even in early stages of disease (Gillespy et al 1986, Sims & Genant 1986). Recent studies have suggested that the techniques may be complementary, MR imaging being used for early diagnosis and CT for assessment of subarticular fractures prior to corrective surgery. MR imaging may also have a screening role in patients at risk (Hernandez 1988).

SPECIFIC INDICATIONS

The hip

CT may be used in a wide range of conditions affecting the hip, including disease of the capsule, inflammatory arthritis and osteoarthrosis (Dihlmann & Nebel 1983).

Calcified loose bodies of several millimetres in size are readily detected by CT and their relationship to the joint cavity demonstrated without intra-articular contrast (Fig. 21.4). The technique is indicated when radiographs or conventional tomograms fail to reveal calcified fragments. If none are

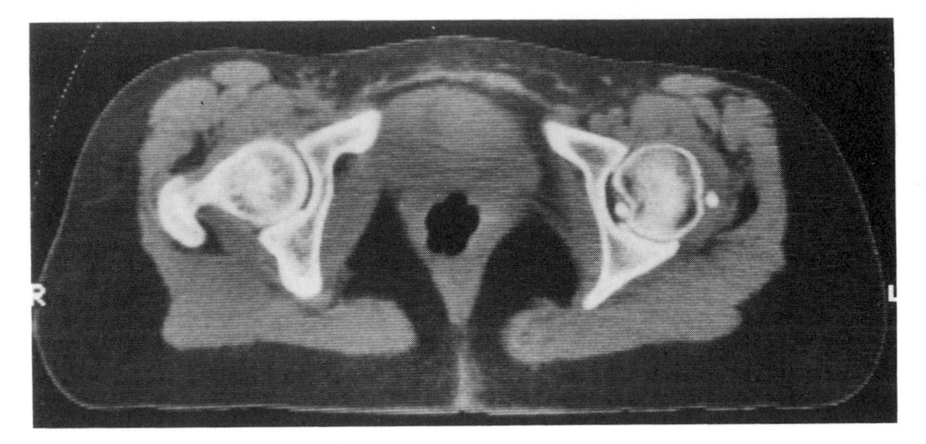

Fig. 21.4 Two loose bodies demonstrated in the left hip joint. These were not detected on conventional radiographs.

seen on CT, despite strong clinical evidence, patients may proceed to arthrography with CT assistance to exclude non-calcified bodies.

Examinations for degenerative disease are of two types. First, areas of joint-space narrowing due to loss of articular cartilage and subarticular cysts may be demonstrated which aids planning of rotation osteotomy. Coronal and sagittal reformatted sections may be valuable in this situation. Secondly, CT is valuable for determining the amount of bone stock in the acetabulum and in the proximal femoral shaft before undertaking prosthetic joint replacement.

In the child CT is most commonly indicated for congenital dislocation of the hip and acetabular dysplasia. The technique demonstrates the position of the femoral head accurately, even when this has not ossified. The configuration of the acetabulum and angle of torsion of the femur are readily demonstrated, the latter with a greater reliability than conventional radiographs and an error of $< 5\%$ (Hernandez 1988). It has been recognized that the technique demonstrates soft-tissue abnormalities which may prevent reduction and is of most use following surgery (Hernandez et al 1982).

Ultrasound may also be used in very young children, although CT has the advantage that it can be used in children in plaster of Paris (Wilson 1988). The radiation dose from CT is higher than that from radiographs but may be limited by reducing tube current, making the dose for an examination in plaster of Paris comparable to that of radiographic examination (Guyer et al 1984).

The shoulder

The main indications are gleno-humeral instability and rotator cuff lesions.

Although the configuration of the bony elements and defects, such as Hill–Sachs and Bankart lesions, may be seen on plain axial scans, most patients require arthrography. However, CT should be a routine part of this procedure in all patients in whom initial arthrographic views have failed to show a definite lesion (Fig. 21.5). This regimen is as easy to perform as a complete arthrogram and is better tolerated by patients (Resnik 1987).

The shoulder joint is a difficult area to assess radiographically but detailed anatomical information is needed for treatment decisions. CT arthrography fulfils these requirements and, in addition to demonstrating bony components and full-thickness rotator cuff tears, the technique shows labral abnormalities, rupture of the long head of the biceps muscle and deformities of the capsule resulting from recurrent injury (Resnik 1987).

CT arthrography of the shoulder is an accurate technique. Labral abnormalities are detected with a 96% sensitivity and diagnoses are made which are not possible either clinically or by conventional radiography (Raffi et al 1987). Care has to be taken in assessing deformation of the capsule because there is a wide variation in normal appearances and partial tears of the rotator cuff can also be difficult to diagnose (Resnik 1987).

MR imaging holds the promise of accurate diagnosis without the need for arthrography and results of early studies are encouraging (Huber et al 1986).

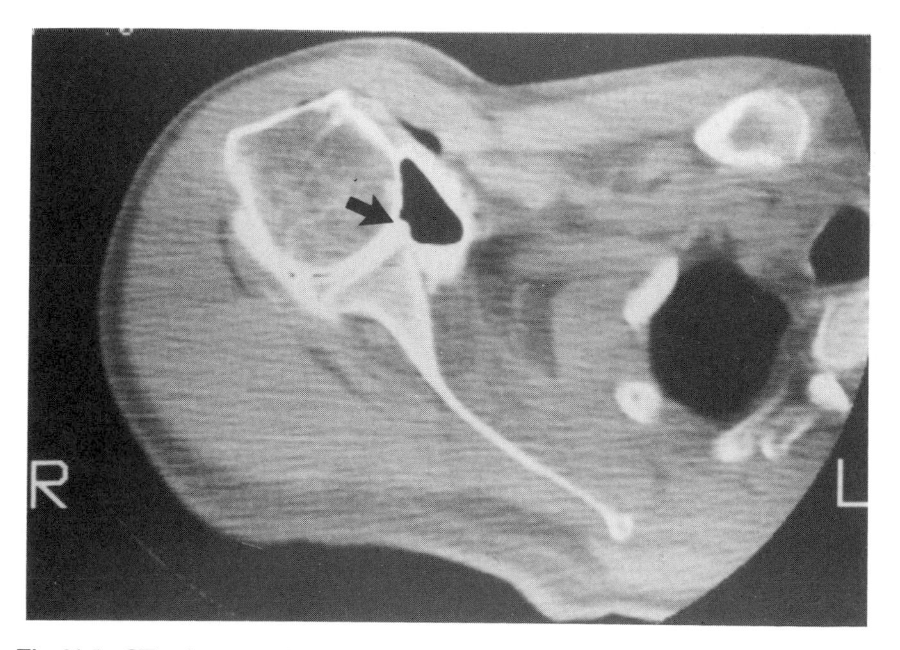

Fig. 21.5 CT arthrogram of the right shoulder. CT provides a confident diagnosis of joint damage and instability. There is deficiency of the anterior glenoid labrum (arrow) and the capsule has been stripped medially from its attachment to the scapula.

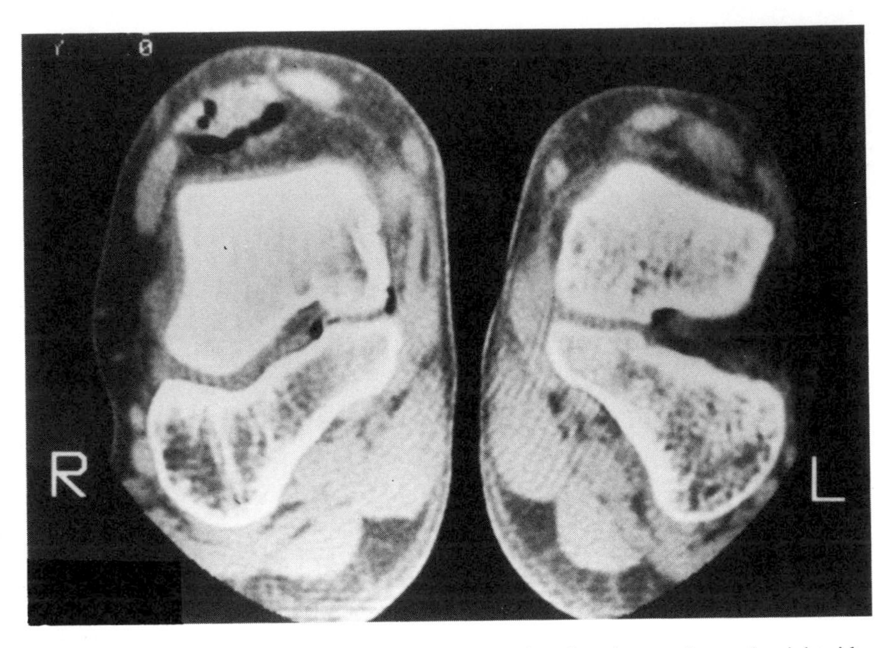

Fig. 21.6 Coronal image of the subtalar joints, following air arthrography on the right side. There is fibrous coalition of the joint on the right.

The ankle

CT is most often required for the diagnosis of tarsal coalition (Fig. 21.6). Calcaneo-navicular fusion may be diagnosed on radiographs but CT is reserved for difficult cases of bony and fibrous coalition. The radiographic diagnosis of talo-calcaneal and talo-navicular fusion is more difficult and CT is therefore frequently required. Both bony and fibrous coalition may be diagnosed and the latter is often suggested by the shape of the opposing bony margins. Lesions may be evident on plain CT scans but arthrography may facilitate the diagnosis of talo-calcaneal fusion (Hernandez 1988).

CT provides a reliable demonstration of anatomy in either coronal or plantar planes. It is suggested that the former is more applicable to talo-calcaneal fusion, whereas the latter should be used for talo-navicular problems (Sarno et al 1984).

CT has also been used to measure the talo-calcaneal angle in congenital club foot. The appearances of tendon injuries have been described (Rosenberg et al 1988). These are also demonstrated by MR imaging but in the ankle joint this technique has the disadvantage of being unreliable for demonstrating articular cartilage (Hajek et al 1986). In practice ultrasound is a more convenient technique for assessing tendon injuries (Wilson 1988).

The knee

CT has been studied as a possible alternative to arthrography or arthroscopy in the diagnosis of meniscal tears. Certainly these lesions can be demonstrated on CT, although horizontal and undisplaced peripheral tears are difficult to detect (Steinbach et al 1987).

CT arthrography may be used to demonstrate chondromalacia, osteochondritis dissecans and abnormalities of the patello-femoral articulation and may be more sensitive than radiographs and arthrograms (Martinez et al 1983). Reformatted CT sections may also be used to demonstrate the cruciate ligaments. In general, the technique is indicated to elucidate any finding on the arthrogram which suggests a synovial or extracapsular mass.

MR imaging has considerable potential for the investigation of the knee, being capable of demonstrating virtually all areas of disease. It seems likely, provided availability is adequate, that MR imaging will become the imaging method of choice after plain radiographs (Mink et al 1987).

CT is frequently used in the detection of soft-tissue sarcoma and although the diagnosis is usually obvious the radiologist should be aware that ruptured popliteal cysts may produce atypical appearances which may mimic neoplasms (Schwimmer et al 1985).

The wrist

CT has been recommended for investigating patients with carpal tunnel syndrome. The cross-sectional area of the tunnel can be measured and the volume of soft-tissue components assessed but measurements have been found to correlate poorly with clinical symptoms (Merhar et al 1986). In practice CT is reserved for lesions which produce equivocal appearances on radiographs, including difficult cases of distal radio-ulnar subluxation (Biondetti et al 1987).

Experience of MR imaging suggests that the technique may be superior to CT for demonstrating the anatomy of the soft tissues around the wrist (Weiss et al 1986).

Other joints

The cartilaginous disc of the temporo-mandibular joint may be demonstrated by CT and damage to this may be diagnosed with a sensitivity comparable to that of arthrography (Thompson et al 1985). MR imaging offers similar advantages without the drawback of ionizing radiation (Helms et al 1986). Neither technique provides a dynamic assessment of temporo-mandibular movement which is possible with fluoroscopy (Lott et al 1988).

Examination of the elbow is required rarely but CT may be used to demonstrate loose bodies, hyperplastic synovium, fracture fragments and osteophytes which are not otherwise detected (Singson et al 1986).

CONCLUSION

The applications of joint CT are wide but, in general, complement conventional radiography and arthrography. In many situations CT may provide unique information which defines the need for surgery and the surgical approach. Although MR imaging is superior to CT in many respects, CT has the advantage of being generally available and it is likely to be several years before MR imaging is used for the assessment of musculoskeletal disease on a routine basis in this country.

REFERENCES

Biondetti P R, Vannier M W, Gilula L A, Knapp R 1987 Wrist: coronal and transaxial CT scanning. Radiology 163: 149–151

Burk D L, Mears D C, Kennedy W H, Cooperstein L A, Herbert D L 1985 Three-dimensional computed tomography of acetabular fractures. Radiology 155: 183–186

Dalinka M L, Arger P, Coleman B 1985 CT in pelvic trauma. Orthopaedic Clinics of North America 16: 471–480

Dihlmann W, Nebel G 1983 Computed tomography of the hip joint capsule. Journal of Computer Assisted Tomography 7: 278–285

Gillespy T, Genant H K, Helms C A 1986 Magnetic resonance imaging of osteonecrosis. Radiologic Clinics of North America 24: 193–208

Griffiths H J, Hamlin D J, Kiss S, Lovelock J 1981 Efficacy of CT scanning in a group of 174 patients with orthopaedic and musculoskeletal problems. Skeletal Radiology 7: 87–98

Griffiths H J, Standertskjold-Nordenstam C G, Burke J, Lamont B, Kimmel J 1984 Computed tomography in the management of acetabular fractures. Skeletal Radiology 11: 22–31

Guyer B, Smith D S, Cady R B, Bassano D A, Levinsohn E M 1984 Dosimetry of computerized tomography in the evaluation of hip dysplasia. Skeletal Radiology 12: 123–127

Hajek P C, Baker L L, Bjorkengren A, Sartoris D J, Neumann C H, Resnick D 1986 High-resolution magnetic resonance imaging of the ankle: normal anatomy. Skeletal Radiology 15: 536–540

Heger L, Wulff K, Seddiqi M S A 1985 Computed tomography of calcaneal fractures. American Journal of Roentgenology 145: 131–137

Helms C A, Gillespy T, Sims R E, Richardson M L 1986 Magnetic resonance imaging of internal derangement of the temporomandibular joint. Radiologic Clinics of North America 24: 189–192

Hernandez R J 1988 Musculoskeletal system. In: Siegel M J (ed) Contemporary Issues in Computed Tomography. Pediatric Body CT. Churchill Livingstone, New York pp 253–292

Hernandez R J, Tachdjian M O, Dias L S 1982 Hip CT in congenital dislocation: appearance of tight iliopsoas tendon and pulvinar hypertrophy. American Journal of Roentgenology 139: 335–337

Huber D J, Sauter R, Mueller E, Requardt H, Weber H 1986 MR imaging of the normal shoulder. Radiology 158: 405–408

Levine E, De Smet A A, Neff J R 1984 Role of radiologic imaging in management planning of giant cell tumour of bone. Skeletal Radiology 12: 79–89

Lott C W, Wilson D J, Juniper R J 1988 Temporomandibular joint arthrography: dynamic study by video recording. Clinical Radiology 39: 73–76

Magid D, Fishman E K, Scott W W et al 1985 Femoral head avascular necrosis: CT assessment with multiplanar reconstruction. Radiology 157: 751–756

Martinez S, Herzenberg J E, Apple J S 1985 Computed tomography of the hindfoot. Orthopaedic Clinics of North America 16: 481–496
Merhar G L, Clark R A, Schneider H J, Stern P J 1986 High-resolution computed tomography of the wrist in patients with carpal tunnel syndrome. Skeletal Radiology 15: 549–552
Mink J H, Reicher M A, Cruez J V 1987 Magnetic resonance imaging of the knee. Raven Press, New York
Raffi M, Firooznia H, Honamo J J, Minkoff J, Golimbu C 1987 Athlete shoulder injuries: CT arthrographic findings. Radiology 162: 559–564
Resnik C S 1987 The shoulder. In: Scott W W, Magid D, Fishman E K (eds) Contemporary Issues in Computed Tomography. Computed Tomography of the Musculoskeletal System. Churchill Livingstone, New York pp 139–154
Rosenberg Z S, Feldman F, Singson R D, Kane R 1988 Ankle tendons: evaluation with CT. Radiology 166: 221–226
Sarno R C, Carter B L, Bankoff M S, Semine M C 1984 Computed tomography in tarsal coalition. Journal of Computer Assisted Tomography 8: 1155–1160
Schwimmer M, Edelstein G, Heiken J P, Gilula L A 1985 Synovial cysts of the knee: CT evaluation. Radiology 154: 175–177
Sims R E, Genant H K 1986 Magnetic resonance imaging of joint disease. Radiologic Clinics of North America 24: 179–188
Singson R D, Feldman F, Rosenberg Z S 1986 Elbow joint: assessment with double-contrast CT arthrography. Radiology 160: 167–173
Smith J, Ludwig R L, Marcove R C 1987 Sacrococcygeal chordoma. Skeletal Radiology 16: 37–44
Steinbach L S, Helms C A, Sims R E, Gillespy T, Genant H K 1987 High resolution computed tomography of knee menisci. Skeletal Radiology 16: 11–16
Thompson J R, Christiansen E, Sauser D, Hasso A N, Hinshaw D B 1985 Dislocation of the temporomandibular joint meniscus: contrast arthrography vs computed tomography. American Journal of Roentgenology 144: 171–174
Weiss K L, Beltran J, Shamam O M, Stilla R F, Levey M 1986 High-field MR surface-coil imaging of the hand and wrist. Radiology 160: 143–146
Wilson D J 1988 Diagnostic ultrasound in the musculoskeletal system. Current Orthopaedics 2: 41–50
Yousem D M, Scott W W 1987 The foot and ankle. In: Scott W W, Magid D, Fishman E K (eds) Contemporary Issues in Computed Tomography. Computed Tomography of the Musculoskeletal System. Churchill Livingstone, New York pp 113–138

22. Pitfalls in CT

Adrian Dixon

INTRODUCTION

Just as in all branches of radiology, even the most experienced CT radiologist can make the most simple of errors. A review of the CT errors made in the author's department shows that approximately half are errors of observation and half are those of interpretation. This chapter will consider ways of minimizing errors. The first section will deal with errors of observation. In the larger second section on errors of interpretation, both false positive and false negative diagnoses need to be considered. Particular emphasis will be placed on the pitfalls peculiar to CT where the axial display of normal anatomical structures can simulate disease processes.

ERRORS OF OBSERVATIONS

Technique

CT will obviously fail to provide the correct diagnosis if the lesion is not covered by the series of scans selected. By and large, the usual error is to examine an insufficient volume of the patient rather than to select an injudicious use of slice intervals. For example, in most institutions, an abdominal examination with reference to the pancreas does not normally include the pelvis. However, clinicians may not always be accurate in coning down their clinical suspicions to one particular area; e.g. a patient referred on account of possible pancreatic disease may actually have a primary pelvic malignancy metastatic to upper abdominal nodes which are not seen on CT. Should this count as a negative CT? In the mind of the clinician it certainly does! Obviously there has to be some compromise. It is impossible to examine the chest, abdomen and pelvis on every patient, even though we are frequently asked so to do! However, the radiologist should carefully attempt to match the volume of the patient examined with the likely disease processes and patterns of spread.

The slice thickness and intervals chosen will only infrequently contribute to errors of observation, provided they are kept within the ranges of the protocols detailed in other chapters. Even when the correct slice thickness

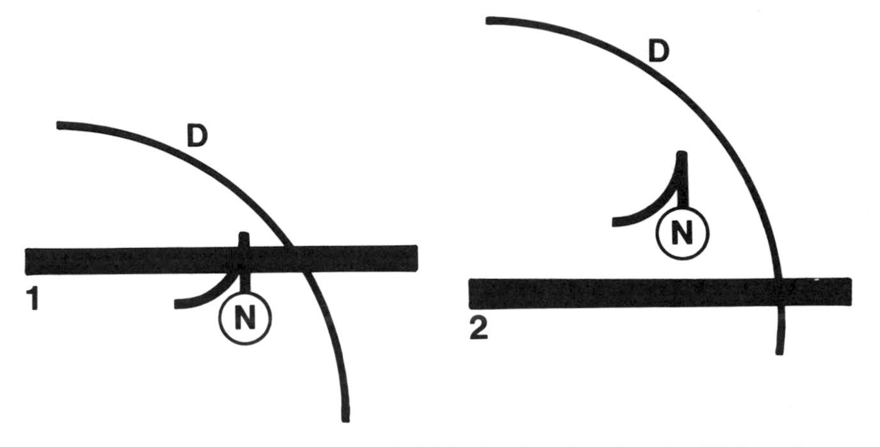

Fig. 22.1 Diagram showing how a nodule (N) in the adrenal can be missed if the patient breathes irregularly. D, Diaphragm. (Reproduced with permission from Churchill Livingstone.)

and intervals are employed, a lesion can be missed if the patient breathes irregularly. This is a particular problem close to the diaphragm; e.g. a nodule within the adrenal gland can be missed if supposedly contiguous slices miss a portion of the gland due to inconsistencies in respiration (Fig. 22.1). In the same way, irregular respiration can also cause problems in the lung and large nodules can be missed with ease (Krudy et al 1982). Great care must be taken to ensure that slices are anatomically contiguous; this, of course, must be done at the time of the examination and before the patient moves out of position.

For many applications it is desirable to zoom in on an organ or site. Most examinations of the adrenal glands and lumbar spine are undertaken in this way but care should be taken as important information may be 'coned off'. The patient with Cushing's syndrome referred for adrenal CT may have liver metastases; likewise the patient referred for lumbar spine CT may turn out to have a lesion peripheral to the field of view used, e.g. carcinoma of the kidney.

It is a moot point how often poor technique and poor patient co-operation contribute to errors. Obviously if the patient cannot keep still, movement blur may mask significant lesions but sometimes movement blur is inevitable, e.g. the patient in pain following trauma. Young children will have to be sedated in order to obtain adequate images but at the other end of the spectrum, advanced age alone is no excuse for poor image quality (Baldwin et al 1987).

Reporting

This should obviously be done in as careful a fashion as possible. It is worth remembering that few radiologists are as familiar with the anatomical features of any one CT slice as they are with those of a chest radiograph. Thus, one could argue that a CT examination, which commonly comprises 30 plus scans should take at least 30 times as long to report as one chest film. This is probably an underestimate because of the wealth of data stored by electronic means.

One of the commonest methods of making an error of observation is to rely on reviewing hard copy images only. This has been emphasized time and time again but still the practice continues. Even if the radiographer is meticulous in the preparation of hard copy film, the data must still be reviewed on the monitor. For example, bone detail will not be adequately displayed on the majority of hard copy images taken to show the soft tissues of the abdomen (Laval-Jeantet et al 1985). Indeed, it is not unknown for the only slice showing the lesion to have been inadvertently omitted from the hard copy series of images.

Despite careful attention to detail, it is still possible for experienced observers to completely miss a lesion. Abnormalities on the edge of the image, such as a soft-tissue deposit in the paraspinal muscles, are extremely difficult to recognize. Sometimes there are mitigating circumstances, such as a gastric air–fluid level artefact obscuring a lesion in the left lobe of the liver. All too often the error is an outright miss and glaringly obvious in retrospect. Dual reporting is probably the best method of preventing these errors.

There are also difficulties in relation to body habitus as the identification of normal structures (and thereby interpretation) is much easier in patients with reasonable depots of fat.

ERRORS OF INTERPRETATION

These errors broadly break down into several groups. The most obvious, and perhaps most widely described, are the normal anatomical variants which may simulate disease. Then there are the more worrying problems of normal structures which can simulate disease and, thereafter, the classification becomes more complex but includes the misinterpretation of the nature of abnormal structures. Such errors can have very serious implications, e.g. assuming a benign hepatic haemangioma to be a metastasis.

Anatomical variants simulating disease

Chest

There is a large range of normal anatomical variants which can cause interpretation problems within the thoracic cage. Most of these are in the mediastinum where abnormal nodes may be simulated by variations in the expected vascular anatomy. Such pitfalls should be prevented by the use of intravenous contrast medium. The vessel should show intense avid opacification whereas most nodes will enhance much more slowly and to a lesser degree. However, nodes involved by highly vascular tumours, e.g. thyroid carcinoma, can enhance in a way which may cause confusion. Perhaps an even more important clue to the presence of an anomalous vessel is the characteristic appearance of a tubular structure present on several contiguous scans. Even if a vessel runs obliquely, e.g. an anomalous right subclavian artery, it should also be readily identified on adjacent scans. It would be very rare for a chain of enlarged nodes to simulate such a perfect tubular structure.

The anomalous vessels that cause most problems in the mediastinum are the azygo/hemiazygos variants and persistence of the left superior vena cava. Variants of the azygos venous system can simulate nodes in the azygo-oesophageal recess and more caudally simulate those in the posterior mediastinum. The azygos system is especially prominent when there is congenital absence of the inferior vena cava or if it is obliterated by pathology which should be discernible in the upper abdomen. In these situations, the azygos system will be prominent throughout and can be traced from the region of the renal veins, posterior to the diaphragmatic crura and into the posterior mediastinum. Opacification will confirm the vascular nature should doubt remain.

Persistence of the left superior vena cava is a relatively obvious anomaly. The left brachiocephalic vein drains into the coronary sinus via the oblique cardiac vein, having passed on the left anterolateral aspect of the aortic arch. There is no normal confluence of the brachiocephalic veins and again, the tubular nature of the vascular anomaly should be apparent on adjacent scans. More difficult is the variant whereby the bulk of blood in the left brachiocephalic vein passes normally to the superior vena cava at confluence but with a small tributary persisting in the course of the 'left superior vena cava'. A large left superior intercostal vein, which drains the second and fourth intercostal veins into the caudal aspect of the left brachiocephalic vein, can also simulate an enlarged node in this region.

Variations in the aortic arch are much more obvious and, just occasionally, it may be difficult on unenhanced scans to sort out such anomalies from thyroid tissue when a retrosternal goitre extends down to the mediastinum.

Abdomen

Splenunculi (accessory spleens) can cause considerable difficulty in the left upper quadrant. They can simulate splenic hilar nodes or even adrenal neoplasms (Fig. 22.2). Although small splenunculi are found in 20–25% of post-mortem examinations they are usually too small to be identified on CT. Nevertheless, they should be considered whenever a mass is identified in this region. Enhancement is helpful since splenunculi should manifest exactly the same enhancement pattern as the adjacent normal splenic parenchyma. The splenunculus which hypertrophies after splenectomy in a

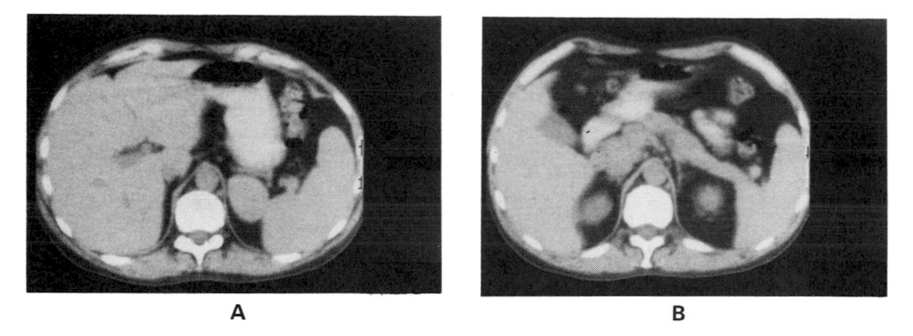

Fig. 22.2 **A** A mass in the left hypochondrium which at first glance might be mistaken for an adrenal mass. **B** In fact a normal adrenal was identified more caudally. This is a splenunculus enlarged by lymphomatous infiltration.

patient with lymphoma is more difficult to assess because although the enhancement pattern may be reassuring, it is more difficult to judge in the absence of a normal spleen (Beahrs & Stephens 1980). If doubt persists, a radionuclide study of the reticulo-endothelial system will confirm the splenic nature of this mass.

In a similar fashion, congenital anomalies of the renal contour may cause problems. In some examples of renal duplication, the upper moiety may remain rather separate simulating an adrenal mass. Renal fusion anomalies, e.g. horseshoe kidney, should be readily recognized because the isthmus runs anterior to the vena cava and aorta providing a very 'clear' demarcation of the para-aortic region. The only difficulty is that the normal shape of the kidney is distorted and malignancies may be more difficult to recognize. Likewise, the anatomy of normal adjacent structures, e.g. para-aortic nodal chain, may be altered and abnormalities such as enlarged nodes should be searched for in areas over and above the usual sites.

The venous abnormalities of the retroperitoneum have been well described and are now familiar (Royal & Callen 1979). The more common ones are the retro-aortic left renal vein, the double inferior vena cava and the left-sided inferior vena cava. It is less well recognized that the ovarian veins may become markedly distended for no apparent reason. All these structures can simulate para-aortic lymphadenopathy. With regard to opacification of venous structures, there was initial enthusiasm for injecting via an appropriate foot vein. Although this does give intense opacification, it is difficult to achieve optimal timing. Furthermore, the streaming of venous flow, especially in large veins, can lead to an inhomogeneous appearance which may simulate thrombus or tumour extension (Glazer et al 1981). Thus, it is better to use a conventional intravenous injection via an arm vein and wait for the circulation to opacify the venous phase. This is especially important for evaluating possible renal tumour extension into the renal veins and inferior vena cava.

The psoas minor is another variant which can cause a problem in the retroperitoneum. This variable muscle which runs anterior to the psoas major can appear totally separate from its larger fellow muscle and thereby simulate a chain of enlarged nodes. Obviously when there is bilateral symmetry this variant is readily recognized.

Normal structures masquerading as disease entities

The most common pitfalls are those artefacts which, when viewed in the axial plane, can simulate disease processes. Sometimes these are machine-related but others are caused by normal structures merely viewed in an unfamiliar projection.

Chest

One of the most surprising artefacts in the early days of body CT was the lung pseudonodule caused by irregularities of the anterior chest wall (Dixon & Wylie 1981). If a small portion of bone (usually the first rib) protrudes down into a more caudal slice, it is possible for that structure to simulate a lung nodule (Fig. 22.3). Since it only occupies a part of the thickness of the slice (the rest being lung parenchyma) the attenuation

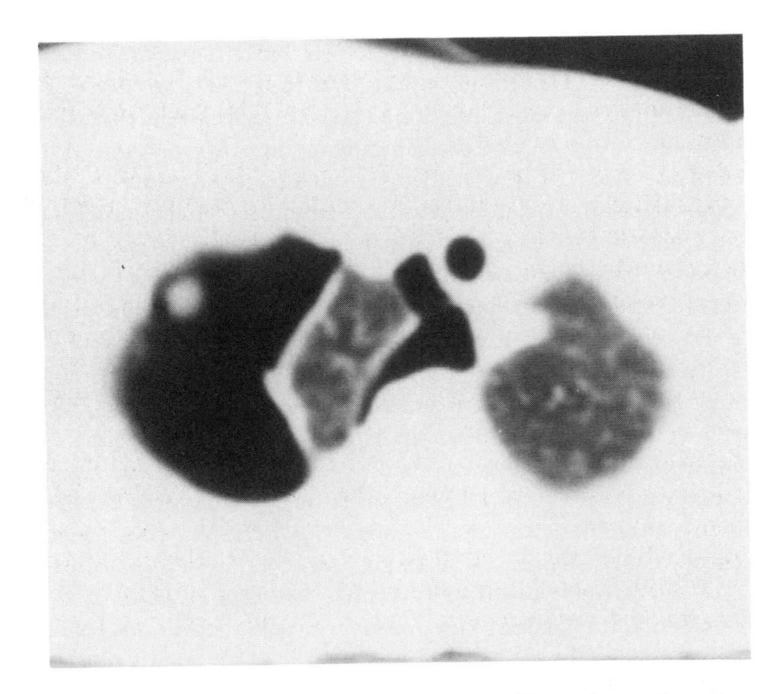

Fig. 22.3 A rib artefact in a patient with a pneumothorax. If superimposed over lung parenchyma such artefacts readily simulate pulmonary nodules. (Reproduced with permission from Churchill Livingstone.)

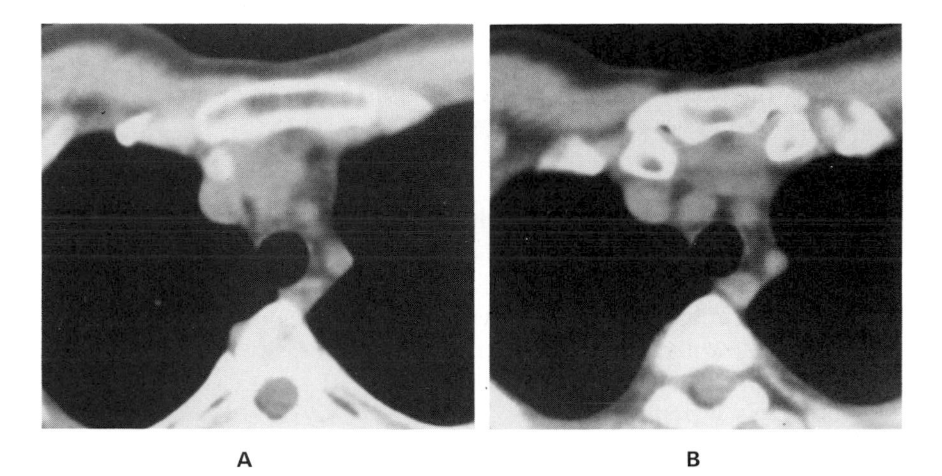

Fig. 22.4 **A** Apparent calcified mediastinal node. **B** A more cranial scan showing that this patient has a prominent medial end of right clavicle. There is minimal pectus excavatum and the bone is very closely applied to the mediastinal structures. The apparent 'node' is due to a small portion of the clavicle being included in the more caudal slice by partial volume averaging.

values may approximate to that of soft tissue due to partial volume averaging. The pseudonodule appears internal to the pleura due to the curvature of the chest wall. Likewise, the inferior aspect of the bulbous medial end of the clavicle can be subject to partial volume averaging thereby simulating a mediastinal node (Fig. 22.4). Such problems are less evident if thin slices are used.

Subpleural lung nodules can be simulated by the margins of the fissures and attachments of the pulmonary ligaments (Proto & Rost 1985). Postural changes may also lead to pseudonodules in the most posterior (dependent) regions of the lungs in the supine position. Controversy persists as to whether these are due to excessive perfusion or inadequate ventilation of the dependent lung parenchyma. Suffice it to say that these 'lesions' are not persistent when the patient is turned into the prone position (Spirt 1980). Such pseudonodules are especially common in children examined under general anaesthesia (Damgaard-Pedersen & Qvist 1980).

Within the mediastinum a most worrying 'lesion' may appear in the subcarinal region due to the most cranial portion of the left atrium being viewed in isolation. This may easily be mistaken for subcarinal lymphadenopathy. The use of intravenous contrast medium should prevent such errors. Inevitably interpretation is more difficult in those patients with little mediastinal fat in whom the normal and abnormal structures are closely grouped together.

The numerous artefacts which can simulate aortic dissection are now well recognized (Godwin et al 1982). However, with an increasing number of cases of suspected aortic dissection being referred for CT it is perhaps useful to review these here. The most frequently occurring artefacts are technical, the commonest is a streak artefact running across the aorta from adjacent structures which are either moving, e.g. the edge of left ventricle giving a streak across the descending aorta, or of much higher attenuation, e.g. the contrast-laden superior vena cava giving a streak across the ascending aorta. Such streak artefacts tend to fan out from a point of origin and thus change in thickness across the aorta. In contrast, a true intimal flap has a constant thickness across the aorta (Gallagher & Dixon 1984). Occasionally dissection can be simulated by an anatomical artefact, such as fluid in the superior pericardial recess overlying the ascending aorta. Although of low attenuation, this rim of fluid can still be mistaken for an unopacifying lumen. Careful scrutiny of adjacent scans should reveal the true extent of the pericardial fluid.

There is plenty of room for error in lesions close to the diaphragm and the crura themselves may cause problems. Retrocrural nodes are often the first sign of disseminated disease and it is recognized that visible nodes here are of more significance than elsewhere in the body. Thus, difficulty arises when the crura appear unduly bulky. This is a common trap when CT slices are obtained on inspiration.

Abdomen

It is in the abdomen that the most serious errors can be made. The variable anatomy and the ever present difficulty of opacifying, and thereby recognizing, all loops of bowel combine to make the abdomen a veritable tiger country!

Correct bowel preparation is crucial and it is worth remembering that it

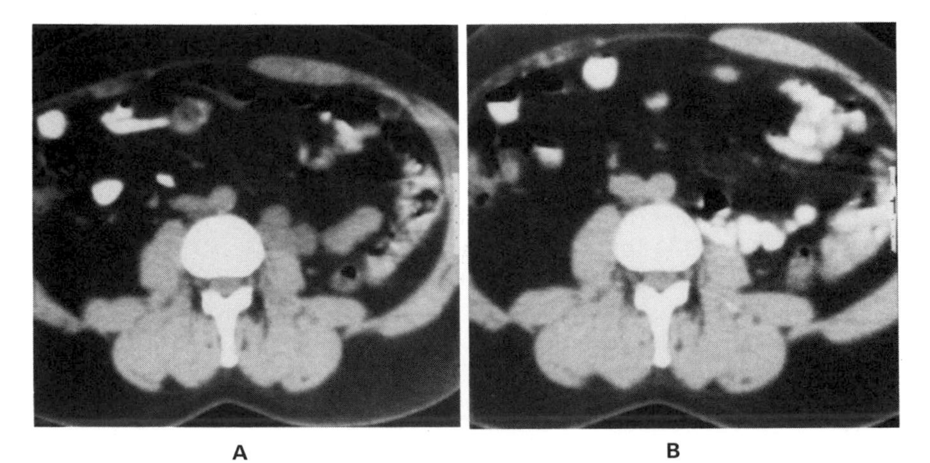

Fig. 22.5 **A** Possible retroperitoneal nodes adjacent to left psoas in a patient who has had a nephrectomy for a renal tumour. **B** A delayed scan with further oral contrast medium shows that the appearances are due to normal bowel.

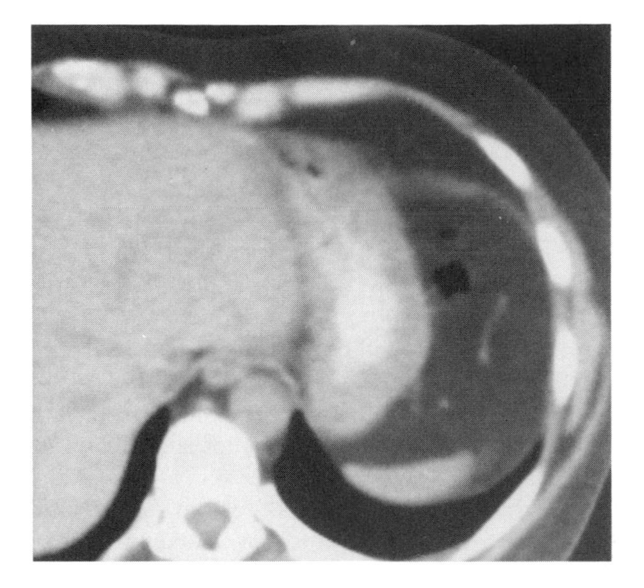

Fig. 22.6 CT scan of a normal stomach showing apparent thickening of the wall.

is much better to give too much oral contrast medium than too little. Underfilled loops of small bowel around the tail of the pancreas, in the left para-aortic region and in the pelvis regularly cause problems in interpretation (Fig. 22.5). So long as these problems are recognized while the patient is in the department, delayed scans following further oral contrast medium will resolve the difficulty. Note that all such errors are likely to result in false positive diagnoses.

In some critically ill patients it may be inadvisable to administer oral contrast medium and gross errors may result, e.g. a subphrenic abscess may be misinterpreted as a normal stomach or vice versa. These patients frequently have a nasogastric tube in situ. Under these circumstances, the administration of air or simple aspiration may allow correct identification of the stomach.

The stomach is a notoriously difficult area in body CT with its immensely variable shape, size and position. The relation of the fundus to the diaphragmatic hiatus is also very variable (Thompson et al 1982). The gastric wall may appear grossly thickened in this region but this thickening is virtually always normal, even when it extends round the stomach curvatures (Fig. 22.6). Whenever doubt persists, a lateral decubitus (left side up) study or prone view following oral effervescent tablets should elucidate the problem. The gastric fundus may fold back on itself in the region of a tortuous splenic artery. In this way the caudal portion of the fundus, which is closely related to the left adrenal gland, may simulate an adrenal mass due to partial volume averaging. A narrow-necked epiphrenic gastric diverticulum which has failed to fill with oral contrast medium is also a potential pitfall as a low attenuation adrenal mass is readily simulated.

It is well known that underfilling of the duodenojejunal flexure with contrast medium can lead to an erroneous diagnosis of a low attenuation pancreatic or juxta-pancreatic mass. It is uncertain whether this underfilling is caused by too long a time delay between glasses of oral contrast medium or whether it is due to the relative trapping of contrast medium in the stomach and second part of the duodenum when the patient is in the supine position. In either case there are numerous methods of proving that this 'mass' of fluid attenuation is merely underfilled bowel.

Similar problems of underfilled bowel loops occur in the pelvis and can readily simulate ovarian masses. Delayed scans with a completely full bladder should help to overcome the problem because normal loops of bowel are displaced cranially whereas, in general, pelvic masses retain a fixed position.

The anatomy of the pelvis is not always easy to follow. Obliquity of the vessels and the curvature of the sacrum create particular problems, especially in the female. The interpretation of anatomy can be very difficult following surgery and it is essential to know the precise operative details. One particular trap is the patient who has undergone a hysterectomy coupled with ovarian conservation. The ovaries are moved on their vascular pedicles from their native sites within the true pelvis to new sites in the false pelvis and are commonly fixed to the anterior aspects of the psoas muscles. This is done partly to prevent problems of dyspareunia and partly to allow intensive radiation treatment without damage to the ovaries (Reed et al in press). Likewise, knowledge of previous gynaecological surgery is essential when interpreting a patient for possible pelvic recurrence following rectal excision.

The spleen is a notoriously difficult organ to evaluate with CT. On the one side of the coin, in non-Hodgkin's lymphoma, splenic involvement will be present in up to one-third of patients in whom the organ appears completely normal at CT. On the other side of the coin, not all areas of inhomogeneity after intravenous enhancement are due to disease and many will be due to areas of poor perfusion and other benign conditions.

The porta hepatis is a difficult region to interpret, largely because the portal vein runs oblique to the axial plane. Thus, partial volume problems may occur and the logical solution, therefore, is to use thin slices. These, coupled with the judicious use of intravenous contrast medium should resolve many difficulties.

CONCLUSION

This section has dealt with just a few of the pitfalls which may trap even the most experienced radiologist and we have all been caught out at one time or another. As knowledge is gained and more of these pitfalls are recognized, errors will only be kept to a minimum by paying close attention to technique, observation and interpretation. Even then we must continue to be on our guard!

REFERENCES

Baldwin J, Sharpe P, Cole S, Dixon A K 1987 Image quality of abdominal computed tomography in the elderly. Age and Ageing 16: 261–264

Beahrs J R, Stephens D H 1980 Enlarged accessory spleens: CT appearance in post-splenectomy patients. American Journal of Roentgenology 135: 483–486

Damgaard-Pedersen K, Qvist T 1980 Paediatric pulmonary CT scanning. Paediatric Radiology 9: 145–148

Dixon A K, Wylie I G 1981 Rib artefact in computed tomography. British Journal of Radiology 54: 78–79

Gallagher S, Dixon A K 1984 Streak artefacts of the thoracic aorta: pseudodissection. Journal of Computer Assisted Tomography 8: 688–693

Glazer G M, Callen P W, Parker J J 1981 CT diagnosis of tumour thrombus in the inferior vena cava: avoiding the false positive diagnosis. American Journal of Roentgenology 137: 1265–1267

Godwin J D, Breiman R S, Speckman J M 1982 Problems and pitfalls in the evaluation of thoracic aortic dissection by computed tomography. Journal of Computer Assisted Tomography 6: 750–756

Krudy A G, Doppman J L, Herdt J R 1982 Failure to detect a 1.5 cm lung nodule by chest computed tomography. Journal of Computer Assisted Tomography 6: 1178–1180

Laval-Jeantet M, Paxton L, Frija J, Preteux F 1985 Observer variation in bone lesion destruction in thoraco-abdominal visceral CT images. European Journal of Radiology 5: 310–313

Proto A V, Rost R C 1985 CT of the thorax: pitfalls and interpretation. Radiographics 5: 693–712

Reed D H, Williams M V, Dixon A K Ovarian conservation at hysterectomy: potential diagnosis pitfall. Clinical Radiology (in press)

Royal S A, Callen P W 1979 CT evaluation of anomalies of the inferior vena cava and left renal vein. American Journal of Roentgenology 132: 759–763

Spirt B A 1980 Value of the prone position in detecting pulmonary nodules by computed tomography. Journal of Computer Assisted Tomography 4: 871–873

Thompson W M, Halvorsen R A, Williford M E 1982 Computed tomography of the gastroesophageal junction. Radiographics 2: 179–193

Index

Abdomen
  anatomical variants simulating disease, 252–254
  normal structures masquerading as disease entities, 256–258
Abdominal abscess, 179–184
  definition, 179–180
  detection, 180–181
  patient monitoring, 183–185
  percutaneous drainage, 181–183
Abdominal malignancy *see* Gynaecological malignancy
Abdominal trauma, 165–177
  CT role in, 165–166
  CT technique, 166–167
  laboratory guidelines for CT, 166
  patient selection and indications for CT, 165–166
Abdominoperineal (AP) resection, 118–119
Abscess
  abdominal *see* Abdominal abscess
  in acute pancreatitis, 82–83
  renal, 147
Acetabular dysplasia, 242
Acquired cystic disease of uraemia, 129–130
ACTH, 153
Adenocarcinoma, 29, 66, 115–119
Adrenal adenoma, 154
Adrenal angiomyolipomas, 160
Adrenal cortex, 153–157
Adrenal disorders, silent, 159–161
Adrenal function, 152
Adrenal gland
  anatomy, 151
  left, 152
  right, 151
  role of CT, 151
Adrenal imaging, 151–163
Adrenal masses, biopsy, 187
Adrenal medulla, 158–159
Adrenal metastases, 161
Adrenocortical tumours, 156
Adrenocorticotrophic hormone (ACTH), 153
Adult polycystic disease, 128–129
Air–fluid collections, 25–26
Aldosteronomas, 154–155
Anaplastic carcinoma, 69
Angiography, 71
Angiomyolipoma, 107, 144–145
Ankle, CT role, 244
Anterior commissure, 6
Aortic dissection, artefacts simulating, 255–256
Appendicitis, 114
Arteriography, 165
Arthrography, 243, 245
Ary-epiglottic folds, 3
Arytenoid cartilage, 5, 9
Asbestos exposure, 28, 29
Atelectasis
  cicatrization, 39
  compressive, 38–39
  rounded, 39
Autoimmune adrenalitis, 157

Bacterial infection, 146
Barium enema examination, 109, 114, 115
Biliary cystadenomas, 105–106
Biopsy *see* Percutaneous biopsy techniques
Bladder carcinoma, 203–215
  accuracy of CT, 209–210, 212–213
  CT findings, 207–209
  CT technique, 205–207
  difficulties of interpretation, 207–209
  lymph-node involvement, 204, 211–213
  patterns of tumour spread, 204–205
  staging methods, 203–204
  TNM classification, 204
Bone biopsies, 187
Bowel, blunt trauma, 173
Brachalgia, 228
Bronchial cancer, 13–21
  CT technique, 14
  direct tumour spread, 18
  distant metastases, 18–19
  histological variants, 13
  incidence of, 13
  non-small-cell, 13

Bronchial cancer (*cont.*)
  pitfalls of CT interpretation, 14
  small-cell, 13
Bronchiectasis, 25
Bronchopleural fistula, 26
Bronchoscopy, 33

Calcaneo-navicular fusion, 244
Calcification, 48–49, 124, 130, 133, 143, 234, 241
Castleman's disease, 50
Catheters in pleural drainage, 27
Cavernous haemangioma, 99–102
Cerebrospinal fluid (CSF), 228
Cervical carcinoma
  CT stage criteria, 193
  FIGO classification, 193–195
Cervical spine
  CT technique, 230
  role of CT, 228
Cervical spondylosis, 228, 230, 233
Chest
  anatomical variants simulating disease, 251–252
  normal structures masquerading as disease entities, 254–256
Chest wall tumours, 30–31
Chondromalacia, 245
Cicatrization atelectasis, 39
Colitis
  granulomatous, 110–113
  ulcerative, 110
Colon carcinoma, 116
Colon wall, normal appearances, 110
Colonic disease, 109–121
  CT role in, 109
  CT technique, 109–110
Colonic lipomas, 116
Colorectal adenocarcinoma, 116
Colorectal carcinoma, 115
  preoperative staging, 117–118
  recurrent, 118–119
Compressive atelectasis, 38–39
Computed myelography, 228, 233
Computed tomographic arterial portography (CTAP), 92–94
Computed tomographic arteriography (CTA), 91–92
Computed tomography (CT)
  errors of interpretation, 251–258
    abdomen, 252–254, 256–258
    chest, 251–252, 254–256
  errors of observation, 249–251
    reporting, 250–251
    technique, 249–250
  interventional, 179–190
  pitfalls in, 249–259
Congenital cysts, 43–45
Conn's syndrome, 154
Cord compression, 233
Cortical disease with hypoadrenalism, 157
Crico-arytenoid joints, 5
Cricoid cartilage, 4, 9
Cricothyroid joint, 4
Crohn's colitis, 110–113
Cushing's syndrome, 153–154
Cystic masses, 43–47
Cystic neoplasms, 45–47
Cyst(s)
  adrenal, 179–198
  bronchogenic, 43, 44
  congenital, 43–45
  dermoid, 59
  foregut, 43–45
  haemorrhagic, 99, 126
  hepatic, 98–102, 129
  multiple, 130–132
  neurenteric, 45
  oesophageal, 45
  pericardial, 44–45
  renal *see* Renal cystic disease
  thymic, 45, 60–61
  see also Pancreas

Degenerative disease, 242
  see also Spine
Delayed high-dose iodine CT (DICT), 90–91
Dermoid cysts, 59
Disc disease *see* Spine
Diverticulitis, 113
Duodenum
  common injury, 171
  rupture of, 172

Echinococcus granulosus, 134
Echinococcus multilocularis, 134
Elbow, CT role, 245–246
Empyema, 25–26
  drainage, 27
Endocrine conditions, 153–159
Endometrial cancer
  CT staging, 195–198
  FIGO classification, 196
EOE-13 (ethiodized oil emulsion 13), 91
Epiglottis, 2
Epithelial neoplasms, 69
Extramedullary haematopoiesis, 43

Fatty masses, 41–43
Focal benign liver disease, 97–108
Focal fatty infiltration, 97–98
Focal nodular hyperplasia, 102–104
Fractures, 237–240

Ganglioneuroma, 159
Gastrinomas, 72–73
Germ-cell tumours, 45, 59, 62
  benign, 59
  malignant, 59–60
Giant-cell carcinoma, 69
Glosso-epiglottic fold, 3
Glottic injuries, 10–11
Glottic tumours, 7, 8
Glottis, 2
Glucagonomas, 73
Goitre, 47–48, 50
Granulomatous colitis, 110–113
Graves' disease, 57
Gynaecological malignancy, 191–202
  CT technique, 191–192

Haemangioma, 61, 99–102
Hepatic adenomas, 107
Hepatic-cell adenomas, 104–105
Hepatic cysts, 129
Hepatic lacerations, 169
Hepatic parenchymal gas, 170
Hepatic specific contrast-enhanced CT, 91
Hepatic trauma, 169–170
Hepatocellular carcinoma, 104, 107
Herniation of abdominal fat, 42
Hilar lymph-node involvement, 16–17
Hip, CT role, 241–242
Hodgkin's disease, 30, 45, 54, 58, 60–61, 141, 217–226
  abdominal nodal involvement, 223
  extranodal disease, 223
  lung involvement, 221–222
  pattern of tumour growth, 217–219
  pulmonary changes in, 220
  role of CT, 222, 225
  staging classification, 219–220
Hydatid disease, 134
Hyoid bone, 2
Hyperaldosteronism, primary, 154–155
Hypervascular neoplasms. 49–50
Hypoadrenalism, chronic primary, 157

Idiopathic atrophy, 157
Incremental dynamic contrast-enhanced CT, 90
Inferior cornua, 4
Inflammatory bowel diseases, 113
Inflammatory diseases, 47, 110–114
Insulinomas, 71–72
Interventional CT, 179–190
Ischaemic colitis, 112
Islet-cell tumours, 71
  clinical syndromes, 71
  localization, 71
  non-functioning, 73–74

Joint disease, 237–247
  equivocal radiographic appearances, 240
  general indications for CT, 237–241
  juxta-articular neoplasms, 240–241
  role of CT, 237
  specific indications for CT, 241–246
  trauma, 237–240

Kidney
  biopsies, 186–187
  multicystic dysplastic, 130–132
  see also Renal
Knee, CT role, 245

Laparotomy, 176
Laryngeal carcinoma, 1
Laryngeal ventricle, 5
Laryngoscopy, 1
Larynx, 1–11
  carcinoma, 6–9
  CT technique, 1–2
  limitations of CT, 10
  nodal involvement, 7
  normal anatomy, 2–6
  trauma, 1, 10–11
  tumour classification, 7
Lipid-rich hyperalimentation fluid, 43
Lipomatous tumours, 107
Liver
  benign lipomatous tumours, 107
  biopsy, 186
  cysts, 98–102
  focal fatty infiltration, 97–98
  fracture, 169–170
  trauma, 169–170
  see also Hepatic
Liver disease *see* Focal benign liver disease
Liver metastases, 87–95, 224
  CT role in, 88–94
  CT screening techniques, 89–94
  imaging techniques, 87–88
Lumbar spine
  CT technique, 229–230
  role of CT, 227
Lung
  abscess, 26–27
  biopsy, 186
  carcinoma
    metastatic small-cell, 93
    non-small-cell, 19
  metastases, 144
  pseudonodule, 254
  see also Pulmonary
Lung disease, 25
Lymphangiography, 225
Lymphangiomas, 46, 61

Lymph nodes
calcification, 48–49
'cystic', 45
Lymph-node involvement, 14–16
bladder carcinoma, 204, 211–213
hilar, 16–17
Hodgkin's disease, 223
lymphoma, 217
mediastinal, 13–18
non-Hodgkin's lymphoma, 223
prostatic carcinoma, 204–205, 211–213
thorax, 220
Lymphography, 212
Lymphoma, 217–226
adrenals in, 160
extranodal, 219
lymph-node involvement, 217

Magnetic resonance (MR) imaging, 10–11
94, 120, 214, 227–229, 237, 241, 243, 245
Mediastinal abscess, 47
Mediastinal biopsies, 186
Mediastinal haemorrhage post-mediastinoscopy, 46
Mediastinal lipomas, 42
Mediastinal lipomatosis, 41
Mediastinal lymphadenopathy, 29
Mediastinal lymph-node involvement, 13–16
Mediastinal lymph-node metastases, 16–18
Mediastinal neoplasms, 42–43
Mediastinal pathology, 41–51
contrast-enhancing masses, 49–50
high attenuation masses, 48–50
unenhanced masses, 48–49
Mediastinal seminomas, 60
Mediastinoscopy, 15
Mediastinum, errors of interpretation, 255
Meningocoele, 47
Mesentery
blunt trauma, 173
metastases, 201
Mesothelioma, 29
Microcystic adenoma, 70
Micrometastases, 217
Morgagni hernia, 42
Mucinous adenocarcinoma, 69
Mucinous cystic neoplasm, 70
Multicystic dysplastic kidney, 130–132
Multilocular cystic nephroma, 132–133
Multiple endocrine neoplasms type I (MEN I), 73
Musculoskeletal neoplasms, 240
Myasthenia gravis, 54–56, 62
Myelography, 227
Myelopathy, 228

Nephritis, acute focal bacterial, 146
Nephrotomography, 129
Nerve root tumours, 46
Neuroblastoma, 159
Neurofibromas, 46
Non-Hodgkin's lymphoma, 58, 74, 141, 217–226
abdominal nodal involvement, 223
pattern of tumour growth, 217–219
role of CT, 222, 225
soft-tissue muscle masses, 224
staging classification, 219–220

Occult cancer, 176
Oesophageal varices, 49
Omental metastases, 201
Oncocytoma, 146
Osteochondritis dissecans, 245
Osteochondromata, 241
Osteonecrosis, 241
Ovarian carcinoma, 199–201
Ovarian lymphatic metastases, 201

Pancreas, 65–76
assessment of resectability, 68
biopsy, 186
common injury, 171
CT technique, 65
duct dilatation, 67
indeterminate mass, 68
involvement of adjacent structures, 67–68
nodal and distant metastases, 68
primary cystic neoplasms of duct-cell origin, 70–71
primary tumour, 66–67
role of CT, 69
solid neoplasms of duct cell origin, 66–69
trauma, CT role in, 171–172
Pancreatic lymphoma and metastases, 74, 224
Pancreatic parenchyma and ducts, 84
calculi, 85
Pancreatitis, 77–86
acute, 77–83
abscess, 82–83
CT role in, 77
effusions, 78–80
haemorrhage, 80–81
oedematous, 78
phlegmon, 82
pseudocyst, 81–82
tissue necrosis, 80
chronic, 83–85
alterations in morphology, 84–85
CT role in, 83–85
fluid collections, 85
pseudoaneurysms, 85

Pancreatitis (*cont.*)
oedematous, 78
Para-aortic lymphadenopathy, 253
Paralaryngeal space, 4
Parapelvic cysts, 127–128
Patello-femoral articulation, 245
Pelvis
CT technique, 191–192
errors of interpretation, 258
see also Gynaecological malignancy
Percutaneous biopsy techniques, 184–188
accuracy of, 185
bleeding, 188
choice of radiological modality, 185–186
complications, 187–188
needle selection, 184–185
quality of tissue removed, 185–186
specific sites, 186–187
Pericardial thickening, 29
Peritoneal tumour implants, 201
Phaeochromocytoma, 158
Phlegmon, 82
Pleural drainage, 26–27
Pleural effusion, 23–25
Pleural malignancy, 29
Pleural plaques, 28
Pleural space, 23–32
fluid detection, 23–27
Pleural thickening, 28
Pleuropulmonary disease, 25
Pneumothorax, 27, 254
in lung biopsy, 188
Polycystic disease, 99
Porta hepatis, 258
Posterior commissure, 6
Post-pneumonectomy space, 29–30
Pre-epiglottic space, 3
Prolapsed calcified thoracic disc, 234
Prostate carcinoma, 203–215
accuracy of CT, 211–213
CT findings, 210–211
CT technique, 205–207
lymph-node involvement, 204–205, 211–213
patterns of tumour spread, 204–205
staging methods, 203–204
TNM classification, 204–205
Pseudoaneurysms, 85
Pseudocysts, 81–82, 85
Pseudomembranous colitis, 112
Psoas minor, 253–254
Pulmonary collapse, 33–40
general observations, 33
left lower lobe, 34, 38
left upper lobe, 34
right lower lobe, 36–38
right middle lobe, 36–38
right upper lobe, 35–36
Pulmonary nodules, 254
Pulmonary parenchymal disease, 221
Pyriform sinus, 3–4
tumours, 7

Radiculography, 227
Radionuclide scintigraphy, 87
Rectal carcinoma, staging, 117
Rectosigmoid carcinoma, 118
Rectus muscle sheath, 175
Renal abscess, 147
Renal adenocarcinoma, 129
Renal artery, 175
Renal carcinoma, 137–141
CT accuracy, 140
CT appearances, 137–138
detection of recurrence, 141
direct tumour extension, 140
nodal involvement, 140
postoperative assessment, 141
staging, 138–140
vascular invasion, 138–140
see also Kidney
Renal contour anomalies, 253
Renal cystic disease, 123–135
benign cortical cysts, 123–124
complicated cysts, 124–127
hyperdense cysts, 126–127
parapelvic cysts, 127–128
thick wall, 124–126
Renal fusion anomalies, 253
Renal injuries, 173–175
Renal laceration, 174
Renal lymphoma, 141–142
CT appearances, 142
Renal masses, 137–149
Renal metastases, 142
Renal neoplasms, smaller than 3 cm in diameter, 138
Renal tumours, benign, 144–147
Renal vein involvement, 139
Retroperitoneal haematoma, 175
Retroperitoneal masses, biopsy, 187
Retroperitoneal spaces, haemorrhage in, 175
Retroperitoneum, venous abnormalities, 253
Rounded atelectasis, 39

Schwannomas, 46
Septations, 124
Shoulder, CT role, 242–243
Silent adenomas, 159
Single photon emission computed tomography (SPECT), 87
Soft-tissue injuries, 10
Soft-tissue pleural lesions, 27–30
Soft-tissue sarcoma, 245
Somatostatinomas, 73

Spine, 227–236
  CT technique, 229–231
  differential diagnosis, 234–235
  interpretation of CT, 231–235
  postoperative problems, 235
  role of CT, 227–229
  see also Cervical spine; Lumbar spine; Thoracic spine
Spleen
  errors of interpretation, 258
  injury, 167–168
Splenunculi, 252
Subglottic injuries, 11
Subglottic tumours, 7
Subglottis, 2
Subpleural lung nodules, 255
Superior cornua, 4
Superior mesenteric artery (SMA), 91–92
Superior thyroid notch, 4
Supraglottic injuries, 10
Supraglottic tumours, 7
Supraglottis, 2

Talo-calcaneal fusion, 244
Talo-navicular fusion, 244
Tarsal coalition, 244
Temporo-mandibular joint, 245
Teratoma, 43
  benign, 59
  malignant, 59
Testicular cancer, 45
Testicular tumours, 57
Thoracic spine, role of CT, 229
Thoracocentesis, 26–27
Thorax, lymph-node involvement, 220
Thymic cysts, 60–61
Thymic function, 53
Thymic lymphoid hyperplasia, 56–57
Thymic rebound hyperplasia, 57, 59
Thymolipoma, 43, 61–62
Thymoma, 45, 54–56
  accuracy of detection, 55–56
  benign, 54
  malignant, 55
Thymus, 53–63
  abnormal, 54–61
  lymphomatous infiltration, 58–59
  normal, anatomy, 53–54
Thyroid
  carcinoma, 48
  cartilage, 4
  cartilage invasion, 8
T lymphocytes, 53
Tracheal injuries, 11
Transitional-cell carcinomas, 142–143
Tuberous sclerosis, 106, 144

Ulcerative colitis, 110
Ultrasound, 26–27, 69, 88, 94, 124, 129, 131, 200, 203, 242
Uterine fluid collections, 198–199

Valleculae, 3
Vena caval involvement, 139
Vestibule, 3
Vipomas, 73
Virilism, 155
Vocal cord mobility, 2
Vocal processes, 5–6, 9

Wilms' tumour, 143–144
Wrist, CT role, 245

Xanthogranulomatous pyelonephritis, 147

Zollinger–Ellison syndrome, 72, 73
Zona glomerulosa (zG), 152
Zona reticularis (zR), 152